Pediatric Craniomaxillofacial Pathology

Editor

SRINIVAS M. SUSARLA

ORAL AND MAXILLOFACIAL SURGERY CLINICS OF NORTH AMERICA

www.oralmaxsurgery.theclinics.com

Consulting Editor
RUI P. FERNANDES

August 2024 • Volume 36 • Number 3

ELSEVIER

1600 John F. Kennedy Boulevard • Suite 1800 • Philadelphia, Pennsylvania, 19103-2899

http://www.oralmaxsurgery.theclinics.com

**ORAL AND MAXILLOFACIAL SURGERY CLINICS OF NORTH AMERICA Volume 36, Number 3
August 2024 ISSN 1042-3699, ISBN-13: 978-0-443-24622-7**

Editor: John Vassallo; j.vassallo@elsevier.com
Developmental Editor: Anita Chamoli

Oral and Maxillofacial Surgery Clinics of North America (ISSN 1042-3699) is published quarterly by Elsevier Inc., 360 Park Avenue South, New York, NY 10010-1710. Months of issue are February, May, August, and November. Business and Editorial Offices: 1600 John F. Kennedy Blvd., Suite 1800, Philadelphia, PA 19103-2899. Periodicals postage paid at New York, NY and additional mailing offices. Subscription prices are $417.00 per year for US individuals, $100.00 per year for US students/residents, $488.00 per year for Canadian individuals, $100.00 per year for Canadian students/residents, $540.00 per year for international individuals, $235.00 per year for international students/residents. For institutional access pricing please contact Customer Service via the contact information below. To receive student/resident rate, orders must be accompanied by name or affiliated institution, date of term, and the *signature* of program/residency coordinator on institution letterhead. Orders will be billed at individual rate until proof of status is received. Foreign air speed delivery is included in all *Clinics* subscription prices. All prices are subject to change without notice. **POSTMASTER:** Send address changes to *Oral and Maxillofacial Surgery Clinics of North America,* Elsevier Periodicals **Customer Service, 11830 Westline Industrial Drive, St. Louis, MO 63146. Tel: 1-800-654-2452 (U.S. and Canada); 314-447-8871 (outside U.S. and Canada). Fax: 314-447-8029. E-mail: journalscustomerservice-usa@elsevier.com (for print support); journalsonlinesupport-usa@elsevier.com (for online support).**

Reprints. For copies of 100 or more, of articles in this publication, please contact the Commercial Reprints Department, Elsevier Inc., 360 Park Avenue South, New York, NY 10010-1710. Tel.: 212-633-3874; Fax: 212-633-3820; Email: reprints@elsevier.com.

Oral and Maxillofacial Surgery Clinics of North America is covered in *MEDLINE/PubMed (Index Medicus), Science Citation Index Expanded (SciSearch®), Journal Citation Reports/Science Edition*, and *Current Contents®/Clinical Medicine.*

Contributors

CONSULTING EDITOR

RUI P. FERNANDES, MD, DMD, FACS, FRCS(Ed)
Clinical Professor and Chief, Division of Head and Neck Surgery, Program Director, Head and Neck Oncologic Surgery and Microvascular Reconstruction Fellowship,

Departments of Oral and Maxillofacial Surgery, Neurosurgery, and Orthopaedic Surgery and Rehabilitation, University of Florida Health Science Center, University of Florida College of Medicine, Jacksonville, Florida

EDITOR

SRINIVAS M. SUSARLA, DMD, MD, MPH, FACS, FAAP
Surgical Director, Craniofacial Center, Division Chief, Craniofacial and Plastic Surgery,

Division Chief, Oral and Maxillofacial Surgery, Seattle Children's Hospital, Associate Professor, University of Washington, Seattle, Washington

AUTHORS

SHAUNAK N. AMIN, MD
Resident Physician, Department of Otolaryngology–Head and Neck Surgery, University of Washington, Seattle, Washington

ERIN E. ANSTADT, MD
Fellow, Division of Plastic Surgery, University of Washington School of Medicine, Craniofacial Center, Seattle Children's Hospital, Seattle, Washington

CHRISTINA M. BECK, MD, PhD
Plastic surgeon, Division of Plastic and Reconstructive Surgery, Department of Pediatrics, University of Washington School of Medicine, Seattle Children's Hospital, University of Washington, Seattle, Washington

APARNA BHAT, DMD, MD
Resident, Department of Oral and Maxillofacial Surgery, University of Washington School of Dentistry, Seattle, Washington

CRAIG BIRGFELD, MD
Associate Professor, Division of Plastic Surgery, Department of Surgery, University of Washington, Seattle, Washington

RANDALL A. BLY, MD
Associate Professor, Division of Pediatric Otolaryngology–Head and Neck Surgery, Department of Otolaryngology–Head and Neck Surgery, University of Washington Medical Center, Seattle Children's Hospital, Seattle, Washington

MARKUS D. BOOS, MD, PhD
Adjunct Associate Professor, Division of Dermatology, Department of Pediatrics, University of Washington School of Medicine, Seattle Children's Hospital, Seattle, Washington

ANDREA B. BURKE, DMD, MD
Assistant Professor, Department of Oral and Maxillofacial Surgery, University of Washington School of Dentistry, Seattle, Washington

PATRICK BYRNE, MD
Chair and Professor, Department of Otolaryngology–Head and Neck Surgery, Cleveland Clinic Foundation, Cleveland, Ohio

LETICIA M. CUELLAR, DMD
Resident, Division of Oral and Maxillofacial
Surgery, Carle Foundation Hospital, Urbana,
Illinois

DAVID J. CVANCARA, BS
Department of Otolaryngology – Head and
Neck Surgery, University of Washington
School of Medicine, Seattle, Washington

JOHN P. DAHL, MD, PhD, MBA
Associate Professor, Division of Pediatric
Otolaryngology-Head and Neck Surgery,
Department of Otolaryngology–Head and Neck
Surgery, University of Washington, Seattle
Children's Hospital, Seattle, Washington

NATALIE DERISE, MD
Clinical Instructor, Department of
Otolaryngology–Head and Neck Surgery,
University of Washington, Seattle, Washington

SEAN EDWARDS, DDS, MD
James Hayward Endowed Clinical Professor of
Department of Oral and Maxillofacial Surgery,
Chief of Pediatric Oral and Maxillofacial
Surgery, Associate Chair of Oral and
Maxillofacial Surgery, Hospital Dentistry,
University of Michigan School of Dentistry,
Ann Arbor, Michigan

MARK EGBERT, DDS
Associate Professor, Department of Oral and
Maxillofacial Surgery, University of Washington
School of Dentistry, Division of Plastic Surgery,
Department of Surgery, University of
Washington School of Medicine, Craniofacial
Center, Seattle Children's Hospital, Seattle,
Washington

RUSSELL E. ETTINGER, MD
Assistant Professor, Division of Plastic
Surgery, University of Washington School of
Medicine, Craniofacial Center, Seattle
Children's Hospital, Seattle, Washington

JASON HAUPTMAN, MD, PhD
Associate Professor, Craniofacial Center,
Department of Neurosurgery, Seattle
Children's Hospital, University of Washington
School of Medicine, Seattle, Washington

AMY LEE, MD
Professor, Department of Neurological
Surgery, University of Washington, Seattle
Children's Hospital, Seattle, Washington

ANDREW D. LINKUGEL, MD
Division of Plastic Surgery, Department of
Surgery, University of Washington School of
Medicine, Craniofacial Surgery Fellow,
Craniofacial Center, Seattle Children's
Hospital, Seattle, Washington

ALEXIS M. LINNEBUR, DMD
Pediatric Craniomaxillofacial Surgery Fellow,
Arnold Palmer Hospital for Children – Orlando
Health, Orlando, Florida

JOSEPH LOPEZ, MD, MBA
Chief of Pediatric Head and Neck Surgery,
Director, Pediatric Head, Neck, and Thyroid
Oncology Center, Clinical Professor, Division
of Pediatric Head and Neck Surgery,
Department of Children's Surgery,
AdventHealth for Children, Florida State
University, AdventHealth for Children's
Hospital, Orlando, Florida

G. NINA LU, MD
Assistant Professor, Department of
Otolaryngology–Head and Neck Surgery,
University of Washington, Seattle,
Washington

CAITLIN B.L. MAGRAW, MD, DDS, FACS
Pediatric Craniomaxillofacial Surgeon, The
Head and Neck Institute, Head and Neck
Surgical Associates, Associate Clinical
Professor, Department of Oral and
Maxillofacial Surgery, Oregon Health and
Sciences University, Portland, Oregon

ASHLEY E. MANLOVE, DMD, MD, FACS
Associate Clinical Professor, Medical Director,
Carle Illinois College of Medicine, Carle Cleft
and Craniofacial Team, Carle Foundation
Hospital, Urbana, Illinois

MICHAEL R. MARKIEWICZ, DDS, MPH, MD
Professor and William M. Feagans Endowed
Chair of Department of Oral and Maxillofacial
Surgery, Associate Dean for Hospital Affairs,
Clinical Professor, Departments of
Neurosurgery and Surgery, University at
Buffalo, Buffalo, New York

SARAH LOREN MOLES, DMD
Fellow, Head and Neck Surgical Oncology and
Microvascular Reconstruction, Providence
Cancer Institute, Portland, Oregon

DOMINIC NISTAL, MD
Resident, Department of Neurological Surgery,
University of Washington, Seattle, Washington

TITO ONYEKWELI, BS
University of Pittsburgh School of Medicine,
Pittsburgh, Pennsylvania

KRISTOPHER T. PATTERSON, BS
School of Medicine, University of Washington,
Seattle, Washington

ERIK N. QUINTANA, DMD
Resident, Division of Oral and Maxillofacial
Surgery, Carle Foundation Hospital, Urbana,
Illinois

CORY M. RESNICK, MD, DMD
Associate Professor, Department of Oral and
Maxillofacial Surgery, Harvard Medical School,
Oral and Maxillofacial Surgeon, Department of
Plastic and Oral Surgery, Boston Children's
Hospital, Boston, Massachusetts

JEREMY S. RUTHBERG, MD
Physician, Department of Otolaryngology–Head
and Neck Surgery, University of Washington
Medical Center, Seattle, Washington

JACOB RUZEVICK, MD
Assistant Professor, Department of
Neurological Surgery, University of
Washington, Seattle Children's Hospital,
Seattle, Washington

BARBARA SHELLER, DDS, MSD
Affiliate Professor, Departments of
Orthodontics and Pediatric Dentistry,
University of Washington School of Dentistry,
Division Chief of Pediatric Dentistry,
Department of Dentistry, Seattle Children's
Hospital, Seattle, Washington

RYAN SMART, DMD, MD
Clinical Assistant Professor, Department of
Surgery, University of North Dakota School of
Medicine and Health Sciences, Grand Forks,
North Dakota

HARLYN K. SUSARLA, DMD, MPH
Affiliate Assistant Professor, Department of
Pediatric Dentistry, University of Washington
School of Dentistry, Pediatric Dentist,
Department of Dentistry, Seattle Children's
Hospital, Seattle, Washington

**SRINIVAS M. SUSARLA, DMD, MD, MPH,
FACS, FAAP**
Surgical Director, Craniofacial Center, Division
Chief, Craniofacial and Plastic Surgery,
Division Chief, Oral and Maxillofacial Surgery,
Seattle Children's Hospital, Associate
Professor, University of Washington, Seattle,
Washington

LINDSEY TEAL, MD, MPH
Resident Physician, Division of Plastic Surgery,
Department of Surgery, University of
Washington Medical Center, Seattle,
Washington

ANTHONY P. TUFARO, DDS, MD
Director of Surgical Oncology, Institute
of Plastic Surgey and Dermatology,
Cleveland Clinic Foundation, Cleveland,
Ohio

Contents

Facial soft tissue lesions in children are often classified based on their structure or cellular origin and can be benign or malignant. This review focuses on common facial soft tissue lesions in children, their clinical morphology, natural history, and medical and surgical management, with an emphasis on those considerations unique to soft tissue lesions present at this anatomic site.

Benign intraoral soft tissue pathology in pediatric patients includes developmental, traumatic, inflammatory, and infectious lesions. Common pathology includes gingival cysts, mucoceles, fibromas, and parulis. Less common lesions include peripheral ossifying fibromas, congenital epulis of the newborn, and congenital mandibular duct atresia. Most of these lesions present at painless masses but can have significant effects on children and their caregivers. Although these lesions are generally harmless, evaluation and treatment is necessary for appropriate management and health of the child.

Pediatric odontogenic cysts and tumors are rare and often associated with developing or impacted teeth. Odontogenic cysts are broadly categorized as inflammatory or developmental while odontogenic tumors are classified histologically as epithelial, mesenchymal, or mixed tumors. This article will discuss the presentation, diagnosis, and treatment of odontogenic cysts and tumors in the pediatric population.

This article provides a comprehensive overview of benign non-odontogenic pathologies. Bone-derived lesions like osteoma, osteoid osteoma, osteoblastoma, and osteochondroma are discussed in detail, emphasizing their radiographic features, locations, and treatment strategies. Cartilage-derived lesions such as chondroma, chondroblastoma, and chondromyxoid fibroma are also examined, noting their typical presentation and management approaches. The article then delves into fibroconnective tissue lesions. Mesenchymal and vascular lesions are detailed regarding their clinical and radiographic characteristics and treatment options. Lastly, nerve-derived lesions like schwannoma and neurofibroma are covered, providing insights into their association with diseases like neurofibromatosis and preferred management strategies.

Pediatric temporomandibular joint (TMJ) disorders represent a broad range of congenital and acquired diagnoses. Dentofacial deformities, including facial asymmetry, retrognathism, and malocclusion, commonly develop. Compared with adult TMJ conditions, pain and articular disc pathology are less common. Accurate diagnosis is paramount in planning and prognostication. Several specific considerations apply in preparation for skeletal correction, including timing in relation to disease progression and growth trajectory, expectation for postcorrection stability, reconstructive technique as it applies to expected durability and need for future revision, management of occlusion, and need for ancillary procedures to optimize correction. This article reviews common conditions and treatment considerations.

Benign and malignant salivary gland disorders are uncommon in the pediatric population; however, these can be frequently seen in pediatric otolaryngology or oral and maxillofacial surgery practices. The astute clinician should be aware of the clinical presentation, diagnosis, and management options for common inflammatory, infectious, benign, and malignant disorders of salivary glands.

Pediatric orbital and skull base pathologies encompass a spectrum of inflammatory, sporadic, syndromic, and neoplastic processes that require a broad and complex clinical approach for both medical and surgical treatment. Given their complexity and often multicompartment involvement, a multidisciplinary approach for diagnosis, patient and family counseling, and ultimately treatment provides the best patient satisfaction and clinical outcomes. Advances in minimally invasive surgical approaches, including endoscopic endonasal and transorbital approaches allows for more targeted surgical approaches through smaller corridors beyond more classic transcranial or transracial approaches.

A wide variety of diagnoses can be approached with a common framework for diagnosis, extirpation, and reconstruction of pediatric cranial vault pathologies. Durability of reconstruction is critical for the range of pediatric patients from infancy to adolescence. Rigid reconstruction, preferably with autologous tissue when possible, promotes brain protection and satisfactory aesthetic outcome. Careful planning can allow for immediate definitive reconstruction of defects without need for further surgical intervention.

Craniomaxillofacial vascular anomalies encompass a diverse and complex set of pathologies that may have a profound impact on pediatric patients. They are subdivided into vascular tumors and vascular malformations depending on biological properties, clinical course, and distribution patterns. Given the complexity and potential for leading to significant functional morbidity and esthetic concerns, a multidisciplinary approach is generally necessary to optimize patient outcomes. This article reviews the etiology, clinical course, diagnosis, and current management practices related to vascular anomalies in the head and neck.

Since 2000, the incidence of head and neck cancer has dramatically increased. At this time, future studies are needed to further elucidate the factors contributing to rising incidence of head and neck cancer in children. This article provides a treatment framework for the pediatric surgical oncologist who manages cancer in children.

Craniofacial fibro-osseous lesions represent a diverse spectrum of pathologic conditions where fibrous tissue replaces healthy bone, resulting in the formation of irregular, woven bone. They are more commonly diagnosed in young people, with treatment strategies dependent on clinical behavior and skeletal maturity. This article discusses the examples of craniofacial fibro-osseous lesions, based on the latest classifications, along with their diagnostic criteria and management.

Odontogenic infections are a broad group of head and neck conditions that arise from the teeth and surrounding periodontium. These largely preventable infections disproportionately affect members of ethnic and racial minorities and low-income/uninsured groups, and result in significant costs to our health care system. Left untreated, odontogenic infections can spread to deep spaces of the head and neck and can result in life-threatening complications. The mainstay of treatment includes timely treatment of the affected teeth. These infections are a global public health concern that could be diminished with improved access to routine dental care.

Facial nerve pathology in children has devastating functional and psychosocial consequences. Facial palsy occurs less commonly in children than adults with a greater proportion caused by congenital causes. Most pediatric patients have normal life expectancy and few comorbidities and dynamic restoration of facial expression is prioritized. This article will focus on the unique aspects of care for facial palsy in the pediatric population.

Pediatric craniomaxillofacial reconstruction must be approached through the lens of growth and durability. A systematic approach of matching defects to donor tissue drives the selection of autologous reconstructive technique. The menu of available methods for reconstruction can be organized in a manner similar to adults, with special considerations for growth and development. Reconstructive surgeons have the opprtunity to promote and maintain young patients' sense of identity during psychosocial development.

ORAL AND MAXILLOFACIAL SURGERY CLINICS OF NORTH AMERICA

SERIES OF RELATED INTEREST

Atlas of the Oral and Maxillofacial Surgery Clinics
www.oralmaxsurgeryatlas.theclinics.com

Dental Clinics
www.dental.theclinics.com

THE CLINICS ARE NOW AVAILABLE ONLINE!
Access your subscription at:
www.theclinics.com

Preface
Pediatric Craniomaxillofacial Pathology

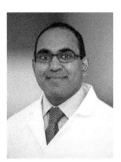

Srinivas M. Susarla, DMD, MD, MPH, FACS, FAAP
Editor

This issue of the *Oral and Maxillofacial Surgery Clinics of North America* focuses on the contemporary management of pathologic lesions involving the craniomaxillofacial region in children and adolescents. Craniomaxillofacial lesions in children can have a multitude of etiologies and can be broadly classified as benign, benign with aggressive features, or malignant. While malignant lesions are, fortunately, uncommon in children, treatment of all types of lesions in this population merits special considerations to account for growth and development, as well as the psychological effects of treatment on children, their families, and care providers.

Optimal treatment of the child with craniomaxillofacial pathology frequently requires collaborative efforts between many specialists, including surgeons as well as primary medical (eg, dermatologists and rheumatologists) and dental (eg, pediatric dentists, orthodontists, prosthetic dentists) providers. In this issue, we are extremely fortunate to have a diverse set of contributors representing the broad spectrum of specialists involved in the care of this unique population. Our expert group of authors has meticulously crafted contributions that cover this expansive topic in a way that is both comprehensive and accessible. It is my hope that this work will be a valuable resource to surgeons, dentists, and medical providers who care for these challenging clinical problems and will foster continued discussions about how we can improve the care that we provide to patients and families.

In addition to our contributors, I would like to recognize the editorial team of *Oral and Maxillofacial Surgery Clinics of North America* for their guidance and support for this issue. Dr Rui Fernandes has been an outstanding friend and mentor; his input regarding the scope of this work was particularly valuable, given his well-recognized expertise in head and neck pathology. John Vassallo's robust experience with the *Oral and Maxillofacial Surgery Clinics of North America* fostered a seamless workflow from project conception through production. Anita Chamoli worked tirelessly to ensure that the process for contributors was straightforward and continually supplied the positive reinforcement needed to ensure prompt production of a high-quality issue.

Finally, I would like to thank my wife, Dr Harlyn Susarla, for her love, support, and partnership. Her devotion to our family is matched by her devotion to the care of pediatric dental patients; she is the apex example of how one achieves work-life balance and is a model to emulate.

Srinivas M. Susarla, DMD, MD, MPH, FACS, FAAP
Craniofaical Center
Seattle Children's Hospital
4800 Sand Point Way Northeast
Seattle, WA 98105, USA

E-mail address:
srinivas.susarla@seattlechildrens.org

Oral Maxillofacial Surg Clin N Am 36 (2024) xi
https://doi.org/10.1016/j.coms.2024.04.002
1042-3699/24/© 2024 Published by Elsevier Inc.

Facial Soft Tissue Lesions in Children

Christina M. Beck, MD, PhD[a], Tito Onyekweli, BS[b], Russell E. Ettinger, MD[c],
Markus D. Boos, MD, PhD[d],*

KEYWORDS

- Melanocytic nevus • Nevus sebaceous • Pilomatricoma • Cyst

KEY POINTS

- Soft tissue growths are common in children and may be more frequently encountered in a head and neck distribution or engender unique management considerations when present in this anatomic location.
- Though melanocytic and epidermal nevi can be either benign or malignant, malignancy in children is exceedingly rare and requires a high degree of suspicion for diagnosis.
- Cystic lesions often require surgical removal to avoid complications including infection, sinus formation, and extension into or destruction of nearby structures.

INTRODUCTION

Facial, head, and neck soft tissue lesions are common in children and can be both congenital and acquired. These lesions are typically classified according to their cellular origin and basic structure (ie, cyst vs nevus) and can be benign or malignant. This review focuses on the most common facial soft tissue lesions in children (excluding vascular anomalies, covered in a separate article in this issue), including their morphology, natural history, and association with extracutaneous co-morbidities. Appropriate medical management and definitive surgical treatments are reviewed.

Soft Tissue Nevi in Children

Table 1 summarizes the clinical features of melanocytic and sebaceous nevi and their initial management with biopsy.

Common acquired melanocytic nevi

Melanocytic nevi, otherwise known as common moles, are ubiquitous findings on the skin of children. They represent benign proliferations of a subtype of melanocytes known as the nevus cell.

Clinical presentation and natural history Common acquired nevi typically present as homogeneously pigmented macules or papules measuring ≤6 mm in diameter, with a well-demarcated border. Common nevi can vary from flesh colored to tan, light brown, or dark brown in color; children with darker hair or darker skin tones typically also have accompanying darker nevi.[1] Melanocytic nevi are more concentrated on chronically sun-exposed areas including the face and neck.[2]

Common acquired nevi appear after 6 months of life and increase in number through childhood.[3] Nevi typically begin as flat macules, called junctional nevi, before progressing along 2 primary pathways: development into a raised, papular or

[a] Division of Plastic and Reconstructive Surgery, Department of Pediatrics, University of Washington School of Medicine, Seattle Children's Hospital, University of Washington, 325 9th Avenue Box 359796, Seattle, WA 98104, USA; [b] University of Pittsburgh School of Medicine, 3550 Terrace Street, Pittsburgh, PA 15212, USA; [c] Division of Plastic and Reconstructive Surgery, Department of Pediatrics, University of Washington School of Medicine, Seattle Children's Hospital, 4800 Sand Point Way Northeast, Seattle, WA 98105, USA; [d] Division of Dermatology, Department of Pediatrics, University of Washington School of Medicine, Seattle Children's Hospital, 4800 Sand Point Way Northeast, OC.9.833, Seattle, WA 98105, USA
* Corresponding author.
E-mail address: markus.boos@seattlechildrens.org

Oral Maxillofacial Surg Clin N Am 36 (2024) 247–263
https://doi.org/10.1016/j.coms.2024.03.001

Table 1
Clinical features of melanocytic and epidermal nevi and indications for biopsy

	Common Acquired Melanocytic Nevus	Congenital Melanocytic Nevus	Spitz Nevus	Sebaceous Nevus
Borders	Well-circumscribed	Geographic	Well-circumscribed	Well-circumscribed
Size	Usually <5 mm	Variable	Usually ≤4-6 mm	Variable
Clinical Features	Tan-brown macule or papule	Variable; features may include hypertrichosis, rugosity, nodules, lesional heterogeneity	Dome-shaped pink-red papule or homogeneously pigmented brown-black papule/thin plaque	Yellow-orange or dark brown alopecic plaque that may thicken and become verrucous with puberty
Indication to Biopsy or Remove	ABCDE criteria, including rapid evolution or other features suspicious for malignancy (ulceration, pain, itch, ugly duckling sign)	Disproportionate growth in thickness or surface area, functional impairment, clinical features concerning for malignancy, cosmetic	Age >12, atypical features including size >1 cm, asymmetry, ulceration, or rapid evolution, pain	Features suspicious for malignancy (ulceration, pain, itch, secondary growth within primary lesion)

"intradermal" lesion, or involution. Intradermal nevi are dome-shaped or pedunculated with a soft, rubbery texture; these nevi are often slightly lighter in color than their junctional counterparts.[4] In contrast, involution is characterized by a gradual fading via atrophy and fibrosis, producing a secondary hypopigmented macule that eventually re-pigments to match an individual's background pigmentation.[4] Apart from children with extremely fair skin that does not tan, non-Hispanic White children typically have higher nevus counts than children with darker skin tones (including children from Black, Asian/Pacific Islander, and Hispanic populations).[3,5–7]

Risk factors and associated considerations An important risk factor for increased number of acquired nevi is acute intermittent and intense sun exposure in childhood.[5] The vast majority of acquired melanocytic nevi do not require active intervention via surgical removal unless they develop atypical features. Nevertheless, over 100 acquired nevi measuring >2 mm were found in a study to represent the strongest clinical risk factor for melanoma, and children with this phenotype warrant regular skin examinations.[8,9]

Atypical/dysplastic nevi "Clinically atypical" or "dysplastic" nevi refer to common acquired nevi that share 1 or more of the classic "ABCDE" criteria of melanoma, though these features may be less striking. Criteria include Asymmetry in color or shape, Border irregularity, Color heterogeneity, and Diameter ≥6 mm. The classic criterion of Evolution used when evaluating melanocytic lesions in adults should also be considered in children, while recognizing that proportional growth is an expected feature of nevi in this population.[3] Atypical nevi are less common in prepubescent children compared to adolescents.[10] Importantly, while atypical nevi are a risk factor for the development of melanoma, they are not typically melanoma precursor lesions themselves.

The scalp is considered a "special site" with a higher incidence of clinically atypical nevi that may prompt concern.[11] Specifically, scalp nevi may be larger than 6 mm and exhibit perifollicular hypopigmentation causing irregular, often scalloped borders. These nevi often display variegated pigmentation, including benign "eclipse" (tan center, brown rim), "reverse eclipse" (brown center, tan rim), or "cockade" (targetoid) nevi.[12,13] In a study, 77% of the scalp nevi developed atypical changes, including an increase in size and color variegation, though these did not prompt removal.[12] Though the appearance and evolution of scalp nevi tend to trigger concern, these nevi are generally appropriate to monitor closely with regular clinic visits (ideally complemented with clinical photography); biopsy or removal should be reserved for nevi that have grossly atypical features or deviate from scalp-specific morphologies described earlier.

Management Prophylactic removal of all atypical nevi that lack worrisome features of melanoma is not warranted; preferred management includes patient education, baseline photography, and serial examinations.[14,15] Worrisome signs for melanoma include lesions that are new, rapidly develop more atypical features, appear distinct from an individual's other nevi, or become symptomatic. The conventional "ABCDE" criteria of melanoma can be used for the diagnosis of melanoma in children, though its use should be augmented with a second set of ABCD criteria to increase diagnostic accuracy. These pediatric "ABCD" criteria include Amelanotic lesions (present in 80% of cases), Bleeding or Bump (papulonodular lesions), Color uniformity, and De novo lesions of any Diameter (including < 6 mm in size). Recent Evolution remains an important characteristic of pediatric melanoma.[16] Children often have multiple nevi with a predominant distinctive clinical appearance ("signature nevus"). As such, 1 method to differentiate a worrisome melanocytic nevus from a benign one is by comparing the morphologic characteristics of the concerning nevus to the patient's other nevi and identifying whether its appearance is comparatively atypical.[17] Worrisome lesions can be sampled via scoop (deep) shave biopsy, punch biopsy, or excisional biopsy of the entire lesion with conservative margins, though the latter 2 are preferred to avoid transection of potentially malignant lesions.

Nevi with mild histologic atypia do not require re-excision, though nevi with severe atypia on histology warrant re-excision with clear margins to exclude the diagnosis of melanoma.[18,19] A melanoma diagnosis should be made via histopathologic evaluation by a dermatopathologist experienced in pediatric melanoma. A complete discussion of diagnosis and management of pediatric melanoma, which may include wide local excision, sentinel lymph node biopsy, and imaging, is beyond the scope of this review.

Congenital Melanocytic Nevi

Congenital melanocytic nevi (CMNs) are melanocytic nevi that are present at birth or within the first weeks of life. They are present in approximately 1% to 3.6% of newborns.[20] CMNs are caused by somatic mutations in melanocytes during embryologic development, with earlier embryologic mutations associated with larger lesions.[21,22]

In contrast to benign acquired nevi, they exhibit significant clinical heterogeneity and exhibit dynamic changes with time.

Clinical presentation and natural history

CMNs typically manifest as darkly pigmented macules, patches, papules, plaques, and/or nodules with clearly defined borders. At birth, they may be homogenously pigmented or have variegated pigmentation, but with age typically become more heterogeneously pigmented and develop progressive secondary features including hypertrichosis, rugosity, and nodularity.[23] (**Fig. 1**) The development of benign proliferations within large CMNs (proliferative nodules) is also common; these are characterized as round or ovoid papules or nodules with a well-defined border, firm, pliable texture, and smooth surfaces that are often less pigmented than the surrounding CMNs.[24,25] The color of CMNs in the first 3 months of life does not reliably indicate the lesion's final color, with lighter-skinned children generally experiencing more spontaneous lightening over time, which is also more common in CMNs of the scalp.[1,3] CMNs occasionally regress under a process termed the "halo phenomenon" in which a depigmented halo around a CMN precedes subsequent involution; rarely they can also regress via a

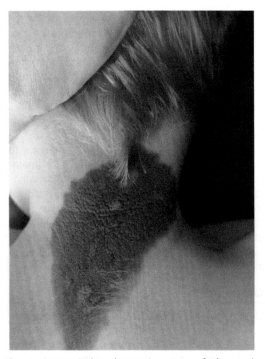

Fig. 1. Congenital melanocytic nevus of the neck. Note the heterogeneous pigmentation, focal areas of nodularity, and hypertrichosis, which are common in these lesions.

process of sclerosis without accompanying pigmentary changes.[26,27]

Classification

CMNs can present as isolated lesions or accompanied by additional, often smaller (satellite) lesions representing additional CMNs. CMNs grow proportionally with the child and are classified based on their projected adult size as small (less than 1.5 cm), medium (>1.5–20 cm), large (>20–40 cm), and giant (>40 cm).[23] Conversion factors can be used to approximate the adult size of a CMN on a newborn; this calculation uses the longest diameter of the nevus and multiplies it by a coefficient dependent on its anatomic location: 1.7 for head location, 3.3 for the legs, and 2.8 for the neck, trunk, buttocks, and arms.[23]

Melanoma and congenital melanocytic nevi

Cutaneous melanoma in CMNs usually presents as a new deep dermal or subcutaneous nodule, with painful, ulcerated, bleeding, and amelanotic nodules engendering heightened concern.[25,28] Any changes observed within a CMN including superficial or deep nodules or focal induration with or without surface changes should prompt biopsy and referral to dermatology for further evaluation.

The risk of melanoma developing within a CMN varies depending on patient characteristics. The incidence of melanoma is estimated at approximately 1% to 2% of all CMNs, and while melanoma has been documented in children with small-sized or medium-sized CMNs, it is a rare event.[29] In contrast, children with a CMN >40 cm and multiple smaller CMNs appear to have a higher incidence of melanoma, estimated in some studies at 10% to 15%.[25] In a cohort of 448 patients in London, children with a giant CMN >60 cm with 1 other CMN of any size, or children with 2 or more CMNs with no single clearly larger nevus had an incidence of melanoma of 8% in childhood.[25] Importantly, primary central nervous system melanoma has been estimated to represent about one-third of all melanomas diagnosed in children with CMNs.[25,28]

Neurologic considerations

The presence of CMNs may be associated with neural melanosis (deposits of melanocytes within the central nervous system [CNS]). Specifically, children with a giant CMN and multiple satellite lesions, or those with multiple medium-sized CMNs, appear to be at elevated risk of accompanying neural melanosis. In a retrospective study, >4 CMNs appeared to impart greatest risk of MRI abnormalities.[30] The authors of this study recommend MRI screening for any child with more than 1 CMN of at least medium size, though this practice has not been universally adopted.[30] Recommendations from a pediatric dermatology working group include MRI of the brain and spine with and without contrast for children with multiple medium CMNs, a giant CMN, or the presence of 10 or more satellite lesions, as well as the presence of any neurologic or developmental abnormalities in a patient with CMNs of any size.[24,31]

Abnormal MRI findings associated with CMNs include parenchymal melanosis and structural abnormalities such as Dandy-Walker complex, hydrocephalus, and non-melanocytic tumors of the CNS.[32] As these findings indicate a risk for neurologic complications including seizure and developmental delay, all children with CMNs and an abnormal MRI should be referred to a neurologist for evaluation and monitoring; neurosurgical consult can also be considered.[24,31] Importantly, abnormal MRI imaging is a strong predictor of melanoma at any site in children with CMNs; screening MRI therefore acts as an important baseline should children develop subsequent neurologic abnormalities.[25] Ongoing radiologic monitoring of children with neurocutaneous melanosis or other intracranial abnormalities should be tailored based on baseline radiologic characteristics and any neurologic or developmental changes.[24,25]

Management

Small and medium CMNs can be monitored annually by a general pediatrician, though referral to dermatology should be considered for those that are symptomatic, changing, or have variegated pigmentation or textural changes.[24] Regular dermatologic follow-up is generally recommended for larger CMNs to facilitate education and monitoring; recommendations include evaluation every 3 months for the first year of life with consideration of less frequent intervals over time, though these children should have at minimum an annual evaluation with a dermatologist.[24]

Surgical guidelines

Conservative management of CMNs with clinical monitoring is recommended, though surgical excision can be considered for small and medium CMNs that are symptomatic, challenging to monitor, or are functionally or cosmetically bothersome to patients.[24] The only absolute indication for surgical intervention is concern for malignancy; studies do not support prophylactic removal of CMNs, regardless of size, as this has not been shown to reduce melanoma risk and may lead to unacceptable scarring, as well as increased risk of pain, anxiety, and complications of multiple episodes of anesthesia.[24,33]

Head and neck CMNs may cause significant cosmetic, psychosocial, and functional impairment (eg, reduced vision, diminished ability to feed) and can be considered a relative indication for surgical intervention.[34] However, surgery at this location also necessitates obvious aesthetic and anatomic considerations so a decision to proceed with surgery should come after thoughtful consultation and discussion between family, patient, and surgeon.[34] Specifically, surgical resection that may result in undesirable cosmesis or occurs in an anatomically sensitive area (ie, alar rim) may not be warrranted.[33,34] Nevertheless, patients undergoing removal of head and neck CMNs often have high (95%) satisfaction rates.[35] Other studies found that surgical removal of CMNs had no effect on quality of life; however, they did find a strong relationship between visibility of CMNs and perceived stigmatization,[36] highlighting the importance of how social support, advocacy groups, and referral to psychology can be helpful for patients with large, visible CMNs.[37]

Surgical technique is highly dependent on anatomic location but generally necessitates full-thickness removal of all dermal layers since melanocytes can be deeply infiltrative and may be found as deep as the subcutaneous plane.[38] Partial-thickness superficial removal techniques such as dermabrasion, split thickness skin grafting, and curettage are not advised due to the associated risks of scarring and repigmentation, often leading to worse cosmetic outcomes.[34] Approaches to CMNs removal include excision with primary closure, serial excision, use of tissue expanders (TE), full-thickness skin grafts, and/or local flaps.[33,38] TE should be employed selectively because of their potential physical and psychological morbidity.[39] In summary, surgeons should approach excision of CMNs with intentional care to ensure that potential benefits outweigh the burdens/outcomes of treatment.

Spitz Nevi

Spitz nevi, also known as "benign juvenile melanoma," are benign melanocytic proliferations defined by their large, spindled cells and epithelioid histology. Spitz nevi exist on a spectrum, ranging from benign Spitz nevi with a regular histologic appearance to atypical Spitz nevi to Spitzoid melanoma.[3]

The incidence of Spitz nevi is estimated at 1.4 to 7 new cases per 100,000 people annually. The majority of these nevi occur in individuals less than 20 years of age, with a mean age of diagnosis of approximately 6 to 7 years.[40–42] Spitz nevi are more common in non-Hispanic White children.[40–42]

Clinical presentation and natural history

The most common anatomic sites for Spitz nevi include the face, head, and neck, accounting for 36% to 38% of all cases.[41,42] Spitz nevi typically appear as 2 main variants: solitary, well-circumscribed pink-red papules, or homogeneously pigmented brown-black papules and plaques.[3,43] (**Fig. 2**) Benign Spitz nevi are typically <1 cm (often 4-6 mm) in size and may exhibit rapid growth before plateauing; over months to years, many Spitz nevi involute spontaneously.[43] Pink-red Spitz nevi may be misdiagnosed as a pyogenic granuloma or hemangioma while darker variants may engender concern for melanoma. Clinically, typical Spitz nevi can be monitored closely with follow-up visits recommended every 3 to 6 months until the lesion involutes or develops stable features of common nevi; ideally, this is performed by a dermatologist or other provider familiar with dermoscopy to aid in clinical surveillance. Caregivers should also be educated about concerning changes that warrant prompt re-evaluation.[3,40,44]

Given their clinical and histologic overlap with melanoma, biopsy with histologic evaluation is recommended for suspected Spitz nevi that newly arise in post-pubertal children (aged 12 years or older), and those with atypical features including size >1 cm, asymmetry, ulceration, or rapid evolution at any age.[3,40,44] These atypical Spitz nevi benefit from more proactive management, though recommendations remain controversial. While all atypical Spitz nevi should be completely excised, some authors recommend excisional margins of 1 cm, while others advocate for more conservative margins, especially in cosmetically sensitive areas.[45] Sentinel lymph node biopsy is not recommended for atypical Spitz nevi, as this is a relatively morbid procedure and lymph node positivity does not appear to confer worse outcomes.[40–42] Instead, patients with atypical Spitz tumors can be followed with periodic clinical examinations and ultrasound of the relevant lymph node basins following excision.[40,41]

Spitzoid melanoma exists on a spectrum with atypical Spitz nevi; this diagnosis is therefore often made based on the degree and number of atypical features present within a given tumor.[46] As such, the expertise of a dermatopathologist skilled in evaluating these tumors histologically should be sought and management undertaken concurrently with an oncologist versed in childhood melanoma. Fortunately, Spitzoid melanoma in children is exceedingly rare.[46]

Nevus Sebaceous of Jadassohn

Nevus sebaceous of Jadassohn (NSJ) is a type of epidermal nevus that arises from postzyogtic activating mutations in the Ras pathway.[47] NSJ affects approximately 0.3% of newborns and is a congenital lesion located most commonly on the scalp (59.3%) and face (32.6%).[48]

Clinical presentation and natural history

NSJs typically present as alopecic, round, or crescentic plaques and their color may vary with an individual's skin tone.[49] In individuals with darker skin tones, NSJs typically appear dark brown, while in individuals with lighter skin tones, they may appear pink or yellow-orange (**Fig. 3**). The natural history of NSJ can be divided into 3 distinct stages.[50] In the prepubertal stage, papillomatous epithelial hyperplasia with immature hair follicles predominates.[50] During this stage, these lesions typically experience proportional growth without significant clinical alteration. As a child enters puberty, NSJs may become thicker with verrucous changes, owing to sebaceous gland hyperplasia.[51]

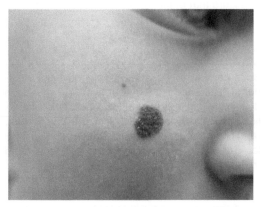

Fig. 2. Spitz nevus of the cheek in a child. This uniformly pigmented dark brown plaque measured 5 mm at widest diameter and was removed given its anatomic location.

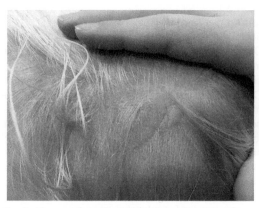

Fig. 3. Nevus sebaceous. Note the yellow-orange color of this alopecic patch on the parietal scalp.

In adulthood, the occurrence of secondary neoplasms within NSJs becomes relatively common, affecting approximately 14% of individuals with NSJs. Among these growths, the majority comprise benign lesions, including trichoblastoma and syringocystadenoma papilliferum.[52] The incidence of malignant transformation within an NSJ remains low at approximately 2%, with basal cell carcinoma representing the most common malignancy.[52,53] Importantly, the overwhelming majority of patients with malignant degeneration of NSJs are adults.[52,53]

Management
Given the low risk of malignant transformation in childhood, the preferred approach to managing NSJs in children involves close observation, with consideration of biopsy if ulceration occurs or papular/nodular lesions develop.[52,54] Superficial removal techniques such as cryoablation, electrodessication, and laser therapy are not recommended due to the tendency of NSJs to recur.[55] Topical 1% sirolimus represents a novel therapy showing promise in flattening pubertal NSJs.[55,56]

Sampling of NSJs via full thickness excisional biopsy is clearly indicated when malignancy is suspected, but no consensus ideal timing exists for elective removal of NSJs if cosmetic concerns predominate. Surgical removal in early childhood affords benefits of greater scalp laxity and the ability to minimize the extent of surgery. Delaying surgery until late childhood/early adulthood can allow patients to assent to the procedure.[57] Importantly, several authors have highlighted challenges in achieving optimal cosmetic results when removing NSJs of the scalp, as this procedure is often accompanied by complications such as widened scars and potential alopecia.[57,58] Nevertheless, even a suboptimal clinical outcome may be preferred relative to the alopecia associated with the primary nevus.

Additional considerations
Nevus sebaceous syndrome denotes the coexistence of extensive NSJs with extracutaneous manifestations. Small, isolated NSJs do not require further evaluation. However, large NSJs of the head and neck, specifically those in a centrofacial location, should raise concern for associated neurologic abnormalities (seizures, hemiparesis, developmental delay).[59] These children should undergo early formal neurodevelopmental testing with their pediatrician, with further evaluation as needed.[60] This high-risk subgroup should also have ophthalmologic examinations to evaluate for colobomas and choristomas and an oral examination to identify associated abnormalities including intraoral verrucous growths, and palatal/dental anomalies.[61–63]

CYSTIC LESIONS IN CHILDREN

Table 2 summarizes the clinical features of cystic lesions, their preferred radiologic evaluation, and management.

Dermoid Cyst
Dermoid cysts are benign neoplasms of ectodermal and mesodermal tissue forming along embryonic fusion lines.[64] They are defined by the presence of these 2 germ cell lineages as opposed to the single ectoderm found in epidermoid cysts.[65,66]

Epidemiology
Dermoid cysts are rare, with an incidence of 3 in 10,000 general pediatric patients, yet they are one of the most common tumors of the head and neck in the pediatric population.[67,68] They are considered congenital, with 40% diagnosed before 1 year of age and 90% diagnosed before age 5.[64,67] There are no known underlying genetic causes or familial inheritance patterns.[67]

Clinical presentation and natural history
The majority of dermoid cysts are found on the head or neck.[69,70] In a case series of 75 pediatric patients, 72 were located on the head, 1 on the neck, and the remaining 2 on the trunk.[67] Within the head, the frontal, occipital, and periorbital regions are the most reported sites of involvement.[66,69,70] Several studies have identified the lateral eyebrow as the most common location.[67,69,71] The parahyoid and suprasternal regions are the 2 most common sites involving the neck.[71]

Clinically, dermoid cysts present as a firm, nonmobile, asymptomatic mass ranging from 0.5 to 5 cm with a mean size of 1.3 cm.[66,67] The majority slowly enlarge over time, but about 30% do not change in size. Rarely, they can grow and then shrink in size or become smaller than at presentation and a small portion of dermoid cysts are identified after trauma to the area.[72] Many dermoid cysts develop deep in the subperiosteal plane and can appear fixed to the underlying bone and firm on palpation.[67] Cranial remodeling, erosion, and intracranial extension can occur.[70] In a series evaluating 655 dermoid cysts, the frontal, occipital, and temporal regions and midline nasal lesions inferior to the nasofrontal junction were the common sites for intracranial extension.[73] In a series of 234 pediatric patients, midline scalp dermoid cysts were found to have a higher probability of intracranial extension, though no association was

Table 2
Clinical features of cystic lesions

	Dermoid Cyst	Pilomatricoma	Branchial Anomalies	Thyroglossal Duct Cyst
Location	Scalp, forehead, lateral brow most common	Most common in periorbital, preauricular regions, cheek	Post and preauricular/parotid region, lateral neck along anterior SCM	Midline from base of the tongue to the thyroid
Appearance	Firm, nonmobile, asymptomatic mass	Hard, well-circumscribed cutaneous or subcutaneous mobile mass	Cystic mass, sinus tract, or fistulae; possible infection	Asymptomatic cystic mass; possible infection
Imaging	Ultrasound or CT in high-risk areas for intracranial extension	Generally not indicated, though ultrasound can be considered to confirm diagnosis	Ultrasound, CT, CT-fistulogram when indicated	Ultrasound
Management	Surgical excision	Surgical excision with involved skin	Surgical excision	Classic or modified Sistrunk procedure

Abbreviations: CT, computed tomography; SCM, sternocleidomastoid muscle.

identified between age or sex and depth of infiltration.[70] Though typically asymptomatic, symptoms associated with dermoid cysts can include yellow discharge, focal pain, headache, pruritis, and infection with purulent discharge.[67,72] Although they have consistent presentation and physical examination findings, dermoid cysts require pathologic evaluation for confirmation of the diagnosis.

Management
Surgical excisional biopsy is recommended to prevent ongoing growth and reduce the potential for bony erosion and intracranial extension, decrease the risk of infection, and to establish diagnosis. Given their origin from embryonic ectoderm, dermoid cysts may extend into the cranium, orbit, paranasal sinus, or temporal fossa.[69] Nasal dermoids should be differentiated from other congenital tumors of the nose including gliomas, encephaloceles, neurofibromas, and vascular malformations. Ultrasound or computed tomography (CT) imaging should be performed if dermoid cysts are located midline, along suture lines, or present with any atypical findings concerning for intracranial, intraorbital, or intranasal extension.[67,73] If ultrasound is inconclusive, or shows high suspicion of high-grade bony erosion, or if the mass is in a high-risk region (midline nasal, frontal, temporal, or occipital region) CT should be performed. If CT shows evidence of intracranial extension, MRI is indicated to determine the extent and depth of dural involvement.

Surgical approach is typically direct excisional biopsy with attempt to remove the entire dermoid cyst and sinus tract, if present, without rupture (**Fig. 4**). When rupture occurs, care is taken to remove all the material from the cavity to reduce the chance of recurrence. If intracranial extension is noted on preoperative imaging, resection should be performed in conjunction with neurosurgery. Rarely, craniotomy, orbitotomy, or open rhinoplasty is performed. A pericranial flap can be utilized if extensive dural resection is required. Recurrence is rare, and long-term follow-up or serial imaging is not generally indicated.

Pilomatricoma

Epidemiology
Pilomatricoma is a skin tumor composed of cells from the hair follicle matrix. They are the second most common superficial tumor in the pediatric population.[74] A histologic evaluation of 140,000 skin tumors from patients of all ages identified pilomatricoma in 1 out of every 824 lesions, with the highest incidence found between 8 and 13 years of age.[75] Age of clinical presentation is bimodally distributed with the highest rate of occurrence between 0 and 20 years of age, and a second less robust peak between 50 and 65 years of age.[76] In a systematic review evaluating 318 pediatric patients with pilomatricomas, there is a slight female predominance (female-to-male ratio 1.65:1).[77] Pilomatricomas are generally considered benign,

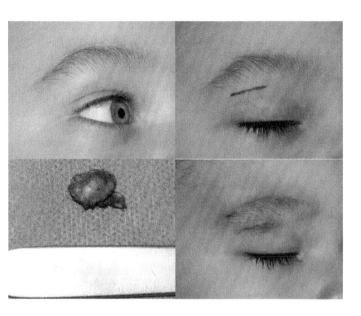

Fig. 4. Surgical excision of a lateral brow dermoid cyst with a linear incision hidden along the inferior brow.

though pilomatrical carcinomas have been rarely reported in the pediatric population.[78]

Clinical presentation and natural history

Given their cellular origin, pilomatricomas are found in hair-bearing regions of the body. A series of 137 pediatric patients found 70% in the head or neck with 22% of the remaining 30% found in the upper extremity.[79] Within the head, the cheek, periorbital, and preauricular regions are the most common sites.[80]

Pilomatricomas present as hard, well-circumscribed cutaneous or subcutaneous nodules (**Fig. 5**).[77] Given their origin in the superficial layers of the skin, pilomatricomas will generally present as more mobile than other masses arising from deeper structures and can aid in the clinical diagnosis and subsequent surgical planning. The majority have normal overlying skin but can present with a blue or red-tinge or with telangiectasias.[77] Central skin tethering with mobilization of the mass can also allude to the superficial tissue origin of a pilomatricoma; as lesions may be calcified, stretching the surrounding skin to demonstrate angulation of the lesion ("tent sign") can help with clinical diagnosis. When evaluating a suspected pilomatricoma, transillumination of the lesion with a handheld otoscope can help secure diagnosis; in contrast to other cystic lesions, pilomatricomas will not allow light to pass through, creating a dark shadow. The size of pilomatricomas within the head and neck ranges between 0.5 and 6 cm with a mean of 1.2 cm.[77] Lesions typically present asymptomatically, but can present with pain, itching, or burning, and rarely ulceration.[77,81] Inflammation and infection of pilomatricomas has also been described. In a series of 228 patients with pilomatricomas, 198 patients experienced a slow rate of growth, 2 had rapid growth, and 23 experienced trauma to the area weeks to years prior to the development of the lesion.[81]

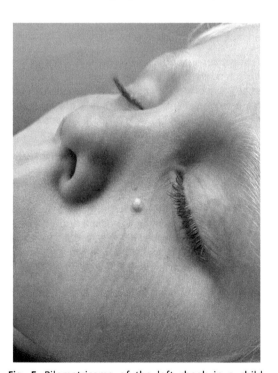

Fig. 5. Pilomatricoma of the left cheek in a child. Given its superficial origin and location, the lesion appears yellow-white in color and on examination the pilomatricoma is firm, mobile, and free tethering to deeper tissues.

Multiple pilomatricomas have been reported as a wide range from 2% to 33%.[75,77,82] Most reports are closer to the lower range with an average of 7.9% of cases in the pediatric population in a large retrospective study.[77] These cases can be random, familial, or associated with an underlying syndrome.[83] Myotonic dystrophy is the most reported association with multiple pilomatricomas, followed by familial adenomatous polyposis (FAP)-related syndromes, Turner, and Rubinstein-Taybi syndromes.[83] Churg-Strauss, Kabuki, and Sotos syndromes and hypercalcemia or sarcoidosis have also been reported on a smaller scale in case reports.[82,84–86] A 2019 review found syndromic patients developed 6 or more lesions 46.3% of the time compared to only 4.5% of the time in sporadic cases.[83]

Diagnosis
Clinical diagnosis based on patient history and examination is achieved in only 12.5% to 55% of cases.[87] Ultrasonography can be helpful to support a diagnosis, in particular for lesions over the parotid gland, and will show an ovoid complex mass between the dermis and subcutaneous fat with thinning of the overlying dermis (Fink, Hughes).[88,89] Hwang and colleagues found ultrasound can increase the accuracy of diagnosis from 33% to 76%.

Management
Management is surgical excision with a goal of complete resection to decrease recurrence (**Fig. 6**). If the lesion is adherent to skin, overlying skin should be removed. Surgical resection during times of acute inflammation or frank infection should be avoided as this can increase recurrence rates due to tissue friability compromising dissection planes. Treatment with incision and curettage or selective debulking has been described for large tumors in cosmetically sensitive areas.[90] Recurrence is rare in the pediatric population and thought to be due to incomplete resection, and limited clinical follow-up is reasonable in most cases.[80,81] However, if pathology demonstrates aggressive or malignant features, patients should be observed for recurrence.[78] Lastly, if >5 pilomatricomas are identified, work up for the aforementioned syndromes should be considered.[83]

Branchial Anomalies

Branchial anomalies result from failure of involution of branchial structures during weeks 3 to 6 of gestation.[91] The remnant tissue forms a cyst, sinus tract, or fistula at the location of the first, second, third, or fourth branchial structure from which it originated.[92]

Epidemiology
Branchial anomalies account for 20% of cervical masses and are the second most common congenital lesion of the head and neck in the pediatric population.[93] Bilateral anomalies account for 1% to 10% of cases.[93,94] Familial inheritance has been described, but there is no predilection for gender or race.[95]

Clinical presentation and natural history
Clinical presentation depends on the branchial structure involved, and the extent of aberrant obliteration during development. Most are diagnosed in the first decade of life with branchial cysts being

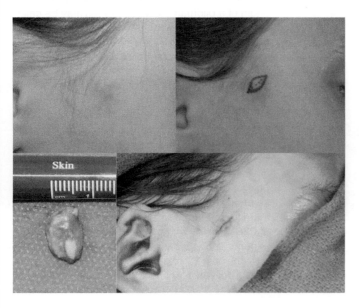

Fig. 6. Pilomatricoma of the right temple in a child. While superficial in origin, this pilomatricoma demonstrates deeper extension manifesting as only slight overlying skin discoloration. On examination, the pilomatricoma is firm, mobile, and demonstrates a focal point of skin tethering denoting the superficial follicular origin of the mass. Surgical excision is conducted with an ellipse of overlying skin incorporating the area of follicular origin.

diagnosed later and more often into adulthood.[94,96] Cysts form when a branchial groove fails to obliterate and have no external or internal opening. Sinus tracts develop when a branchial groove or pouch persists and communicates externally to the neck (branchial cleft sinus) or internally into the mucosa of the upper airway (branchial pouch sinus). Branchial fistulae arise from a connection between a remnant groove and pouch that leads to direct communication between the external skin and mucosa.[93,94] Cysts typically present as asymptomatic lateral neck masses, but can be tender, enlarge with upper respiratory infection, and rarely become infected. Sinus tracts and fistulae can present with recurrent inflammation, drainage, or rarely abscess formation.[96]

First branchial anomalies

First branchial anomalies are the second most common type, making up 4% to 25% of branchial lesions in the pediatric population.[97,98] They can present anywhere from the postauricular and parotid regions to inferior to the mandibular angle, above the hyoid bone in the neck. Symptoms vary based on location. Parotid and postauricular lesions typically enlarge with infection causing erythema and pain. The relationship to the facial nerve varies with the branchial lesions lying superficial, deep, or between branches, with the majority being superficial.[99] Cervical lesions have a range of presentations including overt draining sinus tracts or pin-point depressions that express fluid with compression.[100]

Work classified first branchial cleft anomalies as Type I or Type II.[101] Type I is of ectodermal origin arising from a duplication of the external auditory canal and will be located within the parotid gland or preauricular region with extension into the external auditory canal. Type II lesions contain ectoderm and mesoderm (cartilage), arising from a duplication of the external auditory canal and pinna and will be located posterior to the angle of the mandible with extension into the preauricular area. Given their presentation, first branchial anomalies can mimic a preauricular cyst or sinus tract, epidermal and dermoid cysts, parotid lesions, a mastoid abscess, or postauricular lymphadenopathy (**Fig. 7**).[98]

Second branchial anomalies

Second branchial structure anomalies are the most common and make up 40% to 95% of branchial anomaly lesions.[95] Their course can be from the anterior border of the sternocleidomastoid muscle (SCM), between the external and internal carotid arteries, lateral and superior to the glossopharyngeal and hypoglossal nerves, through the

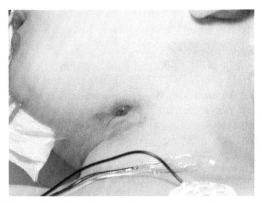

Fig. 7. First branchial cleft anomaly with sinus tract and cyst involving the left lateral neck. (Image courtesy of Jonathan Perkins, DO.)

middle pharyngeal constrictor into the tonsillar fossa.[92] Thus, typical presentations are an asymptomatic neck mass along the upper third of the SCM and draining sinus tracts at the base of the neck. Fistulae are more commonly found on the right, and bilateral fistulae can be associated with branchio-oto-renal syndrome and warrant genetic workup if present.[102]

Third and fourth branchial anomalies

Third and fourth branchial anomalies are extremely rare and predominantly found on the left side of the neck.[97,103] Their courses are similar from the mid to lower third of the anterior border of the SCM, variable involvement of the thyroid, along the carotid sheath over (third) or under (fourth) the superior laryngeal nerve, deep to the glossopharyngeal nerve, piercing the thyroid structures to the piriform sinus.[92] There have been reports of lesions presenting as a lateral neck mass with encroachment on the airway and pyriform sinus fistulae, resulting in suppurative thyroiditis or thyroid abscess.[98,104]

Diagnosis

Imaging is frequently utilized to aid in diagnosis and the extent of branchial lesions. Ultrasound is accurate in the diagnosis of cysts, and of sinuses with the addition of fistulogram studies.[92] CT and MRI are variable in their ability to demonstrate an entire sinus or fistulae tract, but are critical in confirming the relationship of first branchial anomalies with the facial nerve.[92,98] CT fistulography provides more detail than x-ray fistulography in demonstrating the course through critical structures in the neck, including the parotid gland, carotid vessels, and submandibular gland.[105] Esophagogram and direct laryngoscopy/pharyngoscopy is useful in evaluation of third and fourth branchial anomaly sinus and fistula tracts.[92]

Management

Surgical excision is recommended due to a high risk of infection.[93,96] This includes sinus or fistula tract excision with superficial parotidectomy and facial nerve dissection and preservation for first branchial lesions and tonsillectomy for second branchial anomalies. A series of 274 patients with branchial anomaly remnants found a 2.7% recurrence rate after resection of a native lesion, 14% if previous infection was noted, and 21.2% if previous surgical excision was attempted.[106] Sinus tracts recur more often than cysts following excision and recurrence is more common for first, third, and fourth branchial anomalies likely due to incomplete resection.[96] It is reasonable to wait until the patient is 6 months to 1 year of age if there are no recurrent infections, abscess, or airway compromise, although others recommend delaying until age 2 to 3 when adjacent structures are easier to identify.[92] Complications include infection, nerve damage, seromas, and hematomas, with an overall rate of 5%.[97] The risk of facial nerve injury is higher if the nerve is not identified during dissection or if the patient has had multiple infections or prior surgical interventions.[99] An analysis of 895 patients undergoing surgical excision of branchial anomalies found no correlation with depth of excision and complication rate, and a significant increase in post operative infection in patients with a history of developmental delay.[97]

Thyroglossal Duct Cyst

Thyroglossal duct cysts (TDCs) result from remnant embryologic thyroid tissue and are the most common congenital neck mass.[107] During the third week of gestation, thyroid tissue migrates from the foramen cecum at the base of the tongue to its position over the trachea in the neck. The middle portion of the duct involutes at weeks 5 to 10. Failure to do so will result in remnant epithelial tissue causing formation of a cyst.[108]

Clinical presentation and natural history

Clinically, TDCs present as a mass located midline anywhere from the base of the tongue to the thyroid, and occasionally as submental or lower cervical lesions (**Fig. 8**).[109,110] They are tethered to the hyoid bone, thus will move with tongue protrusion and swallowing. Most present asymptomatic in the first decade of life.[111,112] They can become infected with associated erythema and pain, or rupture leading to sinus tract or fistulae formation with ongoing drainage.[111] Lingual remnants may cause stridor, respiratory obstruction,

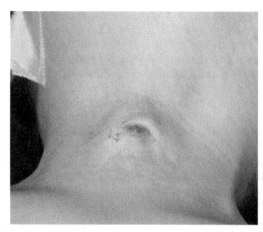

Fig. 8. Midline thyroglossal duct cyst in a child. (Image courtesy of Jonathan Perkins, DO.)

and dysphagia.[109] TDC carcinoma has been identified in 0.7% to 1.5% of thyroglossal duct cysts at a mean age of 40 years, and there have been reports of papillary carcinoma within thyroglossal duct tissue.[113,114]

Diagnosis

Ultrasound is the gold standard imaging modality for diagnosis of TDCs.[108] Computed tomography can be helpful in assessing extent of recurrence or when malignancy or abscess is suspected. Ultrasound-guided fine-needle aspiration cytology can be used to distinguish between TDCs or ectopic thyroid gland and malignancy, however, with low sensitivity, thus is not recommended.[109] Thyroid scan with technetium 99m sodium is used to establish ectopic thyroid tissue when suspected.[109]

Management

Management is surgical excision to prevent infection and sinus or fistulae formation, and to rule out malignancy.[112] The classic and modified Sistrunk procedures have proven to be the gold standard with decreased recurrence from 20% to 49% to 0% to 13.9% compared to simple excision.[108] The modified procedure involves removal of the middle portion of hyoid bone while the classic procedure also carves out a cuff of lingual tissue at the cecum foramen.[115] Complication rates range from 4.4% to 20.9%.[112] Major complications include hematoma or abscess requiring drainage, hypoglossal nerve injury, or violation of the airway; however, the most common reported complication is local skin infection.[112] A review of 340 patients demonstrated there is no indication to wait until a certain age to perform resection.[112]

CLINICS CARE POINTS

- Asymmetry in color or shape, Border irregularity, Color heterogeneity, and Diameter ≥6 mm are features of melanocytic nevi that should engender concern for potential malignancy. In children, additional important criterion suggestive of atypia or malignancy includes Amelanotic lesions, Bleeding or Bump, Color uniformity, De novo lesions of any Diameter (including < 6 mm in size),and recent Evolution.

- When sampling a clinically atypical melanocytic lesion, clinicopathological correlation and involvement of a dermatopathologist with experience in pediatric melanoma is recommended to optimize diagnosis and management.

- Children with giant congenital melanocytic nevi or multiple congenital nevi estimated medium-sized or greater should be monitored closely for development of melanoma and neurocutaneous melanosis and multidisciplinary care should be considered.

- Clinically, typical Spitz nevi can be followed via serial clinical examinations in prepubertal children, though atypical Spitz nevi should be removed or biopsy be done to exclude Spitzoid melanoma.

- Sebaceous nevi have a low risk of malignant transformation in childhood and can be safely monitored in this age group.

- When considering surgical management of soft tissue growths, caregivers should be extensively counseled regarding the risks of post-surgical scarring and recurrence to properly evaluate risks and benefits of a procedure.

- Dermoid cysts should be surgically excised due to their potential for ongoing growth and require appropriate imaging in higher-risk areas such as midline nasal, frontal, temporal, and occipital regions.

- Pilomatricomas require surgical removal due to the risk of infection and low risk of malignancy. The presence of 6 or more pilomatricomas requires genetic evaluation.

- First and second branchial anomalies are far more common than third and fourth and present with a wide range from asymptomatic head and neck masses to draining sinus tracts. Imaging is recommended for surgical planning.

- The classic and modified Sistrunk procedures are the gold standards for removing thyroglossal duct cysts from their location midline on the neck.

DISCLOSURE

The authors have nothing to disclose.

REFERENCES

1. Polubothu S, Kinsler VA. Final congenital melanocytic naevi colour is determined by normal skin colour and unaltered by superficial removal techniques: a longitudinal study. Br J Dermatol 2020; 182(3):721–8.

2. Dodd AT, Morelli J, Mokrohisky ST, et al. Melanocytic nevi and sun exposure in a cohort of colorado children: anatomic distribution and site-specific sunburn. Cancer Epidemiol Biomarkers Prev 2007;16(10):2136–43.

3. Schaffer JV. Update on melanocytic nevi in children. Clin Dermatol 2015;33(3):368–86.

4. Terushkin V, Scope A, Halpern AC, et al. Pathways to involution of nevi: insights from dermoscopic follow-up. Arch Dermatol 2010;146(4):459–60.

5. De Giorgi V, Gori A, Greco A, et al. Sun-protection behavior, pubertal development and menarche: factors influencing the melanocytic nevi development-the results of an observational study of 1,512 children. J Invest Dermatol 2018;138(10):2144–51.

6. Aalborg J, Morelli JG, Byers TE, et al. Effect of hair color and sun sensitivity on nevus counts in white children in Colorado. J Am Acad Dermatol 2010; 63(3):430–9.

7. Asdigian NL, Barón AE, Morelli JG, et al. Trajectories of nevus development from age 3 to 16 years in the colorado kids sun care program cohort. JAMA Dermatology 2018;154(11):1272–80.

8. Chang Y, Newton-Bishop JA, Bishop DT, et al. A pooled analysis of melanocytic nevus phenotype and the risk of cutaneous melanoma at different latitudes. Int J Cancer 2009;124(2):420–8.

9. Youl P, Aitken J, Hayward N, et al. Melanoma in adolescents: a case-control study of risk factors in Queensland, Australia. Int J Cancer 2002;98(1): 92–8.

10. Moustafa D, Duncan LM, Hawryluk EB. A 20-year histopathologic study of pediatric nevi at an academic institution. J Am Acad Dermatol 2021; 84(1):39–40.

11. Hosler GA, Moresi JM, Barrett TL. Nevi with site-related atypia: a review of melanocytic nevi with atypical histologic features based on anatomic site. J Cutan Pathol 2008;35(10):889–98.

12. Gupta M, Berk DR, Gray C, et al. Morphologic features and natural history of scalp nevi in children. Arch Dermatol 2010;146(5). https://doi.org/10. 1001/archdermatol.2010.88.

13. Tcheung WJ, Bellet JS, Prose NS, et al. Clinical and dermoscopic features of 88 scalp nevi in 39 children. Br J Dermatol 2011;165(1):137–43.

14. Bailey KM, Durham AB, Zhao L, et al. Pediatric melanoma and aggressive Spitz tumors: a retrospective diagnostic, exposure and outcome analysis. Transl Pediatr 2018;7(3):20210–310.

15. Pampena R, Kyrgidis A, Lallas A, et al. A meta-analysis of nevus-associated melanoma: prevalence and practical implications. J Am Acad Dermatol 2017;77(5):938–45.e4.

16. Cordoro KM, Gupta D, Frieden IJ, et al. Pediatric melanoma: Results of a large cohort study and proposal for modified ABCD detection criteria for children. J Am Acad Dermatol 2013;68(6): 913–25.

17. Scope A, Dusza SW, Halpern AC, et al. The "ugly duckling" sign: agreement between observers. Arch Dermatol 2008;144(1):58–64.

18. Kim CC, Swetter SM, Curiel-Lewandrowski C, et al. Addressing the knowledge gap in clinical recommendations for management and complete excision of clinically atypical nevi/dysplastic nevi: Pigmented Lesion Subcommittee consensus statement. JAMA Dermatol 2015;151(2):212–8.

19. Soleymani T, Swetter SM, Hollmig ST, et al. Adequacy of conservative 2- to 3-mm surgical margins for complete excision of biopsy-proven severely dysplastic nevi: Retrospective case series at a tertiary academic institution. J Am Acad Dermatol 2020;83(1):254–5.

20. Kanada KN, Merin MR, Munden A, et al. A prospective study of cutaneous findings in newborns in the United States: correlation with race, ethnicity, and gestational status using updated classification and nomenclature. J Pediatr 2012;161(2): 240–5.

21. Kinsler VA, Thomas AC, Ishida M, et al. Multiple congenital melanocytic nevi and neurocutaneous melanosis are caused by postzygotic mutations in codon 61 of NRAS. J Invest Dermatol 2013;133(9): 2229–36.

22. Polubothu S, McGuire N, Al-Olabi L, et al. Does the gene matter? Genotype–phenotype and genotype–outcome associations in congenital melanocytic naevi. Br J Dermatol 2020;182(2):434–43.

23. Krengel S, Scope A, Dusza SW, et al. New recommendations for the categorization of cutaneous features of congenital melanocytic nevi. J Am Acad Dermatol 2013;68(3):441–51.

24. Jahnke MN, O'Haver J, Gupta D, et al. Care of congenital melanocytic nevi in newborns and infants: review and management recommendations. Pediatrics 2021;148(6). e2021051536.

25. Kinsler VA, O'Hare P, Bulstrode N, et al. Melanoma in congenital melanocytic naevi. Br J Dermatol 2017;176(5):1131–43.

26. Margileth AM. Spontaneous regression of large congenital melanocytic nevi, with a halo rim in 17 children with large scalp and trunk nevi during 45 years: a review of the literature. Clin Pediatr (Phila) 2019;58(3):313–9.

27. Ruiz-Maldonado R, Orozco-Covarrubias L, Ridaura-Sanz C, et al. Desmoplastic hairless hypopigmented naevus: a variant of giant congenital melanocytic naevus. Br J Dermatol 2003;148(6): 1253–7.

28. Neuhold JC, Friesenhahn J, Gerdes N, et al. Case reports of fatal or metastasizing melanoma in children and adolescents: a systematic analysis of the literature. Pediatr Dermatol 2015;32(1):13–22.

29. Scard C, Aubert H, Wargny M, et al. Risk of melanoma in congenital melanocytic nevi of all sizes: a systematic review. J Eur Acad Dermatol Venereol 2023;37(1):32–9.

30. Neale H, Plumptre I, Belazarian L, et al. Central nervous system magnetic resonance imaging abnormalities and neurologic outcomes in pediatric patients with congenital nevi: A 10-year multi-institutional retrospective study. J Am Acad Dermatol 2022;87(5):1060–8.

31. Waelchli R, Aylett SE, Atherton D, et al. Classification of neurological abnormalities in children with congenital melanocytic naevus syndrome identifies magnetic resonance imaging as the best predictor of clinical outcome. Br J Dermatol 2015;173(3): 739–50.

32. Rahman RK, Majmundar N, Ghani H, et al. Neurosurgical management of patients with neurocutaneous melanosis: a systematic review. Neurosurg Focus 2022;52(5):E8.

33. Arad E, Zuker RM. The Shifting paradigm in the management of giant congenital melanocytic nevi: review and clinical applications. Plast Reconstr Surg 2014;133(2):367.

34. Ott H, Krengel S, Beck O, et al. Multidisciplinary long-term care and modern surgical treatment of congenital melanocytic nevi - recommendations by the CMN surgery network. J Dtsch Dermatol Ges 2019;17(10):1005–16.

35. Kinsler VA, Birley J, Atherton DJ. Great ormond street hospital for children registry for congenital melanocytic naevi: prospective study 1988–2007. Part 2—evaluation of treatments. Br J Dermatol 2009;160(2):387–92.

36. Masnari O, Neuhaus K, Aegerter T, et al. Predictors of health-related quality of life and psychological adjustment in children and adolescents with congenital melanocytic nevi: analysis of parent reports. J Pediatr Psychol 2019;44(6):714–25.

37. Neuhaus K, Landolt MA, Theiler M, et al. Skin-related quality of life in children and adolescents with congenital melanocytic naevi - an analysis of self- and parent reports. J Eur Acad Dermatol Venereol 2020;34(5):1105–11.

38. Dickie SR, Adler N, Bauer B. Craniofacial, Head and Neck Surgery and Pediatric Plastic Surgery.

In: Losee J, Hoppe R, editors. Plastic SurgeryVol 3, 5th Edition. Philadelphia, PA: Elsevier; 2024.

39. Zhang C, Wu L, Zhao S, et al. Psychosocial experiences in children with congenital melanocytic nevus on the face and their parents throughout the tissue expansion treatment. J Craniofac Surg 2022;33(3):754.

40. Dika E, Ravaioli GM, Fanti PA, et al. Spitz nevi and other spitzoid neoplasms in children: overview of incidence data and diagnostic criteria. Pediatr Dermatol 2017;34(1):25–32.

41. Bartenstein Dw, Fisher Jm, Stamoulis C, et al. Clinical features and outcomes of spitzoid proliferations in children and adolescents. Br J Dermatol 2019;181(2):366–72.

42. Davies OMT, Majerowski J, Segura A, et al. A sixteen-year single-center retrospective chart review of Spitz nevi and spitzoid neoplasms in pediatric patients. Pediatr Dermatol 2020;37(6):1073–82.

43. Argenziano G, Agozzino M, Bonifazi E, et al. Natural evolution of spitz nevi. Dermatology 2011; 222(3):256–60.

44. Tlougan BE, Orlow SJ, Schaffer JV. Spitz nevi: beliefs, behaviors, and experiences of pediatric dermatologists. JAMA Dermatology 2013;149(3): 283–91.

45. Luo S, Sepehr A, Tsao H. Spitz nevi and other spitzoid lesions: part II. natural history and management. J Am Acad Dermatol 2011;65(6):1087–92.

46. Hawryluk EB, Moustafa D, Bartenstein D, et al. A retrospective multicenter study of fatal pediatric melanoma. J Am Acad Dermatol 2020;83(5): 1274–81.

47. Groesser L, Herschberger E, Rütten A, et al. Postzygotic HRAS and KRAS mutations cause nevus sebaceus and Schimmelpenning syndrome. Nat Genet 2012;44:783–7.

48. Jaqueti G, Requena L, Sánchez Yus E. Trichoblastoma is the most common neoplasm developed in nevus sebaceus of Jadassohn: a clinicopathologic study of a series of 155 cases. Am J Dermatopathol 2000;22(2):108–18.

49. Eisen DB, Michael DJ. Sebaceous lesions and their associated syndromes: Part I. J Am Acad Dermatol 2009;61(4):549–60.

50. Kamyab-Hesari K, Seirafi H, Jahan S, et al. Nevus sebaceus: a clinicopathological study of 168 cases and review of the literature. Int J Dermatol 2016; 55(2):193–200.

51. Moody MN, Landau JM, Goldberg LH. Nevus sebaceous revisited. Pediatr Dermatol 2012;29(1): 15–23.

52. Cribier B, Scrivener Y, Grosshans E. Tumors arising in nevus sebaceus: a study of 596 cases. J Am Acad Dermatol 2000;42(2 Pt 1):263–8.

53. Idriss MH, Elston DM. Secondary neoplasms associated with nevus sebaceus of Jadassohn: A study of 707 cases. J Am Acad Dermatol 2014;70(2): 332–7.

54. Barkham MC, White N, Brundler MA, et al. Should naevus sebaceus be excised prophylactically? A clinical audit. J Plast Reconstr Aesthet Surg 2007; 60(11):1269–70.

55. Alkhalifah A, Fransen F, Le Duff F, et al. Laser treatment of epidermal nevi: A multicenter retrospective study with long-term follow-up. J Am Acad Dermatol 2020;83(6):1606–15.

56. Zhou AG, Antaya RJ. Topical sirolimus therapy for nevus sebaceus and epidermal nevus: A case series. J Am Acad Dermatol 2022;87(2):407–9.

57. Goel P, Wolfswinkel EM, Fahradyan A, et al. Sebaceous nevus of the scalp. J Craniofac Surg 2020; 31(1):257–60.

58. Kong SH, Han SH, Kim JH, et al. Optimal timing for surgical excision of nevus sebaceus on the scalp: a single-center experience. Dermatol Surg 2020; 46(1):20–5.

59. Davies D, Rogers M. Review of neurological manifestations in 196 patients with sebaceous naevi. Australas J Dermatol 2002;43(1):20–3.

60. Rizzo R, Pavone P. Nevus sebaceous and its association with neurologic involvement. Semin Pediatr Neurol 2015;22(4):302–9.

61. Chaves RRM, Júnior AACP, Gomes CC, et al. Multiple adenomatoid odontogenic tumors in a patient with Schimmelpenning syndrome. Oral Surgery, Oral Medicine, Oral Pathology and Oral Radiology 2020;129(1):e12–7.

62. Colletti G, Allevi F, Moneghini L, et al. Epidermal nevus and ameloblastoma: a rare association. Oral Surg Oral Med Oral Pathol Oral Radiol 2014; 117(3):e275–9.

63. Friedrich RE, Gosau M, Luebke AM, et al. Oral HRAS mutation in orofacial nevus sebaceous syndrome (schimmelpenning-feuerstein-mims-syndrome): a case report with a literature. Survey. In Vivo 2022;36(1):274–93.

64. Hills SE, Maddalozzo J. Congenital lesions of epithelial origin. Otolaryngol Clin North Am 2015; 48(1):209–23.

65. Pupić-Bakrač J, Pupić-Bakrač A, Bačić I, et al. Epidermoid and dermoid cysts of the head and neck. J Craniofac Surg 2021;32(1):e25–7.

66. Brownstein MH, Helwig EB. Subcutaneous dermoid cysts. Arch Dermatol 1973;107(2):237–9.

67. Orozco-Covarrubias L, Lara-Carpio R, Saez-De-Ocariz M, et al. Dermoid cysts: a report of 75 pediatric patients. Pediatr Dermatol 2013;30(6): 706–11.

68. Ruge JR, Tomita T, Naidich TP, et al. Scalp and calvarial masses of infants and children. Neurosurgery 1988;22(6 Pt 1):1037–42.

69. Pollard ZF, Harley RD, Calhoun J. Dermoid cysts in children. Pediatrics 1976;57(3):379–82.

70. Prior A, Anania P, Pacetti M, et al. Dermoid and epidermoid cysts of scalp: case series of 234 consecutive patients. World Neurosurg 2018;120:119–24.

71. Quintanilla-Dieck L, Penn EB. Congenital neck masses. Clin Perinatol 2018;45(4):769–85.

72. Pryor SG, Lewis JE, Weaver AL, et al. Pediatric dermoid cysts of the head and neck. Otolaryngol Head Neck Surg 2005;132(6):938–42.

73. Overland J, Hall C, Holmes A, et al. Risk of intracranial extension of craniofacial dermoid cysts. Plast Reconstr Surg 2020;145(4):779e–87e.

74. Knight PJ, Reiner CB. Superficial lumps in children: what, when, and why? Pediatrics 1983;72(2):147–53.

75. Moehlenbeck FW. Pilomatrixoma (calcifying epithelioma). a statistical study. Arch Dermatol 1973;108(4):532–4.

76. Julian CG, Bowers PW. A clinical review of 209 pilomatricomas. J Am Acad Dermatol 1998;39(2 Pt 1):191–5.

77. Schwarz Y, Pitaro J, Waissbluth S, et al. Review of pediatric head and neck pilomatrixoma. Int J Pediatr Otorhinolaryngol 2016;85:148–53.

78. Marrogi AJ, Wick MR, Dehner LP. Pilomatrical neoplasms in children and young adults. Am J Dermatopathol 1992;14(2):87–94.

79. Kwon D, Grekov K, Krishnan M, et al. Characteristics of pilomatrixoma in children: a review of 137 patients. Int J Pediatr Otorhinolaryngol 2014;78(8):1337–41.

80. Danielson-Cohen A, Lin SJ, Hughes CA, et al. Head and neck pilomatrixoma in children. Arch Otolaryngol Head Neck Surg 2001;127(12):1481–3.

81. Forbis R, Helwig EB. Pilomatrixoma (calcifying epithelioma). Arch Dermatol 1961;83:606–18.

82. Levy J, Ilsar M, Deckel Y, et al. Eyelid pilomatrixoma: a description of 16 cases and a review of the literature. Surv Ophthalmol 2008;53(5):526–35.

83. Ciriacks K, Knabel D, Waite MB. Syndromes associated with multiple pilomatricomas: When should clinicians be concerned? Pediatr Dermatol 2020;37(1):9–17.

84. Bayle P, Bazex J, Lamant L, et al. Multiple perforating and non perforating pilomatricomas in a patient with Churg-Strauss syndrome and Rubinstein-Taybi syndrome. J Eur Acad Dermatol Venereol 2004;18(5):607–10.

85. Hamahata A, Kamei W, Ishikawa M, et al. Multiple pilomatricomas in Kabuki syndrome. Pediatr Dermatol 2013;30(2):253–5.

86. Gilaberte Y, Ferrer-Lozano M, Oliván MJ, et al. Multiple giant pilomatricoma in familial Sotos syndrome. Pediatr Dermatol 2008;25(1):122–5.

87. Nigro LC, Fuller CE, Rhodes JL. Pilomatrixoma presenting as a rapidly expanding mass of the infant nasion. Eplasty 2015;15:e54.

88. Fink AM, Berkowitz RG. Sonography in preauricular pilomatrixoma of childhood. Ann Otol Rhinol Laryngol 1997;106(2):167–9.

89. Hughes J, Lam A, Rogers M. Use of ultrasonography in the diagnosis of childhood pilomatrixoma. Pediatr Dermatol 1999;16(5):341–4.

90. Bollu BK, Collin M, Shun A. Minimally invasive surgical treatment of pilomatrixoma. ANZ J Surg 2021;91(10):2126–9.

91. Prescher H, Nathan SL, Bauer BS, et al. Branchial cleft anomalies: embryogenesis, clinical features, diagnosis, and management. FACE 2022;3(1):128–37.

92. Goff CJ, Allred C, Glade RS. Current management of congenital branchial cleft cysts, sinuses, and fistulae. Curr Opin Otolaryngol Head Neck Surg 2012;20(6):533.

93. Bajaj Y, Ifeacho S, Tweedie D, et al. Branchial anomalies in children. Int J Pediatr Otorhinolaryngol 2011;75(8):1020–3.

94. Schroeder JW, Mohyuddin N, Maddalozzo J. Branchial anomalies in the pediatric population. Otolaryngol Head Neck Surg 2007;137(2):289–95.

95. Coste AH, Lofgren DH, Shermetaro C. Branchial cleft cyst. In: StatPearls. StatPearls Publishing; 2023. Available at: http://www.ncbi.nlm.nih.gov/books/NBK499914/. [Accessed 16 January 2024].

96. Choi SS, Zalzal GH. Branchial anomalies: a review of 52 cases. Laryngoscope 1995;105(9 Pt 1):909–13.

97. Mattioni J, Azari S, Hoover T, et al. A cross-sectional evaluation of outcomes of pediatric branchial cleft cyst excision. Int J Pediatr Otorhinolaryngol 2019;119:171–6.

98. Teo N, Ibrahim S, Tan K. Distribution of branchial anomalies in a paediatric Asian population. SMEDJ 2015;56(04):203–7.

99. Solares CA, Chan J, Koltai PJ. Anatomical variations of the facial nerve in first branchial cleft anomalies. Arch Otolaryngol Head Neck Surg 2003;129(3):351–5.

100. Prosser JD, Myer CM. Branchial cleft anomalies and thymic cysts. Otolaryngol Clin North Am 2015;48(1):1–14.

101. Work WP. Newer concepts of first branchial cleft defects. 1972. Laryngoscope 2015;125(3):520–32.

102. Maddalozzo J, Rastatter JC, Dreyfuss HF, et al. The second branchial cleft fistula. Int J Pediatr Otorhinolaryngol 2012;76(7):1042–5.

103. Li Y, Lyu K, Wen Y, et al. Third or fourth branchial pouch sinus lesions: a case series and management algorithm. J Otolaryngol Head Neck Surg 2019;48(1):61.

104. Li WX, Dong Y, Zhang A, et al. Surgical treatment of fourth branchial apparatus anomalies: a case series study. J Otolaryngol Head Neck Surg 2020;49(1):79.

105. Sun Z, Fu K, Zhang Z, et al. Multidetector computerized tomographic fistulography in the evaluation

of congenital branchial cleft fistulae and sinuses. Oral Surg Oral Med Oral Pathol Oral Radiol 2012; 113(5):688–94.

106. Deane SA, Telander RL. Surgery for thyroglossal duct and branchial cleft anomalies. Am J Surg 1978;136(3):348–53.

107. Allard RH. The thyroglossal cyst. Head Neck Surg 1982;5(2):134–46.

108. Ross J, Manteghi A, Rethy K, et al. Thyroglossal duct cyst surgery: A ten-year single institution experience. Int J Pediatr Otorhinolaryngol 2017; 101:132–6.

109. Oomen KPQ, Modi VK, Maddalozzo J. Thyroglossal duct cyst and ectopic thyroid: surgical management. Otolaryngol Clin North Am 2015;48(1): 15–27.

110. Santiago W, Rybak LP, Bass RM. Thyroglossal duct cyst of the tongue. J Otolaryngol 1985;14(4):261–4.

111. Thompson LDR, Herrera HB, Lau SK. A Clinicopathologic series of 685 thyroglossal duct remnant cysts. Head and Neck Pathol 2016; 10(4):465–74.

112. Wang Y, Yang G. Optimal age of surgery for children with thyroglossal duct cysts: A single-institution retrospective study of 340 patients. Front Pediatr 2022;10:1038767.

113. Boyanov MA, Tabakov DA, Ivanova RS, et al. Thyroglossal duct cyst carcinoma. Endokrynol Pol 2020;71(3):275–6.

114. Rayess HM, Monk I, Svider PF, et al. Thyroglossal duct cyst carcinoma: a systematic review of clinical features and outcomes. Otolaryngol Head Neck Surg 2017;156(5):794–802.

115. Sistrunk WE. The surgical treatment of cysts of the thyroglossal tract. Ann Surg 1920;71(2):121–2.

Benign Intraoral Soft Tissue Lesions in Children

Ashley E. Manlove, DMD, MD[a],*, Erik N. Quintana, DMD[b,1], Leticia M. Cuellar, DMD[b,1], Alexis M. Linnebur, DMD[c]

KEYWORDS

- Benign soft tissue lesions • Pediatric oral pathology • Pediatric neoplasms • Oral medicine
- Benign oral lesions

KEY POINTS

- Most pediatric intraoral soft tissue pathology is benign.
- Developmental lesions are present at birth or shortly after birth.
- Traumatic lesions develop from acute or chronic injury to tissue.
- Inflammatory lesions usually occur from a chronic irritant such as appliance, plaque, or calculus.
- Intraoral lesions caused by infectious etiology are often managed by the pediatrician.

INTRODUCTION

Oral and maxillofacial surgeons are trained to work up, characterize, diagnose, and treat soft tissue lesions in children. The pediatric population is unique in that a significant amount of growth and development occurs from the neonatal period to childhood to adolescence to adulthood. Treating pediatric patients is a joint endeavor with the child and guardian.

The identification of oral pathology, and surgical intervention, can impact the patient and family for years to come. It is critical to recognize and treat these lesions to the current standard of care. This article broadly classifies benign pediatric soft tissue lesions into developmental, traumatic, inflammatory, and infectious lesions, which offers a useful clinical guide for surgeons.

Developmental pathology includes lesions that result from disturbances of growth and development (**Table 1**). These lesions are present at birth or manifest shortly after birth.

Traumatic lesions develop from acute or chronic injury to the soft tissue of the oral mucosa (**Table 2**). Injury may or may not be known by the child or guardian.

Inflammatory conditions arise from an exuberant host response to a local irritant or cellular injury (**Table 3**).

Intraoral soft tissue pathology caused by infectious etiology includes viral, bacterial, and fungal lesions (**Table 4**). In these instances, there is a distinct cause for the lesion and once the infection resolves, the soft tissue heals.

This article discusses common and uncommon benign intraoral soft tissue lesions in children including the etiology of the lesion, demographics, clinical presentation, histologic findings, and treatment.

DEVELOPMENTAL LESIONS
Epstein's Pearls, Bohn's Nodules, and Gingival Cysts

Cysts of the newborn are common, benign findings of neonates. Epstein's pearls, Bohn's nodules, and gingival cysts are often used interchangeably; however, Epstein pearls and Bohn's nodules only occur on the palate, and gingival cysts of the newborn are on the alveolar mucosa. Palatal cysts arise in 65% to 85% of all newborns, and gingival cysts present in 55% to 85% of neonates.[1]

[a] Carle Illinois College of Medicine, Carle Cleft and Craniofacial Team, Carle Foundation Hospital, Urbana, IL, USA; [b] Division of Oral and Maxillofacial Surgery, Carle Foundation Hospital, Urbana, IL, USA; [c] Arnold Palmer Hospital for Children – Orlando Health, 207 W. Gore Street, 3Road Floor, Suite.302, Orlando, FL 32806, USA
[1] Present address: 3105 Fields South Drive, Champaign, IL 61822.
* Corresponding author. 3105 Fields South Drive, Champaign, IL 61822.
E-mail address: Ashley.Manlove@carle.com

Oral Maxillofacial Surg Clin N Am 36 (2024) 265–282
https://doi.org/10.1016/j.coms.2024.01.005

Table 1
Developmental benign intraoral soft tissue pathology in children

Developmental Lesions	Clinical Pearls
Epstein's pearls	• 1–3 mm white or pink nodules found along the mid-palatine raphe
Bohn's nodules	• Small, white, pink nodules found along the junction of the soft and hard palate
Gingival cyst	• 2 mm small cysts found along the maxillary and mandibular alveolar mucosa
Hemangioma	• Superficial lesions are firm, well-circumcised, and bright to dark red nodular lesions. • Deep lesions have a blue hue and are difficult to palpate • Most commonly found on the lips, buccal mucosa, palate, and tongue
Lymphangioma	• Most frequently occur on the anterior two-thirds of the dorsal tongue. ○ Other locations include lips, palate, gingiva, floor of mouth, buccal mucosa and alveolar ridge • Cavernous lymphangiomas are larger and most common seen on tongue or cheek • Cystic hygromas most common along floor of mouth or tongue • Superficial capillary lymphangiomas present as painless compressible clusters of pebbly translucent vesicles described as frog eggs
Congenital epulis	• 2 cm pedunculated, non-painful, smooth, lobular or multi-lobular polypoidal lesion most commonly found in the lateral incisor or canine region
Melanotic Neuroectroderm Tumor of Infancy	• Rapid, enlarging, pigmented mass most often in the anterior maxilla
Eruption cyst	• Bluish-purple serosanguineous fluid-filled cyst most commonly involving alveolar crest along the central incisor associated with tooth eruption
Dermoid cyst	• Asymptomatic, firm, slow-growing cyst, most commonly found along the floor of the mouth followed by submental space • Variable in size and can range from 1–2 mm to 12 cm • Cause displacement of the tongue altering speech and feeding
Congenital atresia of submandibular duct	• Rare, developmental condition where submandibular duct fails to canalize into the oral cavity • Unilateral or bilateral floor of mouth edema due to failure of saliva to drain mimicking an appearance of ranula
Lipoma	• Soft, nodular, mobile mass with a yellow hue • Asymptomatic, vary in size and are often slow growing

Epstein's pearls are often noted at birth. These lesions are white or pink keratin-filled nodules found along the mid-palatine raphe ranging from 1 to 3 mm in diameter.[1–3] Histologically, these cysts are derived from residual epithelial cells, which are trapped in the formation of the palatine processes during embryogenesis.[1–3] These cysts are self-limiting and they do not require surgical intervention.

Bohn's nodules are similar to Epstein's pearls as they are also present on the palatal mucosa. Bohn's nodules are located at the junction of the hard and soft palate and appear as small, white, pink nodules scattered along that junction.[2] It is

Table 2
Traumatic benign soft tissue pathology in children

Traumatic Lesions	Clinical Pearls
Fibroma	• Well-circumscribed, sessile, pedunculated lesions most commonly found at the buccal mucosa at the level of the occlusal plane • Often asymptomatic but patients may reports pain • Native in tissue color
Mucocele	• Painless, well-circumscribed, dome-shaped mucosal swelling that has a blue hue • Chronic lesions will often wax and wane
Ranula	• Dome-shaped, fluctuant sublingual swelling with a bluish hue • Often found in the lateral aspect of the floor of the mouth • Painless, often wax and wane in size usually with salivation
Iatrogenic ulceration	• Most commonly seen after local anesthesia admission • Found on the tongue, buccal mucosa, and lips

Table 3
Inflammatory benign soft tissue pathology in children

Inflammatory and Local Irritants	Clinical Pearls
Pyogenic granuloma	• Bright red slow-growing, smooth, or lobulated masses which often vary in size most commonly seen on the gingiva, lip, tongue, and buccal mucosa • Seen on facial aspect of gingiva and along maxillary central incisors
Peripheral giant cell granuloma	• Painless, sessile pedunculated bluish-purple mass often 2 cm or less • Radiographically will see "cupping" caused by superficial erosion of underlying alveolar bone
Peripheral ossifying fibroma	• Painless, firm, nodular mass most commonly seen along the anterior maxillary arch • Vary in color from pink to red with and without ulceration

believed that Bohn's nodules are remnants of salivary glands, whereas Epstein's pearls arise from epithelial cells.[2,4] Bohn's nodules are also self-limiting and do not require treatment.

Gingival cysts are small, keratin-filled cysts often noted along the alveolar mucosa in infants and are seen in over half of infants.[5] These cysts arise from the dental lamina and are true cysts lined with epithelium.[2] Gingival cysts are small, around 2 mm, and commonly seen along the maxilla and mandible. These lesions are rarely seen in infants older than 2 to 3 months, as the cysts will spontaneously involute or rupture.[5]

Hemangioma

Hemangiomas are the most common tumor of infancy affecting 4% to 7% of newborns and up to 10% of infants by 1 year of age. Congenital hemangiomas are present at birth, whereas infantile hemangiomas appear after birth, within the first month of life.[2,6–8] They result from endothelial

proliferation and are composed of a collection of endothelial cells and blood vessels. Hemangiomas are more common in females with a ratio up to 5:1.[7,9] Prenatal risk factors include older maternal age, premature infants, placental abnormalities, and multiple gestation.[7,8]

Hemangiomas in the oral cavity occur most commonly on the lips, buccal mucosa, palate, and tongue (**Fig. 1**). Superficial hemangiomas appear red to dark red with a firm nodular well-circumscribed appearance. The lesions blanch with pressure and ulcerations can form. Deep lesions will have a blue hue and may be more difficult to palpate depending on the size.[6,9,10] Hemangiomas undergo a triphasic evolution.

1. *Early proliferative phase* occurs first with rapid growth during months 1–3, and moderate growth during months 5–8 (**Fig. 2**A).

Table 4 Infectious benign intraoral pathology in children	
Infectious Lesions	Clinical Pearls
Parulis	• Small, tender, erythematous swelling associated with a necrotic tooth and a sinus tract • Lesion will most often express purulence on palpation
HSV	• HSV-1 most commonly presents as acute primary herpetic gingivostomatitis • Small, vesicular lesions will develop along the tongue, lips, gingiva, buccal mucosa, soft and hard palate
Hand-foot-mouth	• Small vesicular, erythematous lesions most commonly on the buccal, labial and palatal mucosa which will rupture leaving small ulcerations. • 2–6 mm macular, papular, or vesicular cutaneous rash found along the hand, feet, and abdomen
Thrush/candida	• White plaques most commonly found on the buccal and labial mucosa, soft palate, and tongue • Plaques are easily removed with dry gauze to reveal underlying erythematous mucosa

2. *Plateau phase:* there is no growth and the lesion remains unchanged usually during months 6–12 (**Fig. 2**B).
3. *Involution phase* starts around year 1 and can continue for a few years during which time the lesion becomes softer and the color changes from bright red to gray or purple. The tissue may return to normal, but it is usually an excess of fibrofatty tissue (**Fig. 2**C, D).

Hemangiomas of infancy are characterized by numerous plump endothelial cells and indistinct vascular lumina where they are described microscopically as juvenile or cellular hemangiomas.[2] As the hemangioma involutes, the vascular component will become less prominent and it will contain more fibrofatty connective tissue.[2,6,10]

The primary treatment of infantile hemangiomas is observation because most lesions are small and regress on their own. For large or high-risk hemangiomas, the first-line treatment is oral propranolol (2 mg/kg/day). Another option is oral prednisone (2–4 mg/kg/day). Both medications have side effects and can be managed by the child's pediatrician.[11,12] Surgical treatment during the proliferative or plateau phase is not advised unless the lesion responds poorly to medical management, and early intervention is necessary to prevent complications.[12] Following the involution phase, large lesions may require surgical excision of the fibrofatty tissue to improve esthetics.

Hemangiomas that occur in the head and neck region are categorized as high-risk lesions due to the potential for complications. Oral hemangiomas pose the risk of ulceration, disfigurement,

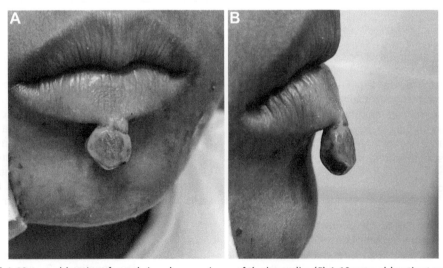

Fig. 1. (*A*) A 10-year-old patient frontal view, hemangioma of the lower lip. (*B*) A 10-year-old patient profile view, hemangioma of the lower lip.

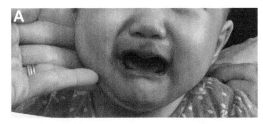

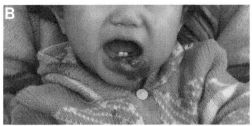

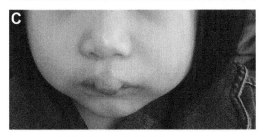

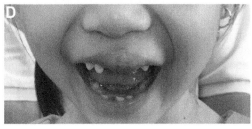

Fig. 2. (*A*) A 6-month-old patient with upper lip hemangioma. (*B*) A 11-month-old patient with large lower lip hemangioma. (*C*) A 3-year-old patient with upper lip hemangioma before complete involution. (*D*) A 5-year-old patient with upper lip hemangioma with residual fibrofatty tissue after involution.

dentofacial abnormalities, scarring, airway obstruction, bleeding, and feeding difficulty.[9,10]

Lymphangioma

Lymphangiomas are developmental malformations within the lymphatic system and can occur anywhere on the mucous membranes or skin where there is lymphatic tissue present. The lymphatic tissue abnormally sequesters altering vascular drainage and leading to lymph accumulation.[13] Lymphangiomas can be categorized as congenital or acquired as well as deep or superficial. Congenital deep lymphangiomas include cavernous lymphangiomas and cystic hygromas. Congenital superficial

lymphangiomas are called capillary lymphangiomas.[14] Acquired lymphangiomas are also referred to as lymphangiectasia and are due to obstruction by an external cause. This section focuses on congenital lymphangiomas.

Lymphangiomas are rare, representing 4% of vascular tumors with an incidence of 1.2–1.8 per 1000 in the head and neck region.[15,16] Oral lymphangiomas occur most frequently on the anterior two-thirds of the dorsal tongue and can cause obstruction.[17] Other common locations include lips, palate, gingiva, floor of the mouth, buccal mucosa, and alveolar ridge.[15]

Oral lesions can be classified into three variants based on size and location: (1) cavernous lymphangioma, (2) cystic hygroma, and (3) superficial capillary lymphangioma. Cavernous lymphangiomas are larger and can be difficult to visualize, often causing mass effects to dense tissues such as the tongue or cheek. This variant is sometimes described as a palpable bag of worms due to the profound collection of lymphatic tissue.[18] Cystic hygromas are thought to arise from the arrested development of lymphatic trunks with failure of the development of the drainage mechanism. Seventy-five to ninety percent of cystic hygromas are found in the cervical region and can present as swelling in the floor mouth or tongue.[19] Both cavernous and cystic lymphangioma variants can cause compressive symptoms leading to dysphagia or airway obstruction.[17] Superficial capillary lymphangiomas present as painless compressible clusters of pebbly translucent vesicles often described as small frog eggs.

Histopathologic examination of lymphatic malformations demonstrates lymphatic vessels varying in size. Superficial capillary variants show a collection of large lymphatic cisterns that link to dilated dermal lymphatic channels with mild to moderate inflammatory infiltrate. Cystic and cavernous lymphangiomas show dilated, irregular vascular spaces within a fibroblastic or collagenous stroma.[14] Lymphangiomas are not encapsulated and the endothelium lining is thin and the spaces contain proteinaceous fluid and occasional lymphocytes. Lymphatic fluid is present with numerous inflammatory cells.[2,16,18]

Treatment of oral lymphangiomas depends on the size of the lesion and its location. For superficial capillary lymphangiomas, treatment is often excision. For deep lesions, conservative management is favored. For nonobstructive and stable small lesions, the lesion is observed for growth. First-line treatment for lesions causing mass effect, obstruction, or dysphagia is surgical excision with attention to preserving vital structures. Deep lymphangiomas are associated with higher

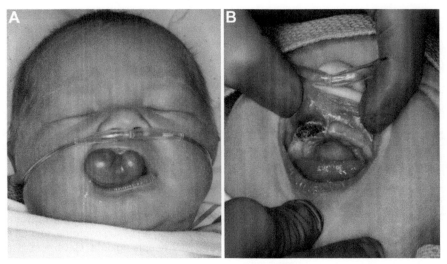

Fig. 3. (*A*) Infant with a large congenital epulis affecting feeding. (*B*) Infant following surgical excision of large congenital epulis.

recurrence rates, likely due to the invasive histologic character of the lesion making complete excision nearly impossible. Adjunctive therapies such as sclerosing agents, serial aspiration, radiotherapy, and cryotherapy have been reported with inconclusive success. Adjunctive treatments are recommended for large lesions or those lesions near vital structures for which surgical resection is not an option.

Recurrence rates are reported to be as high as 10% to 40%.[2,15,16] Facial disfigurement, skeletal discrepancies, malocclusion, speech difficulty, and dysphagia are possible sequelae of both conservative management and surgical excision.

Congenital Epulis

Congenital epulis, also referred to as congenital epulis of the newborn, is an uncommon soft tissue tumor that occurs almost exclusively on the alveolar ridge of newborns. These lesions present two to three times more frequently on the maxillary ridge than on the mandibular ridge. Females have an increased predilection with a ratio of 9:1. Multiple lesions can occur and are reported in 5% to 16% of cases.[20–22] No familiar inheritance has been reported.

The clinical presentation of congenital epulis is a non-painful, smooth, lobular, or multi-lobular polypoid mass that is around 2 cm or less in size, although lesions up to 10 cm have been reported. The lesion can be pedunculated or sessile and pink to red on the alveolar ridge of a newborn[23] (**Fig. 3**). Congenital epulis usually presents lateral to midline in the region of lateral incisor and canine.[20]

Histologic characteristics include large polygonal to rounded-shaped granular cells, and granular eosinophilic cytoplasm within a fibrous connective tissue stroma. The overlying surface epithelium exhibits atrophy of the rete ridges.[20–22,24]

Treatment for congenital epulis depends on the location and size of the lesion. Very small, asymptomatic lesions can be observed and may resolve without treatment. Moderate to large lesions or symptomatic lesions require simple surgical excision with sharp instrumentation or laser. Recurrence is rare, even with incomplete removal.[22,23]

Melanotic Neuroectodermal Tumor of Infancy

Melanotic neuroectodermal tumor of infancy (MNET) is a rare neural crest-derived tumor that occurs in the maxilla. The tumor is often diagnosed within the first year of life.[2,25,26] It is accepted as a benign entity, but it has destructive and locally invasive qualities consistent with malignancy.[2,26]

Clinically, the infant will develop a rapidly enlarging painless mass with pigmentation, most often in the anterior maxilla.[2,26] The tumor can cause facial asymmetry as it grows, and radiographic imaging may show bone loss due to its destructive nature.

Melanotic neuroectodermal tumors are benign but aggressive and destructive; therefore, complete surgical excision is recommended. Wide local excision in neonates can be disfiguring and the size of the tumor-free margin has not been identified. Some surgeons advocate for an aggressive margin up to 1 cm, whereas other surgeons suggest a 0.5-cm margin.[26] Infants diagnosed

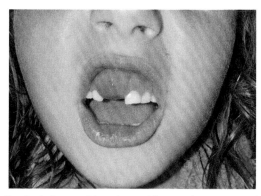

Fig. 4. A 6-year-old patient with eruption cyst associated with right central incisor.

and treated within 2 months of birth had a shorter disease-free survival time and those diagnosed and treated after 4.5 months had a minimal risk of recurrence suggesting that more radical surgery may decrease recurrence rates.[26]

Histologically, melanotic neuroectodermal tumor of infancy is believed to be of neural crest origin and resemble melanocytes. Melanotic neuroectodermal tumor of infancy is a biphasic tumor demonstrating two different cell lineages: epithelial cells resembling melanocytes in conjunction with smaller and neuroblastic cells with a different array of melanin.[2,26]

Surgery is recommended with a local recurrence rate of 10% to 15%.[26] Lower recurrence rates are reported when greater tumor-free margins are achieved.[26]

Eruption Cyst

An eruption cyst, also known as an eruption hematoma, is a developmental odontogenic cyst that occurs before the eruption of a primary or permanent tooth. The cyst is thought to originate from the separation of the epithelium from the crown of the tooth as it erupts into the oral cavity. This separation allows fluid and blood to occupy the follicular space.[27,28] An eruption cyst is believed to be the soft tissue equivalent of a dentigerous cyst.[2] The cyst presents most commonly in the maxilla and involves the central incisor with a blue or purple hue (**Fig. 4**). Studies report conflicting findings for gender predilection. Eruption cysts are commonly encountered in the first or second decade of life.[28,29]

They are true cysts and lined with a thin layer of non-keratinizing stratified squamous epithelium.[30,31]

Treatment is unnecessary as these cysts are self-limiting and resolve as the tooth erupts through the cyst. Most lesions are asymptomatic. If the cyst causes pain and discomfort the crown of the tooth can be surgically unroofed.[2,31,32] Eruption cysts rarely cause complications.[2,30]

Dermoid Cyst

Dermoid cysts are benign developmental lesions of ectodermal origin. Congenital variants are a result of abnormal cell and tissue growth and differentiation during embryogenesis in which epithelial cells are entrapped and filled with keratinous sebum-like material.[33] Traumatic or iatrogenic introduction of entrapped epithelial cells accounts for the acquired variant, which is rare.[33] Dermoid cysts are extremely rare in the oral cavity and account for only 1.6% of all dermoid cysts.[34,35]

Dermoid cysts are true cysts that are typically asymptomatic. The cyst develops midline along the floor of the mouth and can be further classified by location. Sublingual dermoid cysts are the most common followed by submental, multi-space, and submandibular[36] (**Fig. 5**A). The cyst can vary in size from a few millimeters to 12 cm in diameter.[2,34] Dermoid cysts are generally firm, slow-growing, and have the potential to cause displacement of the tongue intraorally which can alter speech and impair feeding.[37]

Treatment of dermoid cysts is surgical removal with complete enucleation. Intraoral versus extraoral removal depends on the location of the dermoid cyst relative to the mylohyoid muscle.

Characteristic histologic findings include a true epithelial cystic lining with ortho-keratinized squamous epithelium, skin appendages, hair follicles, and sebaceous glands along the wall of the cyst. Within the cyst, there is keratin, fat, and sebum due to the presence of sebaceous glands.[2,33,36]

Dermoid cysts can resemble a ranula clinically; therefore, a correct diagnosis is necessary to develop a proper treatment plan. Dermoid cysts cannot be treated with incision and drainage or marsupialization, otherwise the dermoid cyst may recur or be displaced into another deep fascial space in the floor of the mouth.[37] Preoperative imaging such as MRI or CT is recommended for characterization of the lesion. The pathognomonic finding on CT imaging is a thin-walled, unilocular mass filled with homogenous, hypoattenuating material containing multiple hypoattenuating fat nodules (**Fig. 5**B). This appearance is often described as a "sack of marbles."[38] Aspiration cytology may also be helpful to further classify and diagnose the lesion before surgery.[38,39]

Recurrence is rare with complete excision of the dermoid cyst. Risks include obstructive salivary gland sequela and damage to vital structures such as the lingual nerve and Wharton's duct.

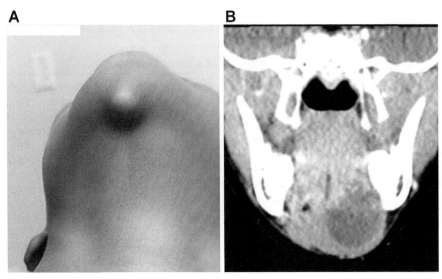

Fig. 5. (*A*) A 12-year-old patient with submental dermoid cyst. (*B*) CT soft tissue window, coronal view, large submandibular epidermoid cyst.

Malignant transformation of the dermoid cyst is reported to be less than 5%.[2,33,39].

Congenital Atresia of Submandibular Duct

Submandibular duct congenital atresia is a rare developmental condition affecting newborns in which the duct does not canalize into the oral cavity.[40] The effect of the failure of the duct to canalize is salivary retention posterior to the imperforate orifice that can cause significant floor-of-mouth swelling that can mimic a ranula (**Fig. 6**A). Since the first published report in 1955, only 30 cases have been published.[41] Submandibular duct atresia is more common in males (73%) and more common unilaterally.[42] The lesion will continue to grow as the infant salivates and the contents distend the mucosa and have no orifice to drain.

Submandibular duct atresia may be more common than reported because the imperforate duct likely spontaneously ruptures with feeding. Treatment starts with observation. If the duct does not rupture and the swelling continues to increase, marsupialization or sialodochoplasty with cannulation of the duct is recommended to avoid airway embarrassment, glandular atrophy, permanent duct dilation, and feeding difficulties[43,44] (**Fig. 6**B). Some authors advocate for the removal of the

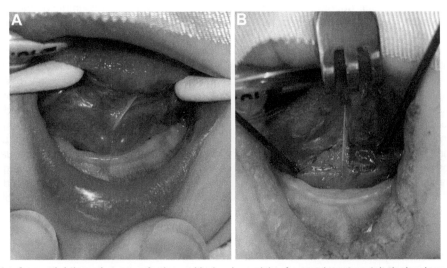

Fig. 6. (*A*) Infant with bilateral atresia of submandibular ducts. (*B*) Infant undergoing sialodochoplasty with cannulation of the submandibular ducts bilaterally.

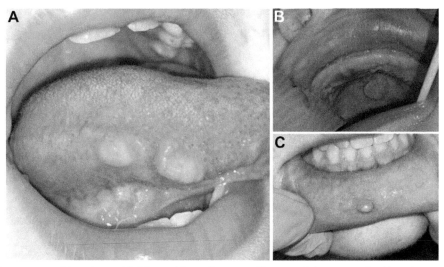

Fig. 7. (*A*) An 8-year-old patient with bilateral lateral tongue fibromas. (*B*) A 7-month-old patient with palatal fibroma. (*C*) A twelve-year-old patient with lower lip fibroma.

affected submandibular gland. The average age of treatment is 4.4 months.[40,42] Of the reported cases, there is no reported recurrence after spontaneous rupture or surgical intervention.

Lipoma

Lipomas are a developmental lesion rarely seen in pediatric patients, although there are reports of lipomas presenting in children as young as 6 weeks of age. The reported incidence of lipomas across all ages is 1.2% to 5% of oral lesions.[45–47] Although lipomas are rare in children, they should be on the differential diagnosis when there is a smooth, round mass with a slight yellow hue. These lesions are most commonly present beneath the buccal mucosa near the buccal fat pad or the tongue. Lipomas may also arise in the floor of the mouth and lip.[45] Lipomas vary in size and typically are slow-growing and are often asymptomatic. Characteristic histology findings for simple lipomas include well-demarcated adipose tissue encapsulated by well-differentiated connective tissue.[48,49]

Treatment of a lipoma includes conservative management with observation or surgical excision for large lesions. For patients who undergo excision, follow-up is recommended to monitor for recurrence.

TRAUMATIC LESIONS
Fibroma

Irritation or traumatic fibromas are one of the most common benign soft tissue lesions in children. Fibromas are typically caused by repeated trauma to the soft tissues of the oral cavity. Common etiologies include malocclusion leading to repeated soft tissue trauma, dental appliances such as braces or space maintainers, and foreign body reaction which is often due to restorative dental work.[50] Fibromas can occur anywhere in the oral cavity, but they are most common along the buccal mucosa at the level of the occlusal plane. Other common areas include the labial mucosa and tongue.[51]

A fibroma presents clinically as a well-circumscribed, sessile, or pedunculated lesion. The color is typically that of the native tissue and the lesion is usually asymptomatic (**Fig. 7**). Some patients may report pain or discomfort due to the size or repeated trauma to the tissue. In this circumstance, the lesion may appear erythematous or ulcerated. Treatment of a fibroma involves simple surgical excision.

Traditional histologic presentation is a fibrous connective tissue stroma covered by stratified squamous epithelium. The fibrous connective tissue stroma blends into the epithelium rather than being an encapsulated lesion. The rete ridges may be blunted or atrophied due to the mass effect of the fibrous stroma. Scattered inflammatory cells such as plasma cells and lymphocytes are often seen and if secondary trauma to the lesion has occurred, hyperkeratosis will be present.[2]

The recurrence rate is reported at 8% to 20% and can be higher if repeated trauma to the area continues, and the cause is not identified and eliminated.[50]

Mucocele

Mucoceles are the most common benign salivary gland lesions found in children. They occur from mucous extravasation following mechanical trauma or chronic irritation to the minor salivary glands. The exact cause of trauma to the tissue is usually not known. The minor salivary glands may rupture or the duct is impaired causing mucin to spill into the submucosa. The mucin prompts an inflammatory response leading to the formation of the lesion.[18,52] The prevalence of mucoceles is reported to be 2.4 cases per 1000 with the highest incidence in the second decade of life.[53,54]

Clinically, a mucocele presents as a painless, well-circumscribed, dome-shaped mucosal swelling that has a blue hue. Many patients seek evaluation after the lesion does not self-resolve with reported duration varying from a few weeks to several years. Painless chronic lesions tend to have a history of recurrent swelling that waxes and wanes. The size of a mucocele varies greatly and can be small (2–5 mm) to large (2–3 cm)[52,54] (Fig. 8).

Mucoceles can present anywhere the minor salivary glands are found; however, the lower lip is the most common site (81%) followed by floor of mouth, anterior ventral tongue, buccal mucosa, palate, and the retromolar trigone.[54] Mucoceles are not common in the upper lip. An upper lip swelling that resembles a mucocele is concerning for a salivary gland tumor.[2]

Treatment of mucoceles includes surgical excision, as most lesions do not resolve on their own. Other treatment modalities discussed in the literature include marsupialization, cryotherapy, intralesional steroids, and sclerosing agents.[53,55] Surgical excision of the mucocele should include the lesion as well as adjacent inflamed minor salivary glands to decrease the risk of recurrence.

Mucoceles are pseudocysts, lacking an epithelial lining. Histologic examination of a mucocele shows subepithelial vesicles containing mucin and attenuated epithelium with an associated inflamed granulation tissue response with no evidence of extension of subepithelial separation at the periphery of the lesion.[54]

Recurrence rates vary widely from 3% to 40%.[52,56] A study of mucoceles in the pediatric population reported a recurrence rate of 8%.[52,56] Potential complications include numbness to the lip due to damage to the mental nerve, scarring, esthetic changes, and damage to adjacent salivary glands.[55,57]

Ranula

A ranula occurs when there is extravasation of saliva and mucin in the submucosa of the floor of the mouth, often involving the sublingual or submandibular gland. The cause of a ranula is thought to be secondary to ductal injury or sialolith obstruction leading to an inflammatory response to the retention of mucus.[18] In the pediatric population there is a slight female predilection with a ratio of 1.15 to 1.[18,58]

Ranulas present as a smooth, dome-shaped, fluctuant sublingual swelling with a bluish hue in the lateral aspect of the floor of the mouth. Ranulas tend to be larger than mucoceles and can displace the tongue if large. They are usually painless and can wax and wane in size, usually with salivation. A plunging ranula occurs when the mucin tracts inferior to the mylohyoid muscle and penetrates the deep fascial planes. Plunging ranulas can cause obvious cervical swelling, with or without floor-of-mouth swelling[57,59,60] (Fig. 9). Imaging is necessary to support the diagnosis of a plunging ranula if there is no floor-of-mouth swelling, as

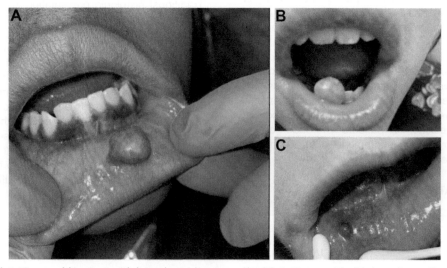

Fig. 8. (A) A 13-year-old patient with large lower lip mucocele. (B) A 11-year-old with large lower lip mucocele. (C) A 10-year-old patient with small lower lip mucocele.

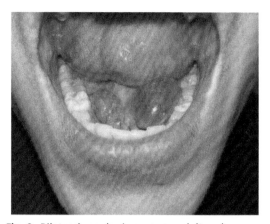

Fig. 9. Bilateral ranulas in a young adult male.

cervical swelling and the absence of floor-of-mouth swelling do not allow for a clinical diagnosis. A ranula on CT imaging will show a "tail sign" which presents as the lesion extends into the sublingual space[61] (**Fig. 10**).

Surgical treatment is necessary for ranulas. Smaller lesions less than 1.5–2 cm can be treated with marsupialization. Marsupialization carries a high risk for recurrence (61%–89%) for larger lesions.[57,58] Therefore, large ranulas are treated with excision of the offending gland with a recurrence rate of 1% to 8.5%.[59,61]

Ranulas are also pseudocysts, lacking an epithelial lining. Histology characteristics of ranulas include a vascular fibrous connective tissue wall containing chronic inflammatory cells, foamy histiocytes, macrophages filled with mucin, and occasional ruptured ductal epithelium.[2,57,60]

Risks of marsupialization include recurrence and the need for further surgery. Excision of the sublingual or submandibular gland has associated risks including hemorrhage, obstructive sialadenitis, hypoglossal nerve injury, lingual nerve injury, and facial muscle weakness with marginal mandibular nerve injury. Recurrence rate varies greatly.

Traumatic ulceration

Soft tissue trauma due to parafunctional habits, oral appliances, or following local anesthesia administration is seen in children. Traumatic ulcerations are most common on the tongue, buccal mucosa, and lips (**Fig. 11**). A thorough clinical examination is necessary as clinical diagnosis can be difficult. Typically, traumatic ulcerations are self-limiting.

Trauma after local anesthesia is most common after inferior alveolar nerve blocks. Causes include iatrogenic trauma such as biting or burns from hot food. Incidence is reported to be as high as 18% among children less than 4 years of age, 16% in children ages 4 to 7 years, 13% in 8 to 11-year-old children, and 7% in children 12 years of age and older.[62] This is a clinical diagnosis obtained with a thorough history and examination. Treatment is palliative. Perioperative education following local anesthesia administration can help prevent these traumatic lesions.

INFLAMMATORY LESIONS

Pyogenic granuloma, peripheral giant cell granuloma, and peripheral ossifying fibroma are soft tissue inflammatory lesions that appear similar on

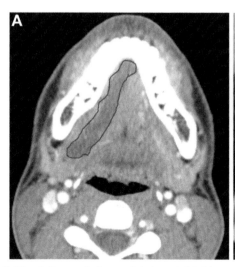
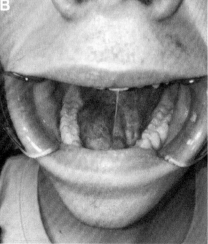

Fig. 10. (*A*) CT soft tissue window, axial view, right side ranula with tail sign. (*B*) Clinical presentation of ranula on the right.

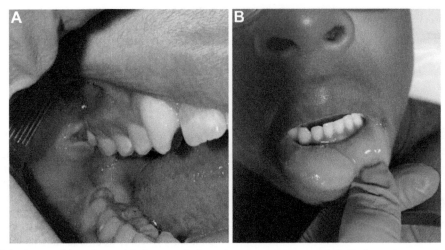

Fig. 11. (A) 12-year-old patient with iatrogenic buccal mucosa trauma. (B) Soft tissue trauma to lower lip following dentist appointment.

examination and thus require histologic examination for definitive diagnosis.

Pyogenic Granuloma

Pyogenic granulomas are reactive, inflammatory, gingival lesions composed of excess granulation tissue. Pyogenic granulomas are not granulomas and arise secondary to local irritants, such as plaque or calculus buildup, food impaction, poorly adapted restorations, foreign body, or orthodontic appliances.[18,63] Pyogenic granulomas occur most frequently on the gingiva (75%–85%) followed by lip, tongue, and buccal mucosa. These lesions tend to occur on the facial surface of the gingiva and are more common on maxillary anterior teeth. The lesion can extend from the facial surface into the interdental space toward the palate (**Fig. 12**A).[2,64] Prevalence is greater in young females in their second decade of life due to hormonal influences.[2,64,65]

Pyogenic granulomas are slow-growing, smooth, or lobulated masses that are bright red on clinical examination. They can vary in size from a few millimeters up to several centimeters in diameter. Chronic lesions tend to present less red and more pink or purple in coloration (**Fig. 12**B). The surface of the lesion is friable and bleeds easily.[18,65,66] Patients often complain about frequent bleeding or rapid growth and bite trauma.

Treatment for pyogenic granulomas includes complete surgical excision to the periosteum. For lesions excised from the gingiva with an identified irritant, remove the nidus, or advise the patient to follow up with a dentist for a prophylactic evaluation to decrease the risk of recurrence.

Histologic evaluation of pyogenic granulomas shows granulation-like tissue with an ulcerated surface epithelium. There are also lobular endothelial channels, red blood cells, and scattered inflammatory cells, such as neutrophils, plasma cells, and lymphocytes. Chronic lesions will show sclerotic changes.[2,18,64]

A complete excision of the lesion is typically curative. Recurrence can be secondary to the irritant still being present or hormonal stimulation. Recurrence rates are reported from 3% to 16%.[2,66]

Peripheral Giant Cell Granuloma

Peripheral giant cell granulomas, also known as giant cell epulis, are a lesion that is not a true granuloma. Like the pyogenic granuloma, this lesion is also often caused by local irritation or trauma. The lesion occurs more frequently in the mandible than the maxilla and develops on the gingiva or the edentulous alveolar ridge. Peripheral giant cell granulomas present more often in females and can occur at any age. Prevalence in children under 10-year-old is reported at 9.5%.[2,67,68]

Classic clinical findings include a painless, sessile, or pedunculated mass with or without surface ulceration. Peripheral giant cell granulomas usually measure 2 cm or less. The lesions tend to resemble pyogenic granulomas in children but are often more of a blue–purple coloration compared with the bright red friable pyogenic granuloma.[18,67] The peripheral giant cells that make up the lesion can cause superficial erosion of underlying alveolar bone and is termed "cupping"[69](**Fig. 13**).

Treatment of peripheral giant cell granulomas is complete surgical excision including the underlying periosteum or periodontal ligament. The specimen

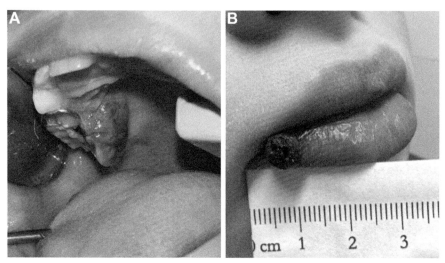

Fig. 12. (*A*) A child with pyogenic granuloma extending to palate secondary to orthodontic space maintainer. (*B*) A 10-year-old patient with lower lip pyogenic granuloma.

must be submitted for histologic evaluation (**Fig. 14**).

Peripheral giant cell granulomas are thought to be the soft tissue counterpart of the central giant cell granuloma because they present with similar histologic findings. Histologic examination shows multiple osteoclast-like multinucleated giant cells within a hemorrhagic background with mesenchymal cells. There is a dense connective tissue stroma composed of spindle-shaped fibroblast with hemosiderin deposits sometimes found at the peripheral margin.[2,70,71]

Recurrence rates following excision of peripheral giant cell granulomas are reported to be 0% to 18%. Lower recurrence rates are associated with curettage in addition to sharp excision, peripheral osteotomy, and removal of irritants.[2,68]

Peripheral Ossifying Fibroma

Peripheral ossifying fibromas occur on the gingiva, predominately in teenagers and young adults. These lesions occur nearly two-thirds of the time in females, and two-thirds of the time in the anterior maxillary arch.[72–74] Peripheral ossifying fibromas are thought to develop from the superficial periodontal ligament and often emerge from the interdental papilla.[75,76] Calculus, dental

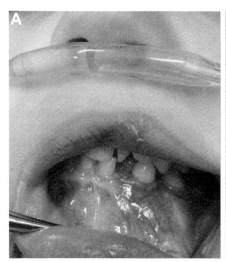
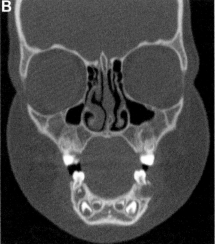

Fig. 13. (*A*) A 4-year-old boy with left mandibular peripheral giant cell granuloma lateral to mandible. (*B*) CT bone window, coronal view showing alveolar erosion, and cupping phenomenon secondary to peripheral giant cell granuloma.

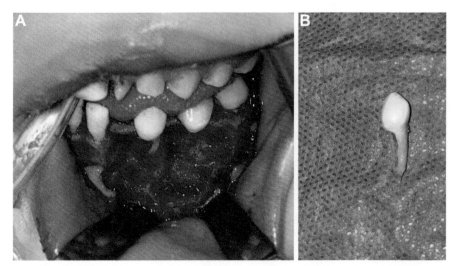

Fig. 14. (*A*) Intraoperative photo of peripheral giant cell granuloma causing erosion of the alveolar bone and teeth. (*B*) Peripheral giant cell granuloma causes erosion of teeth including primary tooth M.

restorations, and orthodontic appliances can lead to chronic irritation and the development of peripheral ossifying fibromas.[73]

Peripheral ossifying fibromas present as a painless, firm, nodular mass arising from the interdental papilla. The color can vary from mucosa pink to red with or without ulceration. Peripheral ossifying fibromas are typically less than 2 cm in size; however, larger lesions have been reported.[76]

Treatment of peripheral ossifying fibromas requires complete surgical excision with excision of the periosteum or associated periodontal ligament. In cases of recurrent lesions, extraction of affected teeth may be necessary.

Histopathologic examination features a nonencapsulated mass with fibrovascular proliferation and deposits of mineralized products. The mineralized product can consist of lamellar or woven bone, cementum-like material, or dystrophic calcifications. Surface epithelium may be ulcerated.[2,72,77]

Complete surgical excision including excision of the periosteum is critical to reduce the risk of recurrence. Recurrence rates are reported to be 8% to 20%.[2,18,72,75,76]

INFECTIOUS LESIONS
Parulis

A parulis develops as a sequela of a necrotic tooth. A soft tissue sinus tract forms through the soft tissue as the chronic infection at the apex of the root destroys the cancellous bone and takes the path of least resistance, perforating the cortical bone. The infection forms a "gum boil" or small subperiosteal abscess that ruptures creating the parulis.[78]

On examination, a parulis presents as a small erythematous swelling that is tender to palpation. These lesions typically measure less than 5 mm with a central sinus tract that expresses purulence near the apex of a non-vital tooth. Parents may report a history of "gum boil" or "whitehead" in the oral cavity. Diagnosing a parulis and identifying the offending tooth can be done with a clinical examination and imaging. If the offending tooth is not obvious, place a gutta-percha cone in the tract until resistance is felt and obtain a periapical image.

Definitive treatment involves addressing the necrotic tooth with either pulpectomy, root canal treatment, or extraction depending on the restorability of the tooth. The chronic infection resolves and the parulis will heal once the infectious source is removed. Antibiotics are adjunctive treatment for immunocompromised pediatric patients or those with systemic signs of infection such as fever or spread of the infection into adjacent soft tissue planes.

Histologic findings of the parulis include edematous tissue and vascular engorgement surrounded by diffuse infiltration of polymorphonuclear leukocytes. The surface epithelium has varying degrees of intra- and extracellular edema, invasion by leukocytes with collections or linear tracts of neutrophils that extend to the base of the specimen.[2]

Recurrence is not a concern following appropriate treatment of the necrotic tooth.

Herpes Simplex Virus

An estimated 3.7 billion people globally less than the age of 50 years (67%) have herpes simplex virus (HSV) type 1 (HSV-1), making it one of the most prevalent orofacial infections.[79,80] There are two strains: HSV-1 and HSV type 2 (HSV-2). HSV-1 is responsible for oral lesions as well as genital herpes, whereas HSV-2 causes only genital herpes. HSV-1 can cause a wide spectrum of clinical manifestations including ulcerative lesions intraorally and along the cutaneous vermillion border (cold sores). Primary HSV-1 infections are acquired through direct contact with a lesion or with infected body fluids of shedding virus.

HSV infection progresses through three phases: primary infection, latency, and recurrent infection. The primary infection may be subclinical.[81] Primary herpetic gingivostomatitis is the most common primary presentation of HSV-1 in children (25%–30%).[82] During the initial infection, the virus enters the sensory nerve terminals and travels along the nerves to the ganglion where it remains during the latency phase until reactivation.[79]

The initial infection of HSV-1 is usually subclinical with flu-like symptoms. Following an incubation period of 2 to 20 days, small vesicular lesions erupt.[82] Lesions can develop along the tongue, lips, gingiva, buccal mucosa, and soft and hard palate. Patients often complain of pain associated with the lesions and these lesions rupture and coalesce to form shallow, irregular ulcers.[82] The ulcers heal slowly over 10 to 14 days without scarring.

Treatment for primary herpetic gingivostomatitis is not necessary as the lesions resolve spontaneously. Recent data show that antiviral medications if administered early, can be beneficial.[82]

HSV-1 infected cells show specific features including acantholytic epithelial cells known as Tzanck cells.[2] Biopsy or surgical intervention is not necessary.

Hand-Foot-Mouth

Hand-foot-mouth (HFM) disease is one of the most common presentations of enterovirus infection. Coxsackievirus A16 is the most common cause of HFM disease; however, other strains of coxsackievirus and enteroviruses also cause HFM.[2] Most cases are reported in infants in children with outbreaks common in daycares, schools, summer camps, and within families. Enterovirus is spread by oral ingestion of the shed virus from the gastrointestinal tract, respiratory tract, oral secretions, or vesicle fluid.[83]

HFM disease presents first with constitutional symptoms including myalgia, fever, and mouth or throat pain. Lesions in the mouth start as vesicles with an erythematous rim which rupture leaving small ulcerations on the buccal, labial, and palatal mucosa as well as the tongue. The ulcerations do cause significant discomfort. Oral lesions are often noted before the development of cutaneous lesions.[83] Cutaneous rash can be macular, papular, or vesicular 2 to 6 mm in diameter. The lesions are not typically painful and rupture after about 10 days leaving shallow non-painful ulcerations on the hands and feet and sometimes trunk

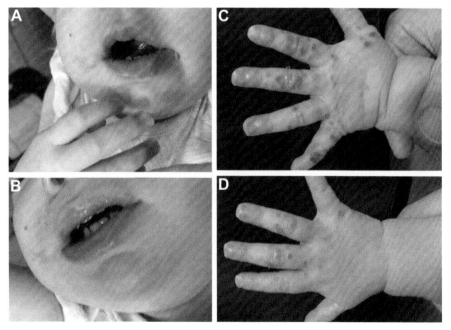

Fig. 15. (*A*) Fever, oral pain, and discomfort from oral lesions; no cutaneous lesion on hands yet. (*B*) Erythema and edema along the lips. (*C*) Shallow cutaneous non-painful ulcerative lesions of the left hand. (*D*) Shallow cutaneous non-painful ulcerative lesions of the right hand.

(Fig. 15). Treatment of HFM disease is supportive as the lesions are self-limiting.

Histologically, patients will develop an intraepithelial vesicle. As the vesicle enlarges, it migrates through the epithelial basal layer forming a subepithelial vesicle leading to necrosis, rupture, and shallow ulcerations that do not scar.[83]

Thrush/Candida

Thrush, also known as pseudomembranous candidiasis, is usually associated with *Candida albicans*. *C albicans* is a naturally occurring fungus that lives on the body and in oral flora. The presence of candida is not pathogenic; however, overproduction of candida or diminished host immunity can lead to infection.[2,84] Pseudomembranous candidiasis is reported to occur in 1% to 37% of infants, likely due to an immature immune system.[84]

Clinically, patients will present with white plaques overlying oral mucosa, most often on the buccal and labial mucosa, soft palate, and tongue.[84] The plaques are easily removed with a dry gauze and the underlying mucosa is erythematous.[84] The white plaques are composed of an assortment of fungal hyphae, inflammatory cells, and desquamated epithelial cells.[2]

Patients with candidiasis often have mild symptoms and may experience a burning sensation. Management is tailored by identifying the etiology and eliminating the underlying cause.[84] Antifungals are the first line of treatment for thrush. In the pediatric population, nystatin and fluconazole are effective in treating oral candidiasis. In immunocompromised children, fluconazole is safe and more effective.[2,84]

If left untreated, thrush can lead to fatal, disseminated disease in severely immunocompromised patients.[84] Thrush will recur if the underlying etiology is not identified and treated.

DISCLOSURE

The authors have nothing to disclose.

REFERENCES

1. Lewis DM. Bohn's nodules, Epstein's pearls, and gingival cysts of the newborn: a new etiology and classification. J Oklahoma Dent Assoc 2010;101(3):32–3.
2. Neville BW, Damm DD, Allen CM, et al. Oral and maxillofacial pathology. 4th edition. MO, USA: Saunders Elsevier; 2016.
3. Marini R, Chipaila N, Monaco A, et al. Unusual symptomatic inclusion cysts in a newborn: a case report. J Med Case Rep 2014;8(1). https://doi.org/10.1186/1752-1947-8-314.
4. Diaz de Ortiz LE and Mendez MD, Palatal and gingival cysts of the newborn. [Updated 2023 Mar 24]. In: StatPearls [Internet]. Treasure Island (FL): StatPearls Publishing; 2024. Available at: https://www.ncbi.nlm.nih.gov/books/NBK493177/.
5. Jorgenson RJ, Shapiro SD, Salinas CF, et al. Intraoral findings and anomalies in neonates. Pediatrics 1982;69(5):577–82.
6. Figueiredo LM, Trindade SC, Sarmento VA, et al. Extensive gingival hemangioma in a 10-year-old boy treated by sclerotherapy: a case report. J Oral Maxillofac Surg 2012;70(11):2585–9.
7. Fevurly RD, Fishman SJ. Vascular anomalies in pediatrics. Surg Clin North Am 2012;92(3):769–x.
8. Haggstrom AN, Drolet BA, Baselga E, et al. Prospective study of infantile hemangiomas: clinical characteristics predicting complications and treatment. Pediatrics 2006;118(3):882–7.
9. Barrón-Peña A, Martínez-Borras MA, Benítez-Cárdenas O, et al. Management of the oral hemangiomas in infants and children: scoping review. Med Oral Patol Oral Cir Bucal 2020;25(2):e252–61.
10. Cawthorn TR, Fraulin FOG, Harrop AR. Infantile hemangiomas of the lip: complications and need for surgical intervention. Plast Reconstr Surg Glob Open 2019;7(6):e2308.
11. Chamli A, Aggarwal P, Jamil RT, et al. Hemangioma, In: StatPearls [Internet]. Treasure Island (FL): StatPearls Publishing; 2024. Available at: https://www.ncbi.nlm.nih.gov/books/NBK538232/.
12. Krowchuk DP, Frieden IJ, Mancini AJ, et al. Clinical practice guideline for the management of infantile hemangiomas. Pediatrics 2019;143(1):e20183475.
13. Colletti G, Biglioli F, Poli T, et al. Vascular malformations of the orbit (lymphatic, venous, arteriovenous): Diagnosis, management and results. J Cranio-Maxillo-Fac Surg 2019;47(5):726–40.
14. Miceli A and Stewart KM, Lymphangioma. [Updated 2023 Aug 8]. In: StatPearls [Internet]. Treasure Island (FL): StatPearls Publishing; 2024. Available at: https://www.ncbi.nlm.nih.gov/books/NBK470333/.
15. Hasan S, Ahmad SA, Kaur M, et al. Lymphangioma of the lower lip-A diagnostic dilemma: report of a rare case with a brief literature review. Case Rep Dent 2022;2022:7890338.
16. Grasso DL, Pelizzo G, Zocconi E, et al. Lymphangiomas of the head and neck in children. Acta Otorhinolaryngol Ital 2008;28(1):17–20.
17. Chouchene F, Masmoudi F, Baaziz A, et al. Oral manifestations and dental care management of a young patient with lymphangioma of the tongue: a case report. Clin Case Rep 2021;9(7):e04537.
18. Marx RE, Stern D. Oral and maxillofacial pathology, a rationale for diagnosis and treatment. 2nd edition. Chicago, IL: Quintessence publishing; 2012.

19. Stal S, Hamilton S, Spira M. Hemangiomas, lymphangiomas, and vascular malformations of the head and neck. Otolaryngol Clin North Am 1986; 19(4):769–96.

20. Ritwik P, Brannon RB, Musselman RJ. Spontaneous regression of congenital epulis: a case report and review of the literature. J Med Case Rep 2010;4:331.

21. Kumar RM, Bavle RM, Umashankar DN, et al. Congenital epulis of the newborn. J Oral Maxillofac Pathol 2015;19(3):407.

22. Babu E, Kamalasanan G, Prathima GS, et al. Congenital epulis of the newborn: a case report and literature review. Int J Clin Pediatr Dent 2021; 14(6):833–7.

23. Kayıran SM, Buyukunal C, Ince U, et al. Congenital epulis of the tongue: a case report and review of the literature. JRSM Short Rep 2011;2(7):62.

24. Jain N, Sinha P, Singh L. Large congenital epulis in a newborn: diagnosis and management. Ear Nose Throat J 2020;99(7):NP79–81.

25. Glickman A, Karlis V. Pediatric benign soft tissue oral and maxillofacial pathology. Oral Maxillofac Surg Clin North Am 2016;28(1):1–10.

26. Chaudhary A, Wakhlu A, Mittal N, et al. Melanotic neuroectodermal tumor of infancy: 2 decades of clinical experience with 18 patients. J Oral Maxillofac Surg 2009;67(1):47–51.

27. Dhawan P, Kochhar GK, Chachra S, et al. Eruption cysts: a series of two cases. Dent Res J 2012;9(5): 647–50.

28. Şen-Tunç E, Açikel H, Sönmez IS, et al. Eruption cysts: a series of 66 cases with clinical features. Med Oral Patol Oral Cir Bucal 2017;22(2):e228–32.

29. Aguiló L, Cibrián R, Bagán JV, et al. Eruption cysts: retrospective clinical study of 36 cases. ASDC (Am Soc Dent Child) J Dent Child 1998;65(2):102–6.

30. Bodner L, Goldstein J, Sarnat H. Eruption cysts: a clinical report of 24 new cases. J Clin Pediatr Dent 2004;28(2):183–6.

31. Killey HC, Kay LW, Seward GR. Benign cystic lesions of the jaws, their diagnosis and treatment. 3rd Edition. New York, NY: Churchill Livingstone, Medical Division of Longman, Inc; 1977.

32. Bilodeau EA, Hunter KD. Odontogenic and developmental oral lesions in pediatric patients. Head Neck Pathol 2021;15(1):71–84.

33. Dillon JR, Avillo AJ, Nelson BL. Dermoid cyst of the floor of the mouth. Head Neck Pathol 2015;9(3):376–8.

34. Le V, Byrne H, Kearns G, et al. Management of a large sublingual dermoid cyst. Arch of Pedia Surg 2021;5(1):104–108DOI.

35. Hamada M, Okawa R, Masuda K, et al. Sublingual dermoid cyst in young child. Children 2023;10(2): 254.

36. Sahoo NK, Choudhary AK, Srinivas V, et al. Dermoid cysts of maxillofacial region. Med J Armed Forces India 2015;71(Suppl 2):S389–94.

37. Puricelli E, Barreiro BOB, Quevedo AS, et al. Occurrence of dermoid cyst in the floor of the mouth: the importance of differential diagnosis in pediatric patients. J Appl Oral Sci 2017;25(3):341–5.

38. Patel H, Mayl J, Chandra B, et al. Dermoid of the oral cavity: case report with histopathology correlation and review of literature. J Radiol Case Rep 2016; 10(12):19–27.

39. Ohta N, Watanabe T, Ito T, et al. A case of sublingual dermoid cyst: extending the limits of the oral approach. Case Rep Otolaryngol 2012;2012: 634949.

40. Hoffrichter MS, Obeid G, Soliday JT. Bilateral submandibular duct atresia: case report. J Oral Maxillofac Surg 2001;59(4):445–7.

41. Hseu A, Anne P, Anne S. Congenital atresia of Wharton's duct. J Clin Diagn Res 2016;10(2):MD01–2.

42. Rosow DE, Ward RF, April MM. Sialodochostomy as treatment for imperforate submandibular duct: a systematic literature review and report of two cases. Int J Pediatr Otorhinolaryngol 2009;73(12):1613–5.

43. Scher LB, Scher I. Case of imperforate submandibular ducts in an infant. Br Dent J.

44. Pownell PH, Brown OE, Pransky SM, et al. Congenital abnormalities of the submandibular duct. Int J Pediatr Otorhinolaryngol 1992;24(2):161–9.

45. Naruse T, Yanamoto S, Yamada S, et al. Lipomas of the oral cavity: clinicopathological and immunohistochemical study of 24 cases and review of the literature. Indian J Otolaryngol Head Neck Surg 2015; 67(Suppl 1):67–73.

46. de Visscher JG. Lipomas and fibrolipomas of the oral cavity. J Maxillofac Surg 1982;10(3):177–81.

47. Morais HGF, Costa CSO, Gonçalo RIC, et al. A 14-year retrospective study focusing on clinical and morphological features of oral cavity lipomas: A review of main topics. J Stomatol Oral Maxillofac Surg 2023;124(3):101387.

48. Ashika BK, Bagchi A, Chawla R, et al. Intraoral lipoma: a case report. J Pharm BioAllied Sci 2023; 15(Suppl 2):S1338–40.

49. Egido-Moreno S, Lozano-Porras AB, Mishra S, et al. Review of literature and report of two clinical cases. J Clin Exp Dent 2016;8(5):e597–603.

50. Lalchandani CM, Tandon S, Rai TS, et al. Recurrent irritation fibroma-"what lies beneath": a multidisciplinary treatment approach. Int J Clin Pediatr Dent 2020;13(3):306–9.

51. Asundaria RR, Tavargeri A. Excision of traumatic fibroma of the tongue in a pediatric patient: a case report. Int J Clin Pediatr Dent 2023;16(1):166–9.

52. Mínguez-Martinez I, Bonet-Coloma C, Ata-Ali-Mahmud J, et al. Clinical characteristics, treatment, and evolution of 89 mucoceles in children. J Oral Maxillofac Surg 2010;68(10):2468–71.

53. Yagüe-García J, España-Tost AJ, Berini-Aytés L, et al. Treatment of oral mucocele-scalpel versus

CO2 laser. Med Oral Patol Oral Cir Bucal 2009;14(9): e469–74.

54. Chi AC, Lambert PR 3rd, Richardson MS, et al. Oral mucoceles: a clinicopathologic review of 1,824 cases, including unusual variants. J Oral Maxillofac Surg 2011;69(4):1086–93.

55. Sadiq MSK, Maqsood A, Akhter F, et al. The effectiveness of lasers in treatment of oral mucocele in pediatric patients: a systematic review. Materials 2022;15(7):2452.

56. Hashemi M, Zohdi M, Zakeri E, et al. Comparison of the recurrence rate of different surgical techniques for oral mucocele: a systematic review and Meta-Analysis. Med Oral Patol Oral Cir Bucal 2023; 28(6):e614–21.

57. Baurmash HD. Mucoceles and ranulas. J Oral Maxillofac Surg 2003;61(3):369–78.

58. Packiri S, Gurunathan D, Selvarasu K. Management of paediatric oral ranula: a systematic review. J Clin Diagn Res 2017;11(9):ZE06–9.

59. Bachesk AB, Bin LR, Iwaki IV, et al. Ranula in children: retrospective study of 25 years and literature review of the plunging variable. Int J Pediatr Otorhinolaryngol 2021;148:110810.

60. Jing F, Wu F, Wen Y, et al. Plunging ranula presenting as a giant anterior cervical cystic mass: a case report and literature review. Case Rep Oncol 2023; 16(1):670–5.

61. Gontarz M, Bargiel J, Gąsiorowski K, et al. Surgical treatment of sublingual gland ranulas. Int Arch Otorhinolaryngol 2022;27(2):e296–301.

62. College C, Feigal R, Wandera A, et al. Bilateral versus unilateral mandibular block anesthesia in a pediatric population. Pediatr Dent 2000;22(6):453–7.

63. Kamal R, Dahiya P, Puri A. Oral pyogenic granuloma: various concepts of etiopathogenesis. J Oral Maxillofac Pathol 2012;16(1):79–82.

64. McNamara KK, Kalmar JR. Erythematous and vascular oral mucosal lesions: a clinicopathologic review of red entities. Head Neck Pathol 2019; 13(1):4–15.

65. Jafarzadeh H, Sanatkhani M, Mohtasham N. Oral pyogenic granuloma: a review. J Oral Sci 2006; 48(4):167–75.

66. Bawazir M, Islam MN, Cohen DM, et al. Gingival fibroma: an emerging distinct gingival lesion with well-defined histopathology. Head Neck Pathol 2021;15(3):917–22.

67. Katsikeris N, Kakarantza-Angelopoulou E, Angelopoulos AP. Peripheral giant cell granuloma. Clinicopathologic study of 224 new cases and review of 956 reported cases. Int J Oral Maxillofac Surg 1988;17(2):94–9.

68. Chrcanovic BR, Gomes CC, Gomez RS. Peripheral giant cell granuloma: an updated analysis of 2824 cases reported in the literature. J Oral Pathol Med 2018;47(5):454–9.

69. Tandon PN, Gupta SK, Gupta DS, et al. Peripheral giant cell granuloma. Contemp Clin Dent 2012; 3(Suppl 1):S118–21.

70. Cahuana-Bartra P, Brunet-Llobet L, Suñol-Capella M, et al. Expansive oral giant cell granuloma in a pediatric patient. Int J Clin Pediatr Dent 2023; 16(2):405–8.

71. Shadman N, Ebrahimi SF, Jafari S, et al. Peripheral giant cell granuloma: a review of 123 cases. Dent Res J 2009;6(1):47–50.

72. Buchner A, Hansen LS. The histomorphologic spectrum of peripheral ossifying fibroma. Oral Surg Oral Med Oral Pathol 1987;63(4):452–61.

73. Mergoni G, Meleti M, Magnolo S, et al. Peripheral ossifying fibroma: A clinicopathologic study of 27 cases and review of the literature with emphasis on histomorphologic features. J Indian Soc Periodontol 2015;19(1):83–7.

74. Cuisia ZE, Brannon RB. Peripheral ossifying fibroma–a clinical evaluation of 134 pediatric cases. Pediatr Dent 2001;23(3):245–8.

75. Cavalcante IL, Barros CC, Cruz VM, et al. Peripheral ossifying fibroma: A 20-year retrospective study with focus on clinical and morphological features. Med Oral Patol Oral Cir Bucal 2022;27(5):e460–7.

76. Lázare H, Peteiro A, Pérez Sayáns M, et al. Clinicopathological features of peripheral ossifying fibroma in a series of 41 patients. Br J Oral Maxillofac Surg 2019;57(10):1081–5.

77. Abitbol TE, Santi E. Peripheral ossifying fibroma–literature update and clinical case. Periodontal Clin Invest 1997;19(1):36–7.

78. Chen K, Liang Y, Xiong H. Diagnosis and treatment of odontogenic cutaneous sinus tracts in an 11-year-old boy: a case report. Medicine (Baltim) 2016;95(20):e3662.

79. Agrawal AA. Gingival enlargements: differential diagnosis and review of literature. World J Clin Cases 2015;3(9):779–88.

80. Herpes simplex virus. World Health Organization; 2023. https://www.who.int/news-room/fact-sheets/detail/herpes-simplex-virus. [Accessed 15 November 2023].

81. Miller CS, Redding SW. Diagnosis and management of orofacial herpes simplex virus infections. Dent Clin North Am 1992;36(4):879–95.

82. Kolokotronis A, Doumas S. Herpes simplex virus infection, with particular reference to the progression and complications of primary herpetic gingivostomatitis. Clin Microbiol Infect 2006;12(3):202–11.

83. Saguil A, Kane SF, Lauters R, et al. Hand-foot-and-mouth disease: rapid evidence review. Am Fam Physician 2019;100(7):408–14.

84. Fotos PG, Vincent SD, Hellstein JW. Oral candidosis. Clinical, historical, and therapeutic features of 100 cases. Oral Surg Oral Med Oral Pathol 1992;74(1): 41–9.

Pediatric Odontogenic Cysts and Tumors

Sarah Loren Moles, DMD[a,1], Caitlin B.L. Magraw, MD, DDS, FACS[b,c],*

KEYWORDS

- Odontogenic cyst • Odontogenic tumor • Maxilla • Mandible • Pediatric • Impacted teeth

KEY POINTS

- Appreciate the presentation of odontogenic cysts and tumors in the pediatric population.
- Recognize the biologic behavior of various odontogenic cysts and tumors.
- Understand treatment recommendations of odontogenic cysts and tumors in the pediatric population.

INTRODUCTION

Pediatric odontogenic cysts and tumors are rare and often associated with developing or impacted teeth. This article will discuss the presentation, diagnosis, and treatment of odontogenic cysts and tumors in the pediatric population.

ODONTOGENIC CYSTS

Odontogenic cysts are broadly categorized as inflammatory or developmental (**Box 1**).

Periapical (Radicular) Cyst

A periapical (radicular) cyst is an inflammatory lesion that forms at the apex of an endodontically compromised tooth (**Fig. 1**). These lesions are thought to arise from the proliferation of epithelial nests present in the periodontal ligament.[1,2]

Periapical cysts represent 52% to 68% of odontogenic cysts and most commonly present in the third decade of life with less than 1% of periapical cysts occurring in the pediatric population.[3] Underreporting of pediatric periapical cysts is likely associated with eventual resolution of the lesion once the primary tooth is lost. Periapical cysts can occur anywhere within the tooth-bearing alveolus, but in the pediatric population are most commonly associated with mandibular primary molars.[4,5] Pulpitis and associated symptoms are the most common presentation. Vitality testing indicates a nonvital tooth.

Treatment of periapical cysts starts with identifying and managing the source of inflammation. Endodontic therapy or extraction should be considered. Any periapical cyst that remains after successful primary treatment should undergo definitive removal of the lesion. With complete excision and removal of the source, recurrence is essentially zero.

Buccal Bifurcation Cyst

A buccal bifurcation cyst (BBC) is an inflammatory odontogenic cyst that is most commonly associated with mandibular first molars in the pediatric population, aged 4 to 14.[6] The first reported BBC was in 1983 by Stoneman and Worth[7] and was recognized by the World Health Organization (WHO) in 1992 as a "mandibular infected buccal cyst."[8] The exact pathogenesis is uncertain, but these lesions are often seen associated with buccal enamel extensions into the bifurcation of the mandibular first and less commonly second permanent molars. Others speculate partial exposure of the crown during eruption leads to inflammation and epithelial proliferation leading to cyst formation.[6]

[a] Head and Neck Surgical Oncology and Microvascular Reconstruction, Providence Cancer Institute, Portland, OR, USA; [b] The Head and Neck Institute, Head and Neck Surgical Associates, Portland, OR, USA; [c] Department of Oral and Maxillofacial Surgery, Oregon Health and Sciences University, Portland, OR, USA
[1] Present address: 1500 SW 5th Avenue, Unit 2606, Portland, OR 97201.
* Corresponding author. 1849 NW Kearney Street, Suite 300, Portland, OR 97219.
E-mail address: caitlin.magraw@gmail.com

Oral Maxillofacial Surg Clin N Am 36 (2024) 283–294
https://doi.org/10.1016/j.coms.2024.01.006

Box 1
Categorized of odontogenic cysts

Odontogenic Cysts

    Odontogenic Inflammatory cysts

        Periapical (Radicular) cyst

        Buccal bifurcation cyst

    Odontogenic Developmental cysts

        Dentigerous cyst

        Odontogenic keratocyst

        Lateral periodontal cyst

        Calcifying odontogenic cyst

        Glandular odontogenic cyst

Odontogenic Tumors

    Epithelial Odontogenic Tumor

        Ameloblastoma

        Adenomatoid odontogenic tumor

        Calcifying epithelial odontogenic tumor

        Squamous odontogenic tumor

        Adenoid Ameloblastoma

    Mixed Epithelial and Mesenchymal Odontogenic Tumor

        Odontoma

        Ameloblastic fibroma

        Primordial odontogenic tumor

    Mesenchymal Odontogenic Tumor

        Odontogenic myxoma

        Cementoblastoma

        Central and peripheral odontogenic fibroma

Patients present with dull or aching discomfort on the buccal aspect of the associated dentition. Buccal edema and foul-tasting discharge may also be present.[9] Examination findings include deep probing depths and pocket formation in the buccal sulcus. Radiographically, BBCs are well-circumscribed unilocular radiolucencies involving the buccal bifurcation and often show displacement of the roots toward the lingual cortex.

Treatment of BBCs includes enucleation of the lesion. Historically, the need for extraction of the associated tooth has been debated.[7] However, recent reports have indicated the tooth may be maintained with irrigation of the periodontal pocket after excision and close clinical follow-up.[10,11]

Dentigerous Cyst

A dentigerous cyst is defined as a lesion originating from separation of the dental follicle from the crown of an unerupted tooth.[9] This occurs when fluid accumulates between the reduced enamel epithelium and the enamel of the developing tooth. The exact pathogenesis is unknown. These lesions are favored to be developmental in origin; however, an inflammatory type has also been described with increased incidence in the pediatric population.[12–14] While dentigerous cysts are the most common developmental cyst, accounting for approximately 20% of all cystic lesions of the jaws, only 4% to 9% of these cysts occur in the first decade of life.[15]

Small developmental dentigerous cysts are typically asymptomatic and noted on routine radiographic examination. They present as unicystic, well-circumscribed, radiolucent lesions originating from the cementoenamel junction of an impacted or developing tooth (**Fig. 2**). Neville and Damm[9] described 3 radiographic variants: central, lateral, and circumferential. Radiographically, it can be difficult to distinguish a large dental follicle from a small dentigerous cyst. In a developing tooth, the dental follicle is considered normal in size if less than 4 mm from the developing tooth.[16] These cysts can become large, cause tooth displacement, root resorption of adjacent dentition, and bone resorption with expansion.

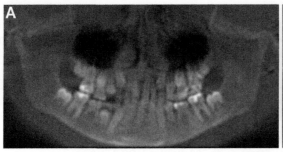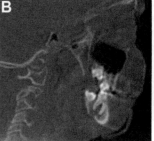

Fig. 1. (*A*) Tru-pan reconstruction with periapical cyst associated with endodontically compromised mandibular first permanent molar in an 11-year-old patient presenting as a neck mass. (*B*) Axial cone beam computed tomography (CBCT) with radiolucent lesion of the left mandible with cortical destruction.

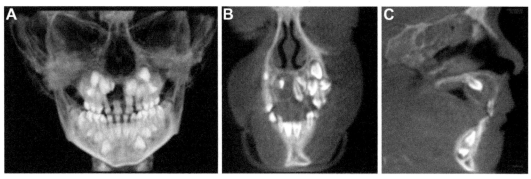

Fig. 2. A 5-year-old patient with dentigerous cyst assoicated with impacted supernumerary maxillary tooth. (*A*) Three dimensional CBCT reconstruction with radiolucency and disturbed eruption of permanent dentition. (*B*) Coronal CBCT and (*C*) Sagittal CBCT with expansile, radiolcuent lesion associatd with crown of impacted tooth.

Incisional biopsy of large lesions is recommended prior to definitive treatment to rule out other odontogenic cysts or tumors. After a diagnosis of dentigerous cyst is obtained, enucleation of the cyst and removal of the associated tooth is often the treatment of choice. Large dentigerous cysts with expansion are amendable to marsupialization allowing for decompression prior to removal. If the associated tooth is determined to be in an ideal position for future eruption, the tooth may be left in place after removal of the cystic lesion. If maintained, these teeth may require additional intervention such as expose and bonding for assisted orthodontic eruption. Fujii and colleagues[17] identified factors favoring the eruption of impacted teeth associated with dentigerous cysts without orthodontic traction including the age of the patient (<10 years), depth of impaction in relationship to the adjacent cementoenamel junction and cusp tip (<5.1 mm), angulation less than 25%, and space to tooth ratio greater than 1:1. The potential for eruption of an impacted tooth associated with a dentigerous cyst can be identified within 3 months of marsupialization and orthodontic traction should be considered if progress toward eruption has not occurred within that time.

Eruption Cyst

An eruption cyst or eruption hematoma is the soft tissue variant of a dentigerous cyst. The lesion develops from the separation of the dental follicle from the crown of a deciduous or permanent tooth as it erupts through the alveolar soft tissues. Eruption cysts are typically seen in children under the age of 10 associated with maxillary and mandibular primary central incisors and permanent first molars.[9] The pathogenesis of eruption cysts is not well understood but it has been suggested that stimulation of soft tissue, early caries, trauma,

infection, and inadequate space for eruption are all possible contributing factors.[18,19]

Eruption cysts appear as soft, fluctuant lesions of the alveolar soft tissue, overlying the crown of an erupting primary or permanent tooth, often with a bluish-purple color. The darker lesions represent blood within the cystic cavity secondary to surface trauma. Because these lesions are soft tissue in nature, radiographs are of limited utility, demonstrating evidence of an erupting tooth; there should not be an associated intraosseous component to the lesion radiographically. Most eruption cysts do not require intervention as they resolve with the eruption of the associated dentition, leading to under reported incidence. If the lesion increases in size, becomes symptomatic, or secondarily infected, an incision can be made at the alveolar crest within the cystic cavity, allowing for marsupialization and continued eruption.

Odontogenic Keratocyst

A dental cyst with keratinization was first described in the 1930s though the term "odontogenic keratocyst (OKC)" was not utilized until 1956. Over the years, OKCs have been under debate as to their classification as an odontogenic cyst or tumor. In 2005, the WHO updated their classification to a benign cystic neoplasm as a keratocystic odontogenic tumor (KCOT). This change in nomenclature was largely based on molecular studies suggesting the pathophysiology of the lesion was not characteristic of other cystic lesions. The OKC shows increased expression of proliferating cell nuclear antigen (PCNA) and Ki-67.[9] Greater than 30% of isolated OKCs and 85% of lesions associated with nevoid basal cell carcinoma (NBCC) also show mutation in the PTCH1 gene, associated with the Hedgehog signaling pathway. Despite these differences, KCOT was reclassified in the 2017 WHO update as an odontogenic cyst and has remained as such in 2022.

OKCs have been identified in a wide age range from infancy to late adulthood, with approximately 60% in patients 10 to 40 year old. Small lesions are asymptomatic and found on routine radiographic examination. Large lesions may also be asymptomatic but expansion, pain, swelling, and drainage are not uncharacteristic. This is thought to be secondary to the inflammatory nature of the keratinized material produced within the OKC. Approximately 75% of lesions occur in the mandible with an increased incidence in the posterior molar/ramus region.[20] Radiographically, OKCs are well-defined unilocular or multilocular radiolucencies with a propensity for anterior posterior growth. A total of 50% of cases are associated with an impacted tooth. The lumen of these lesions may contain clear fluid or "cheesy material" consistent microscopically of keratinaceous debris.[9]

The thin, friable epithelial lining of these cysts makes complete removal difficult with enucleation and curettage alone leading to high recurrence rates, ranging from 5% to 62% depending on treatment technique. Most recurrences occur within 5 years of treatment. For large lesions, marsupialization and decompression have shown to aid in definitive management. By decompressing these lesions, the cystic lining increases in thickness, decreases the size, and potentially provides a barrier between the lesion and surrounding vital structures, ultimately aiding in complete surgical excision. Adjuncts to enucleation and curettage have been utilized to aid in decreasing the recurrence rate of OKCs including peripheral osteotomy, modified Cornoys, and 5-fluorouracil (**Fig. 3**).[21]

OKC Association with Nevoid Basal Cell Carcinoma Syndrome

Nevoid basal cell carcinoma (NBCCS) or Gorlin–Goltz syndrome is an inherited autosomal dominant condition caused by a mutation in the PTCH1 gene. The diagnosis of NBCCS is made when 2 major criteria or 1 major and 2 minor criteria are identified (**Box 2**). The incidence of OKCs in NBCCS patients has been reported as 66% to 86%.[22] The clinical presentation differs between family members and different families (**Fig. 4**). Often, the presence of multiple OKCs is the first presenting sign and should warrant further workup for NBCCS.

Lateral Periodontal Cyst

Lateral periodontal cysts (LPC) account for less than 2% of all odontogenic cysts, with only a few

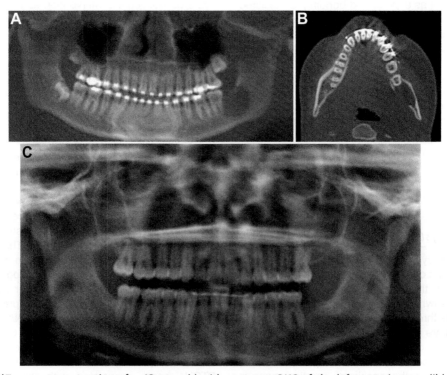

Fig. 3. (A)Tru-pan reconstruction of a 13-year-old with recurrent OKC of the left posterior mandible (*B*) with lingual cortex destruction. Treated with enucleation and curettage with peripheral ostectomy and 5-FU. (*C*) Panoramic 1 -year follow-up without recurrence.

documented cases in the pediatric population.[23,24] These lesions arise from the rests of dental lamina. A botryoid cyst is a multilocular variant of the LPC whereas the gingival cyst is the soft tissue variant.

LPCs are asymptomatic and found on routine imaging. Radiographically they appear as well-circumscribed radiolucent lesions located lateral to the root of a vital tooth. Greater than 75% of these lesions occur in the mandible involving the lateral incisors, canines, and first premolars. These lesions are rarely larger than 1 cm in greatest dimension. Conservative excision of the LPC with preservation of the adjacent tooth structure is recommended. Recurrence is rare with incidence most common in the botryoid variant.[25]

Calcifying Odontogenic Cyst

The calcifying odontogenic cyst (COC) was first described by Gorlin and colleages[26] in 1962 and since that time has been reclassified between an odontogenic cyst and neoplasm. In 2017, COCs were defined as a benign cyst of odontogenic origin, characterized by "ameloblastoma-like epithelium" containing ghost cells that may calcify.[27] In 2022, the definition has excluded ameloblastoma-like epithelium and instead is now defined as "a developmental odontogenic cyst characterized histologically by ghost cells, which often calcify."[28] COCs account for approximately 5% to 7% of all odontogenic cysts and typically present in the third to fourth decade. However, they are also known to occur in the pediatric population, especially when associated with odontomas.

COCs present as an asymptomatic swelling, though they have been known to cause pain and displacement of adjacent teeth.[29] There is equal prevalence in the maxilla and mandible and more than 65% occur anterior to the canines. Radiographically, COCs are unilocular, well-defined, predominately radiolucent lesions with foci of

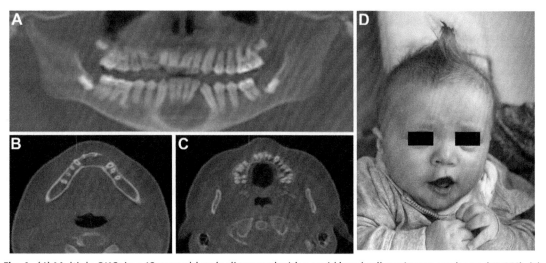

Fig. 4. (A) Multiple OKCs in a 13-year-old male diagnosed with nevoid basal cell carcinoma syndrome (NBCCS). (B) Axial CBCT of anterior mandibular and (C) maxillary radiolucencies. (D) A 4-month-old with NBCCS exhibiting macrocephaly, left minor form cleft lip, and palmar pits.

radiopacity. Approximately one-third are associated with impacted teeth or odontomas.[26] Treatment for COCs is conservative enucleation and curettage with excellent prognosis and low recurrence rates.[3,30]

Glandular Odontogenic Cyst

Glandular odontogenic cysts (GOC) are rare but locally aggressive lesions that primarily present in middle-aged adults, in the fifth to sixth decade. GOCs account for less than 1% of all odontogenic cysts and though rare, can occur within the pediatric population. To date, approximately 10 cases of GOCs within the pediatric population have been reported.[31–33] GOCs are predominately identified in the mandible with increased predilection for the anterior jaws. Many mandibular lesions also cross midline.[34]

Small, unilocular lesions are considered amendable to enucleation and curettage. Larger, multilocular lesions are believed to be more aggressive and treatment recommendations include peripheral ostectomy, marginal resection, and segmental resection.[3] Recurrence rate has been documented as 29% to 50% with enucleation alone, noting increased recurrence rates in large multilocular lesions.

ODONTOGENIC TUMORS

Pediatric odontogenic tumors make up one-third of the tumors found in the maxillofacial region and are more common after age 6 when secondary tooth development begins. Odontogenic tumors are classified histologically as epithelial, mesenchymal, and mixed epithelial and mesenchymal odontogenic tumors (see **Box 1**).

Ameloblastoma

Ameloblastoma is the most common odontogenic tumor in the head and neck; however, it is rare in the pediatric population with only 10% to 15% of cases present under the age of 13.[35,36]

There are 3 histologic subtypes of ameloblastoma: unicystic, solid or multicystic, and peripheral, all arising from odontogenic epithelium.

Within the pediatric population, there is a much higher percentage of unicystic ameloblastomas compared to adults. Most of these lesions involve unerupted dentition. Clinically, these lesions often present as slow-growing expansion with associated asymmetry, usually without pain or paresthesia. Radiographically, unicystic ameloblastomas appear similar to dentigerous cysts as a well-circumscribed radiolucency often associated with the crown of an unerupted tooth. Solid or multicystic ameloblastomas are rare in the pediatric population. Radiographically, they present as multilocular radiolucent lesions. Large loculations have classically been described as "soap bubble" appearance with smaller loculations as a "honeycomb" pattern.[9] Peripheral ameloblastomas are also rare in the pediatric population. Peripheral lesions present as painless, sessile, or pedunculated gingival lesions, clinically similar to a fibroma or pyogenic granuloma.

The solid or multicystic variant has several histologic subtypes including follicular, plexiform, acanthomatous, granular cell, desmoplastic, and basal cell. These variants have little impact on the lesion behavior or treatment recommendations. Three histologic variants for the unicystic ameloblastoma include luminal, intraluminal, and mural. Unicystic ameloblastomas of the luminal variant are considered less aggressive and treatment recommendations include enucleation and curettage with peripheral ostectomy. Other unicystic and conventional ameloblastomas have more aggressive clinical features requiring en bloc resection with 1 cm margin and 1 uninvolved anatomic margin. Peripheral ameloblastomas show low recurrence rates with local excision.

Even though ameloblastomas are benign lesions, approximately 2% metastasize. Ameloblastoma most commonly metastasizes to the lungs but have also been reported to the cervical nodes, vertebrae, kidneys, and heart.[35] Metastatic lesions are reported with long-standing or incomplete excision of maxillofacial lesions and diagnosed 3 to 45 years after initial treatment.[9] Metastatic lesions are benign in nature and not radiosensitive therefore surgical excision is recommended.

Ameloblastic carcinomas are lesions showing features of malignancy in the primary tumor, recurrence, or metastasis. Malignant lesions have been reported in patients from age 6 to 61. Radiographically, ameloblastic carcinoma presents ill-defined margins and cortical destruction. An oncologic resection of these lesions is required.

Adenomatoid Odontogenic Tumor

Adenomatoid odontogenic tumors (AOT) account for approximately 5% of all odontogenic tumors and is often referred to as a "two-thirds tumor." This is due to two-third of cases presenting in the maxilla, two-third in young females, two-third associated with an unerupted tooth, and two-third of affected teeth are canines.[37] AOTs are uncommon in patients older than 30 years of age.

Most AOTs are small and rarely larger than 3 cm in greatest dimension.[9] These lesions are often asymptomatic and identified on imaging when utilized to determine cause of delayed eruption.

Radiographically, AOTs are unilocular radiolucencies associated with an impacted tooth, most commonly a permanent canine. These lesions may be impossible to differentiate from a dentigerous cyst on radiographic examination.

AOTs are formed by a thick, fibrous capsule with varying central densities. Histologically, the 2022 WHO update emphasized that some odontogenic lesions including odontomas, adenoid ameloblastomas, and calcifying epithelial odontogenic tumors may contain areas similar to AOTs. Therefore, to avoid misdiagnosis due to histologically similar presentations, clinicoradiographic evaluation is necessary. Due to its thick cystic lining, AOTs are enucleated easily and recurrence is rare, even with incomplete excision.[38]

Calcifying Epithelial Odontogenic Tumor

Calcifying epithelial odontogenic tumors (CEOT), also known as Pindborg tumors, were first described by Jens Jorgen Pindborg, a Dutch pathologist, in 1955.[39] These lesions are rare, accounting for approximately 1% of all odontogenic tumors. Philipsen and Reichart[40] completed a review of 181 cases of CEOTs with age range of 8 to 92 year old. Less than 15 cases were reported under the age of 20. The vast majority of CEOTs are of the intraosseous variant with only 6% of Pindborg tumors accounting for the peripheral variant.[41]

Intraosseous or central CEOTs are slow-growing masses that present as asymptomatic swelling or expansion, often in the posterior mandible. Radiographically, CEOTs may be unilocular or multilocular with well-defined scalloped margins. CEOTs may be entirely radiolucent, but varying degrees of calcification have been reported. They have been described as having a "snowflake" pattern and are often associated with an impacted tooth.[9] The extraosseous or peripheral variant is most commonly located in the anterior gingiva, presenting as a sessile gingival mass.

The treatment of CEOTs has been debated. While some advocate for enucleation and curettage, conservative treatment has resulted in recurrence rate of approximately 15% to 20%. If there is thinning of the cortical borders or less confined lesions typically seen in the maxilla, a more aggressive resection is recommended. Given the infiltrating nature of these tumors, surgical removal with 1 cm of clinically and radiographically normal bone is recommended.[42]

Squamous Odontogenic Tumors

Squamous odontogenic tumors (SOT) are extremely rare lesions, especially in the pediatric population, most commonly presenting in the third decade.[42] Only 1 case has been described associated with primary dentition.[43] There is no gender predilection, and the maxilla and mandible are affected equally. They present as painless or mildly painful gingival swelling with possible tooth mobility. Radiographically SOTs present as triangular radiolucencies associated with the lateral root surface that rarely exceed 1.5 cm. Conservative excision and curettage is recommended.

Odontoma

Odontomas are the most common odontogenic tumor in the pediatric population. They are typically detected in the first 2 decades with a mean age of 14. Odontomas are considered hamartomatous developmental malformations of dental tissue as opposed to true neoplasms. Two subtypes of odontomas include compound and complex lesions, both formed from enamel and dentin. Compound odontomas are a congregate of small tooth-like structures while complex odontomas are a haphazard arrangement of dental tissues without resemblance to a formed dental structure.

Complex odontomas most commonly develop in the posterior molar region of either jaw and often interfere with molar eruption. Compound odontomas are commonly found in the anterior maxilla. Both compound and complex lesions are typically asymptomatic and found on radiographic examination. Compound odontomas can be diagnosed by their radiographic appearance of small tooth-like structures surrounded by a thin radiolucent rim. Complex odontomas present radiographically as a dense, radiopaque mass with the same density as a tooth. These lesions can be confused radiographically with other radiopaque lesions such as an osteoma.

Both compound and complex odontomas are treated with surgical excision with excellent prognosis. If associated with an impacted tooth and the lesion can be removed without damaging the underlying dentition, the tooth may be maintained. Depending on its position and stage of development, the associated dentition may require additional intervention to assist with eruption.

Ameloblastic Fibroma

Ameloblastic fibromas (AF) represent approximately 2% of all odontogenic tumors and are most commonly found in the pediatric population. The mean age range is 6 to 12 year old with few cases after age 25.[37] AFs have a slight male predilection and are often found on routine imaging. They are typically asymptomatic, slow-growing, expansile lesions with approximately 70% located in the posterior mandible.[9] Radiographically, AFs are well-defined unilocular or multilocular radiolucencies with 75% associated with an impacted tooth.

Definitive treatment for AFs has been debated similar to that of the CEOT. Recurrence rates have been reported anywhere from 0% to 43% with conservative enucleation and curettage.[9,44] It is believed most recurrences are associated with incomplete removal of the original lesion. Because of this, primary enucleation and curettage is the recommended initial treatment with more aggressive resection reserved for large destructive lesions on initial presentation or recurrent AFs. It is important to note that approximately 35% of ameloblastic fibrosarcomas develop in the presence of a recurrent AF.[9,45–49]

Primordial Odontogenic Tumor

Primordial odontogenic tumor (POT) was first described by Mosqueda-Taylor et al[50] in 2014 and was included as an isolated entity in the WHO classification of 2017. A 2020 systematic review identified 16 cases and 3 molecular studies.[51] The mean age was 11.6, ranging from 2 to 18 year old. All cases were identified in the posterior region of the jaws with increased incidence in the mandible. Radiographically, POTs are well-defined, radiolucent, unilocular lesions associated with an unerupted tooth. They often cause tooth displacement, root resorption, and cortical destruction.[51] Clinically these lesions appear as a solid, multilobulated, glossy white mass. The term "POT" was selected due to the histologic features that closely resemble the early (primordial) stages of tooth development.[50] Treatment includes complete excision with extraction of the associated dentition. To date, only 1 recurrence has been reported in the literature for which the patient underwent a segmental mandibular resection.[52]

Odontogenic Myxoma

Odontogenic myxomas (OM) are rare, benign but aggressive lesions that are formed from the odontogenic ectomesenchyme. OMs account for less than 12% of pediatric odontogenic tumors.[35] Overall, myxomas have a predilection for the posterior mandible although several reports have suggested increased frequency in the maxilla in the pediatric population.[53,54] The age distribution ranges from 5 to 65, mean of 25 to 30.

Small lesions may be asymptomatic and discovered on routine imaging with larger lesions associated with slow, painless expansion. Radiographically, OMs may appear as unilocular or multilocular radiolucencies that displace adjacent structures or cause root resorption (**Fig. 5**). The margins are often scalloped and large OMs may have a "soap bubble" appearance similar to an ameloblastoma. On gross examination, OMs appear as a solid, gelatinous mass.

Because OMs are not encapsulated and show aggressive infiltration into surrounding tissues, surgical resection with 1 to 1.5 cm clinical and radiographically normal-appearing bone with 1 uninvolved anatomic border is recommended (**Fig. 6**). Recurrence rates have been reported as high as 25%; however, this number represents conservative treatment with enucleation and curettage.[55] In the pediatric population, many have advocated for less aggressive surgical intervention due to concern for interference with facial growth. However, the aggressive nature of OMs can lead to seeding of the tumor into adjacent and often unresectable anatomic spaces.[37,55] Therefore, wide surgical excision remains the recommend surgical intervention for both pediatric and adult populations.

In 2014, Kadlub and colleagues[56] suggested an infantile variant of OM. They reported 4 cases of OM in patients under the age of 2 who presented with rapidly expanding paranasal swelling associated with nasal or lacrimal duct obstruction. These lesions were all clinically, radiographically, and histologically similar to the traditional OM but showed rapid growth with a maxillary predilection.

Cementoblastoma

Cementoblastomas are benign tumors arising from cementoblasts and represent less than 1% of all odontogenic tumors. Approximately 80% of cementoblastomas are associated with mandibular posterior dentition and identified in the second or third decade; only 5 cases have been reported associated with primary dentition.[57]

Patients often present with a nonspecific, dull, aching discomfort in the region of a cementoblastoma. The involved dentition responds normal to vitality testing. Cementoblastomas are not classically described as aggressive tumors; however, expansion, displacement of adjacent teeth, maxillary sinus involvement, and extension into the pulp chamber of the associated dentition are commonly seen. These tumors are radiopaque and fused with an associated tooth root, obscuring the periodontal ligament space. They also typically present with a radiolucent rim surrounding the extent of the mass.

Treatment of cementoblastomas consists of excision and extraction of the associated tooth. An alternative to extraction includes excision of the cementoblastoma with root amputation,

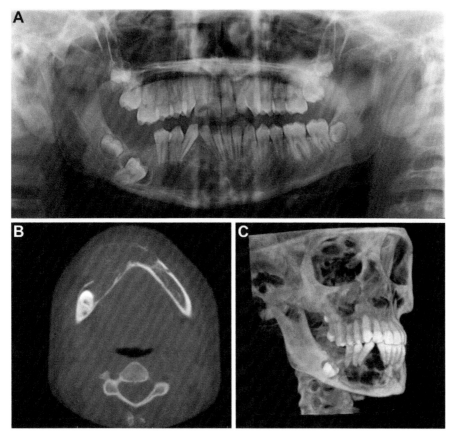

Fig. 5. (*A*) Multilocular radiolucency of mandible with "soap bubble" appearance. (*B*) Axial CBCT with buccal expansion, cortical destruction, and root displacement of an odontogenic myxoma. (*C*) Three-dimensional reconstruction of CBCT.

followed by endodontic therapy of the associated tooth. Recurrence is not expected with complete surgical excision.

Odontogenic Fibroma

Central and peripheral odontogenic fibromas are uncommon tumors. The central variant has been reported in patients 4 to 80 year old with a mean of 40. There is a female predilection with equal distribution in the maxilla and mandible. A third of central odontogenic fibromas are associated with an unerupted tooth. Small lesions are asymptomatic while large lesions may cause expansion and tooth mobility. Radiographically, the central variant appears as a well-defined, unilocular, radiolucent

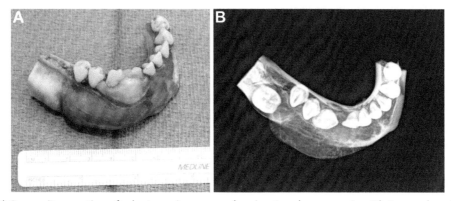

Fig. 6. (*A*) Composite resection of odontogenic myxoma showing 1 cm bone margin with 1 normal anatomic soft tissue margin. (*B*) Intraoperative radiograph of specimen showing margins free of tumor.

lesion, often causing root divergence or resorption. Treatment includes complete excision with aggressive curettage because the lesion is not encapsulated. Recurrence is rare with complete excision.[35]

The peripheral odontogenic fibroma presents as a slow-growing, sessile, gingival mass with normal overlying mucosa. They have been reported in a wide age range but are most commonly identified in the second to fourth decade on the buccal mandibular gingiva. Radiographic examination often identifies calcification within the soft tissue mass and may show a "cupping" appearance to the underlying alveolus. Treatment includes local surgical excision with low recurrence following complete excision.

SUMMARY

Odontogenic cysts and tumors are rare in the pediatric population and treatment requires understanding of the biology of the pathologic entity as well as dental development and craniomaxillofacial complex growth. In general, conservative management leads to excellent results since children heal well. Long-term follow-up is important to monitor growth, ensure eruption of permanent dentition, and to evaluate for recurrence.

CLINICS CARE POINTS

- Pediatric odontogenic cysts and tumors are rare and often associated with developing or impacted teeth.

- Odontogenic cysts are broadly categorized as inflammatory or developmental while odontogenic tumors are classified histologically as epithelial, mesenchymal, or mixed tumors.

- Treatment of odontogenic cysts and tumors requires understanding of the biology of the pathologic entity as well as growth and development.

- Long-term follow-up is important to monitor growth and development of the craniomaxillofacial complex, ensure eruption of permanent dentition, and to evaluate for recurrence.

DISCLOSURE

The authors have nothing to disclose.

REFERENCES

1. Lin LM, Huang GT, Rosenberg PA. Proliferation of epithelial cell rests, formation of apical cysts, and regression of apical cysts after periapical wound healing. J Endod 2007;33(8):908–16.
2. Nair PN. New perspectives on radicular cysts: do they heal? Int Endod J 1998;31(3):155–60.
3. Arce K, Streff CS, Ettinger KS. Pediatric Odontogenic Cysts of the Jaws. Oral Maxillofac Surg Clin 2016;28(1):21–30.
4. Shetty S, Angadi PV, Rekha K. Radicular cyst in deciduous maxillary molars: a rarity. Head Neck Pathol 2010;4(1):27–30.
5. Mass E, Kaplan I, Hirshberg A. A clinical and histopathological study of radicular cysts associated with primary molars. J Oral Pathol Med 1995;24(10):458–61.
6. Ramos LM, Vargas PA, Coletta RD, et al. Bilateral buccal bifurcation cyst: case report and literature review. Head Neck Pathol 2012 Dec;6(4):455–9.
7. Stoneman DW, Worth HM. The mandibular infected buccal cyst-molar area. Dent Radiogr Photogr 1983;56:1–14.
8. Kramer IRH, Pindborg JJ, Shear M. Histological typing of odontogenic tumors. World Health Organization. 2nd edition. Berlin: Springer; 1992. p. 40–2.
9. Neville BW, Damm DD, Allen CM, et al. Oral & maxillofacial pathology. 4th edition. Missouri: WB Saunders, Elsevier; 2016. p. 604–5.
10. Iatrou I, Theologie-Lygidakis N, Leventis M. Intraosseous cystic lesions of the jaws in children: a retrospective analysis of 47 consecutive cases. Oral Surg Oral Med Oral Pathol Oral Radiol Endod 2009;107:485–92.
11. Corona-Rodriguez J, Torres-Labardini R, Velasco-Tizcareno M, et al. Bilateral buccal bifurcation cyst: case report and literature review. J Oral Maxillofac Surg 2011;69:1694–6.
12. Main DM. Epithelial jaw cysts: 10 years of the WHO classification. J Oral Pathol 1985;14(1):1–7.
13. Benn A, Altini M. Dentigerous cysts of inflammatory origin: a clinicopathologic study. Oral Surg Oral Med Oral Pathol Oral Radiol Endod 1996;81(2):203–9.
14. Bloch-Jorgensen K. Follicular cysts. Dental Cosmos 1928;70:708–11.
15. Deboni MC, Brozoski MA, Traina AA, et al. Surgical management of dentigerous cyst and keratocystic odontogenic tumor in children: a conservative approach and 7-year follow-up. J Appl Oral Sci 2012;20(2):282–5.
16. Daley TD, Wysocki GP. The small dentigerous cyst: a diagnostic dilemma. Oral Surg Oral Med Oral Pathol Oral Radiol Endod 1995;79(1):77–81.
17. Fujii R, Kawakami M, Hyomoto M, et al. Panoramic findings for predicting eruption of mandibular premolars associated with dentigerous cyst after marsupialization. J Oral Maxillofac Surg 2008;66(2):272–6.
18. Anderson R. Eruption cysts: a retrograde study. ASDC (Am Soc Dent Child) J Dent Child 1989;57(2):124–7.

19. Aguilo L, Cibrian R, Bagan JV, et al. Eruption cysts: retrospective clinical study of 36 cases. ASDC (Am Soc Dent Child) J Dent Child 1998;65(2):102–6.

20. Brannon RB. The odontogenic keratocyst. A clinico-pathologic study of 312 cases. Part I. Clinical features. Oral Surg Oral Med Oral Pathol 1976;42(1):54–72. https://doi.org/10.1016/0030-4220(76)90031-1.

21. Singh AK, Khanal Nikita, Chaulagain Rajib, et al. How effective is 5-Fluorouracil as an adjuvant in the management of odontogenic keratocyst? A systematic review and meta-analysis. Br J Oral Maxillofac Surg 2022;60(Issue 6):746–54.

22. Noike J, Kawahara R, shimizu T, et al. Clinial study of 14 cases of nevoid basal cell carcinoma syndrome in 10 families. Jpn J Oral Maxillofac Surg 2013; 59(6):432–7.

23. Govil S, Gupta V, Misra N, et al. Bilateral lateral peri-odontal cyst. BMJ Case Rep 2013;2013:1–3.

24. Yang Y, Xia X, Wang W, et al. Uncommon fusion of teeth and lateral periodontal cyst in a Chinese girl: a case report. Oral Surg Oral Med Oral Pathol Oral Radiol Endod 2011;112(4):e18–20.

25. Kaugars GE. Botryoid odontogenic cyst. Oral Surg Oral Med Oral Pathol 1986. https://doi.org/10.1016/0030-4220(86)90320-8.

26. Gorlin RJ, Pindborg JJ, Odont, et al. The calcifying odontogenic cyst–a possible analogue of the cutaneous calcifying epithelioma of Malherbe. An analysis of fifteen cases. Oral Surg Oral Med Oral Pathol 1962;15:1235–43.

27. El-Naggar AK, John KC, Grandis JR, et al. WHO classification of head and neck tumours. 4th edition. Lyon: IARC; 2017.

28. WHO Classification of Tumours Editorial Board. Head and neck tumours. In: WHO classification of tumours series, vol. 9, 5th ed. Lyon (France): International Agency for Research on Cancer; 2022.

29. Fregnani ER, Pires FR, Quezada RD, et al. Calcifying odontogenic cyst: clinicopathological features and immunohistochemical profile of 10 cases. J Oral Pathol Med 2003;32(3):163–70.

30. Jonhson IIIA, I Fletcher M, Gold L, et al. Calcifying odontogenic cyst: a clinicopathologic study of 57 cases with immunohistochemical evaluation for cytokeratin. J Oral Maxillofac Surg 1997;55:679–83.

31. Tavargeri AK, Anehosur V, Niranjan KC, et al. Case report of a rare glandular odontogenic cyst in a child: A diagnostic dilemma. Int J Health Sci 2019;13(3):53–5.

32. Noffke C, Raubenheimer EJ. The glandular odontogenic cyst:Clinical and radiological features:Review of the literature and report of nine cases. Dentomaxillofac Radiol 2002;31:332–8.

33. Faisal M, Ahmad SA, Ansari U. Glandular odontogenic cyst literature review and report of a paediatric case. J Oral Biol Craniofac Res 2015;5:219–25.

34. Mascitti M, Santarelli A, Sabatucci A, et al. Glandular odontogenic cyst: review of literature and report of a new case with cytokeratin-19 expression. Open Dent J 2014;8:1–12.

35. Abrahams JM, McClure SA. Pediatric Odontogenic Tumors. Oral Maxillofac Surg Clin 2016;28(1):45–58.

36. Bansal S, Desai RS, Shirstat P, et al. The occurrence and pattern of ameloblastoma in children and adolescents: an Indian institution study of 41 years and review of the literature. Int J Oral Maxillofac Surg 2015;44:725–31.

37. Marx RE, Stern D. Oral and maxillofacial pathology: a rationale for diagnosis and treatment. Hanover Park: Quintessence Co; 2003. p. 609–12.

38. Rick GM. Adenomatoid odontogenic tumor. Oral Maxillofac Surg Clin 2004;16:333–53.

39. Pindborg JJ. Calcifying epithelial odontogenic tumors. Acta Pathol Microbiol Scand Suppl 1955; 111:71.

40. Philipsen HP, Reichart PA. Calcifying odontogenic tumor: biological profile based on 181 cases from the literature. Oral Oncol 2000;36:17–26.

41. Badni M, Nagaraja A, Kamath V. Squamous odontogenic tumor a case report and review of literature. J Oral Maxillofac Pathol 2012;16:113–7.

42. Vinayakrishna K, Soumithran CS, Sobhana CR, et al. Peripheral and central aggressive form of Pindborg tumor of mandible - A rare case report. J Oral Biol Craniofac Res 2013 Sep-Dec;3(3):154–8.

43. Philipsen HP, Reichart PA. Squamous odontogenic tumor (SOT): a benign neoplasm of the periodontium. A review of 36 reported cases. J Clin Periodontol 1996;23:922–6.

44. Pereira K, Bennett K, Elkins T, et al. Ameloblastic fibroma of the maxillary sinus. Int J Pediatr Otorhinolaryngol 2004;68:1473–7.

45. Soluk-Tekkesin M, Wright JM. The World Health Organization Classification of Odontogenic Lesions: A Summary of the Changes of the 2022 (5th) Edition. Turk Patoloji Derg 2022;38(2):168–84.

46. Sabu AM, Gandhi S, Singh I, et al. Ameloblastic Fibrodentinoma: A Rarity in Odontogenic Tumors. J Maxillofac Oral Surg 2018 Dec;17(4):444–8.

47. Ramakrishnan DS, Gouthaman SS, Muthusekhar MR. Ameloblastic fibrosarcoma transformation from ameloblastic fibroma. Natl J Maxillofac Surg 2022; 13(Suppl 1):S145–9.

48. El-Mofty SK. Odontogenic carcinosarcoma. In: El-Naggar AK, Chan JKC, Grandis JR, Takata T, et al, editors. World Health Organization classification of head and neck tumours. 4th edition. Lyon: IARC Press; 2017. p. 213.

49. Bregni RC, Taylor AM. Ameloblastic fibrosarcoma of the mandible: report of two cases and review of the literature. J Oral Pathol Med 2001;30:316–20.

50. Mosqueda-Taylor A, Pires FR, Aguirre-Urízar JM, et al. Primordial odontogenic tumour: clinicopathological analysis of six cases of a previously undescribed entity. Histopathology 2014;65(5):606–12.

51. Bologna-Molina R, Pereira-Prado V, Sánchez-Romero C, et al. Primordial odontogenic tumor: A systematic review. Med Oral Patol Oral Cir Bucal 2020;25(3):e388–94.

52. Almazyad A, Collette D, Zhang D, et al. Recurrent Primordial Odontogenic Tumor: Epithelium-Rich Variant. Head Neck Pathol 2022;16(2):550–9.

53. Mckenzie J, Charles ZY, Simpson E, et al. Pediatric Odontogenic Myxoma: A Case Report and a Systematic Review of the Literature. FACE 2022;3(4):517–26.

54. Ana Cláudia Garcia Rosa AC, Abdalla Rosa Cristiano, Zambaldi da Cruz Eduardo, et al,

André Machado de Senna. Odontogenic myxoma in childhood. Human Pathology Reports 2023;32.

55. King T, Lewis J, Orvidas L, et al. Pediatric maxillary odontogenic myxoma: a report of 2 cases and review of management. J Oral Maxillofac Surg 2008;66:1057–62.

56. Kadlub N, Mbou VB, Leboulanger N, et al. Infant Odontogenic Myxoma: a specific entity. J Cranio-Maxillo-Fac Surg 2014;42(8):2082–6.

57. Schafer T, Singh B, Myers D. Cementoblastoma associated with a primary tooth: a rare pediatric lesion. Pediatr Dent 2001;23:351–3.

Benign Non-Odontogenic Pathology in Children

Aparna Bhat, DMD, MD[a], Ryan Smart, DMD, MD[b,*], Mark Egbert, DDS[a,c,d], Srinivas M. Susarla, DMD, MD, MPH[a,c,d]

KEYWORDS

- Bone-derived lesions • Cartilage-derived lesions • Fibroconnective tissue lesions
- Mesenchymal tissue lesions • Vascular tissue lesions • Nerve-derived lesions
- Radiographic features • Surgical management

KEY POINTS

- Pediatric non-odontogenic pathology of the craniofacial skeleton is rare, however, diverse in nature.
- Non-odontogenic pathology can be categorized by tissue of origin.
- There are key radiographic makers and clinical examination findings that help ultimately guide appropriate treatment.

INTRODUCTION

Non-odontogenic pathology is a broad term, encompassing various lesions. This article seeks to define some of the more commonly seen diagnoses of benign non-odontogenic pathology. These lesions will be categorized based upon tissue of origin. The main categories include lesions derived from bone, cartilage, fibroconnective tissue, mesenchymal tissue, vascular tissue, and nervous tissue.

Bone-Derived Lesions

Osteoma

An osteoma is a slow-growing, benign lesion best characterized by the proliferation of either compact or cancellous bone. These can be categorized as peripheral, central, or extra skeletal depending upon their origin.[1,2] Peripheral osteomas are derived from periosteum, central osteomas are derived from endosteum, and extra skeletal osteomas are derived from soft tissue,

most commonly, muscle tissue.[2] Osteomas are often located within the craniofacial skeleton. While osteomas are typically solitary lesions, in cases of multiple osteomas, one must consider Gardner syndrome—an autosomal dominant disease characterized by multiple osteomas, gastrointestinal polyps, and mesenchymal tumors of the soft tissue.[2] Radiographically, osteomas are represented by a radiopaque, well-circumscribed lesion, with a sclerotic border (**Fig. 1**). As these lesions are often slow growing and asymptomatic, they are conservatively managed with monitoring. If the lesions begin to cause pain, they can be excised via enucleation or resection.[1,2]

Osteoid osteoma

While the origin of osteoid osteomas is unclear, they are noted to most commonly present in the second decade of life and are typically associated with pain relieved by aspirin or non-steroidal anti-inflammatory drugs (NSAIDs).[3,4] Radiographically, osteoid osteomas are characterized by a

[a] Department of Oral and Maxillofacial Surgery, University of Washington School of Dentistry, 1959 NE Pacific Street, B-307, Seattle, WA 98195, USA; [b] Department of Surgery, University of North Dakota School of Medicine and Health Sciences, Private clinic 2585 23rd Avenue South, Fargo, ND 58103, USA; [c] Division of Plastic Surgery, Department of Surgery, University of Washington School of Medicine, 1959 Northeast Pacific Street, B-307, Seattle, WA 98195, USA; [d] Craniofacial Center, Seattle Children's Hospital, 4800 Sand Point Way Northeast, Seattle, WA 98015, USA
* Corresponding author.
E-mail address: ryan.smart@yahoo.com

Oral Maxillofacial Surg Clin N Am 36 (2024) 295–302
https://doi.org/10.1016/j.coms.2024.01.007
1042-3699/24/© 2024 Elsevier Inc. All rights reserved.

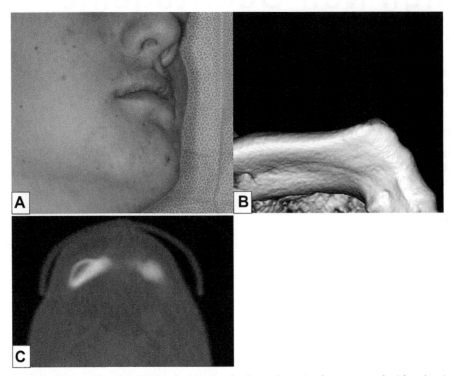

Fig. 1. Patient is a 14-year-old male with family history of colon polyposis who presented with enlarging mass to the right chin. Biopsy was consistent with osteoma. Genetic screening for Gardner syndrome was negative. (*A*): Clinical photo showing increased fullness to the right chin. (*B*): 3 dimensional (3D) reconstruction of computed tomography (CT) maxillofacial showing mass to the right chin. (*C*): CT maxillofacial showing well-circumscribed bony lesion to the right chin.

radiolucent lesion with a surrounding zone of reactive sclerosis. These lesions typically occur in the appendicular skeleton and are less commonly seen in the craniofacial region. Lesions are managed by monitoring and analgesia, as these lesions tend to spontaneously regress over a 2 to 6 year span.[4] For lesions resistant to conservative management, en-bloc resection can be considered, though in recent years, providers have opted for a minimally invasive approach, such as laser ablation or cryoablation.[3,4]

Osteoblastoma

An osteoblastoma is a primary bone tumor, derived from osteoblasts, which is typically associated with the axial skeleton, though 10% to 15% of cases are associated with the head and neck, most commonly in the posterior mandible.[5] These lesions are associated with localized pain and tenderness. Radiographically, osteoblastomas have a mixed radiolucent-radiopaque pattern, with a surrounding radiolucent margin.[5,6] Treatment involves surgical resection, though some providers have noted success with thorough enucleation.[5–7]

Osteochondroma

An osteochondroma is a benign neoplasm of bone and cartilaginous tissue, typically found in the long bones. In the head and neck region, it can be associated with the coronoid process or the condyle of the mandible, though incidence is rare.[8] Lesions are associated with symptoms of facial asymmetry, malocclusion, and limited mouth opening. Radiographically, osteochondromas are seen as radiopaque lesions with a well-defined cortical border. Treatment involves surgical excision via mandibular condylectomy or coronoidectomy.[8,9]

Cartilage Derived

Chondroma

Chondromas are benign tumors derived from chondrocytes which produce hyaline cartilage. While typically seen in the hands and feet, cases have been associated in the head and neck region. These lesions are slow growing and often asymptomatic, and radiographically appear as well-defined areas of radiolucency with possible internal calcification. These lesions are difficult to distinguish from low-grade chondrosarcomas and as such, aggressive management is pursued with wide surgical resection with 1 cm margins.[10,11]

Chondroblastoma

Chondroblastoma is a rare benign tumor derived from chondroblasts, typically seen in long bones; however, some cases have been reported associated with the squamous portion of the temporal bone and the temporomandibular joint.[12–14] These lesions are typically slow growing with symptoms including limited mouth opening and swelling. Radiographically, these lesions appear as well-circumscribed radiopacities. Treatment consists of surgical excision.[12–14]

Chondromyxoid fibroma

Chondromyxoid fibroma is a benign cartilage-producing tumor that is most often noted in the long bones of young adults. In rare occurrences, this lesion is noted in the head and neck. Radiographically, these lesions can be identified as a well-circumscribed radiopacity, or erosion of the surrounding bone. Treatment consists of complete surgical excision.[15,16]

Fibroconnective Tissue

Fibrous dysplasia

Fibrous dysplasia is a benign disease that involves normal fibrous tissue that is replaced with abnormal bone. This condition is mainly associated with the ribs, long bones, and craniofacial skeleton.[17] The etiology of fibrous dysplasia is unclear, but fibrous dysplasia has been associated with McCune–Albright syndrome (MAS) and Jaffe–Lichtenstein syndrome (JLS). While these are 3 separate disease processes, MAS and fibrous dysplasia have been associated with activating mutations in the GNAS gene.[18] MAS includes endocrine-related features such as

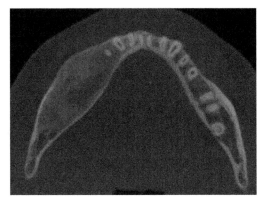

Fig. 2. Patient is a 13-year-old female with no significant medical history with biopsy-proven fibrous dysplasia of the right posterior mandible.

hyperparathyroidism, acromegaly, and precocious puberty, in addition to café au lait macules and polyostotic fibrous dysplasia. In comparison, JLS is associated with polyostotic fibrous dysplasia and café au lait macules, but without endocrine features. Fibrous dysplasia of the facial bones is often slow growing and asymptomatic. Radiographically, fibrous dysplasia appears as patchy radiopacities within the normal bone (**Fig. 2**); however, it can be difficult to distinguish a clear margin between affected and unaffected tissue. Confirmation of the disease is possible via biopsy; however, treatment is only indicated if patients become symptomatic.[17] In most cases, providers manage fibrous dysplasia by monitoring the lesions radiographically and clinically to intercept complications such as impingement of cranial nerve foramina to avoid cranial neuropathies. If treatment is indicated, resection is preferred.

Cherubism

Cherubism is a benign pathologic condition involving slow, painless expansion of the maxilla and mandible. This is associated with a mutation in the protein SH3BP2, and is typically seen to arise in patients who are 2 to 5 years old, and the lesions continue to progress until puberty, after which time they may regress. Radiographically, these lesions are radiolucent, well-defined lesions within either the maxilla or mandible. On clinical examination, it may be possible to detect a bony expansion with the jaw bones. Given that the lesions tend to resolve after puberty, treatment is usually relegated to conservative management with periodic monitoring.[19]

Ossifying fibroma

Ossifying fibromas are divided into 2 subcategories—juvenile ossifying fibroma (JOF) and peripheral ossifying fibroma. This section will discuss JOF. JOF are benign fibro-osseous lesions defined by the ability to form bone.[20] These lesions are noted to have an early onset, typically noted in the first 2 decades of life, are mostly seen in males, and have a rapid growth pattern.[20,21] The most common location for JOF are around the paranasal sinuses, and these lesions are typically asymptomatic.[10] Radiographically, these lesions are seen as well-defined areas of radiolucency with internal calcifications (**Fig. 3**). Treatment involves thorough enucleation if caught early; however, if the lesion is fast growing, this may require surgical resection.[20,21] With lesions that exhibit an aggressive growth pattern, post-operative interferon alpha therapy may decrease recurrence rates after enucleation/curettage or resection.[22]

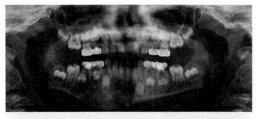

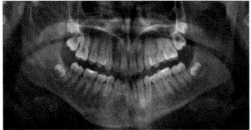

Fig. 3. (Top): Patient is a 14-year-old male with history of recurrent juvenile ossifying fibroma to the right anterior mandible, subsequently treated with enucleation and curettage, followed by interferon alpha treatment. (Bottom): Patient after 7 years of follow-up with good bony fill to the right anterior mandible.

Non-ossifying fibroma

Non-ossifying fibromas are benign lesions typically present in the long bones, with rare occurrence in the craniofacial skeleton. These lesions typically present in the first decade of life, however, are typically slow growing and asymptomatic.[23] Radiographically, the lesions present as well-circumscribed radiolucent lesions with a sclerotic margin. Treatment is varied, as some report that the lesion will ossify and resolve with time, while others have achieved success with enucleation and curettage.[23]

Desmoplastic fibroma

Desmoplastic fibromas are rare, benign fibrous lesions that typically affect the pelvis, long bones, and are rarely seen in the facial bones. These lesions are often misdiagnosed as non-ossifying fibromas; however, a key distinguishing factor is the aggressive nature of desmoplastic fibromas (**Fig. 4**). The lesion starts as a slow-growing, asymptomatic lesion, however, can expand rapidly and invade the surrounding soft tissue.[24] Radiographic features include radiolucency with poorly defined borders, and with more aggressive lesions, cortical erosion is seen. Treatment options include enucleation and curettage, or surgical resection (see **Fig. 4**).

Mesenchymal Tissue

Central giant cell lesion

Central giant cell lesions (CGCL) are benign lesions composed of fibroblasts and multinucleated giant cells that are often seen in the jaws, and typically occur prior to the fourth decade of life.[25] These lesions can be locally aggressive, exhibiting rapid growth, tooth disruption, and destruction of cortical bone. CGCL have also been associated with Noonan syndrome, which is typically also characterized by craniofacial dysmorphia, short stature, and cardiac anomalies.[26] Radiographically, CGCL are classically noted to be multilocular radiolucent lesions, often described as having a soap-bubble–like appearance but may present as a mere radiolucent lesion (**Fig. 5**). Treatment is dependent on the size and clinical features of the lesion. For smaller, asymptomatic lesions, enucleation and curettage is preferred. For larger, more aggressive lesions, some providers opt for resection. Post-operatively, after resection, some providers have opted for interferon alpha 2a therapy[22] to prevent recurrence, as some studies have proposed a relationship between CGCL and proliferative vascular lesions. Given that interferon therapy has been associated with inhibition of angiogenesis via inhibition of fibroblast growth factors, this therapy has been thought to reduce recurrence. Another proposed therapy is that of receptor activator of nuclear factor kappa beta ligand (RANK-L) inhibitors, such as denosumab, given that CGCL contain stromal cells which express RANK-L. While this treatment was noted to have 100% success after 12 months of denosumab therapy, there was an increased rate of recurrence, with only 22% of patients noted to be disease free at 5 years post-therapy.[27]

Lipoma

Lipomas are benign lesions of adipose tissue often found in soft tissue and are usually asymptomatic. In rare cases, these lesions can also be found within the oral cavity. There have also been some reports of lipoma associated with cleft palate. Radiographically, the lesions are radiopaque, with well-defined borders. These lesions, if symptomatic, are treated via excision.[28]

Vascular Tissue

Hemangioma

Hemangiomas are benign lesions of vascular origin. A type of hemangioma, infantile hemangioma, is noted to be one of the most common lesions seen in infants. These lesions can grow rapidly, in the first few months of life. These lesions are typically seen in soft tissues of the head and neck and appear as a smooth mass. Treatment is varied depending upon symptoms. Beta blockers can be used for treatment, and in some cases, infantile hemangiomas are noted to spontaneously resolve.[29] For

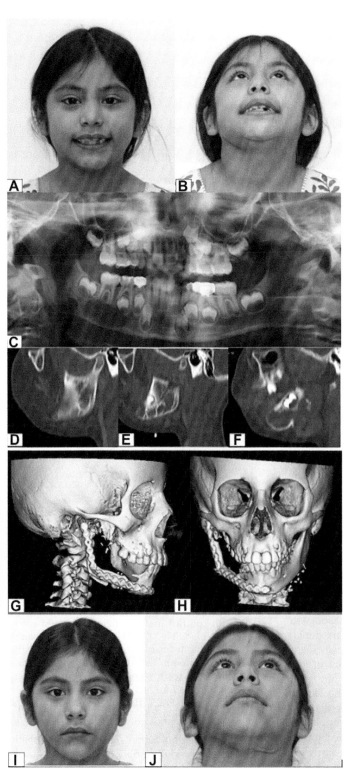

Fig. 4. Patient is a 7-year-old female with biopsy-proven desmoplastic fibroma of the right mandible treated via surgical resection and reconstruction with 2 segment-free fibula flap. (*A*, *B*): Clinical photos showing frontal and submental views of the lesion. (*C-F*): Panoramic radiograph and CT imaging showing extent of well-circumscribed radiolucent lesion to the right posterior mandible extending up the right ramus of the mandible. (*G*, *H*): 3D reconstruction of CT imaging, obtained 9 months post-operatively, showing reconstruction using 2 segment-free fibula flap. (*I*, *J*): Clinical photos at 9 month post-operative visit showing frontal and submental views.

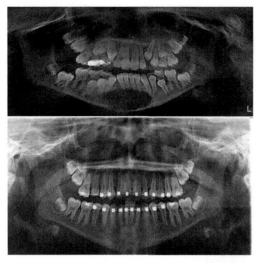

Fig. 5. Patient is a 10-year-old male with biopsy-proven central giant cell lesion, treated with interferon therapy followed by enucleation, autogenous stem cell transplantation, and bone grafting (Top): Preoperative panoramic radiograph showing radiolucent lesion to the anterior mandible. (Bottom): Panoramic radiograph obtained 2 years post-operatively showing bony fill to anterior mandible with no signs of recurrence.

larger lesions that are symptomatic, surgical resection may be more appropriate.

Vascular malformations

Vascular malformations are rare but abnormal communications between vascular tissue. These are characterized by the speed of blood flow, as high-flow and low-flow lesions.[30] High-flow lesions include arteriovenous malformations (AVM), while low-flow lesions include lymphatic or venous malformations. Vascular malformations are congenital and are often asymptomatic. Low-flow lesions may exhibit stasis, thereby resulting in propensity toward clotting. High-low lesions are associated with changes in hormone levels, such as during puberty. As such, these lesions are typically diagnosed in the second and third decades of life. When present, the most common symptoms of AVM include spontaneous oral bleeding, loose teeth, and pain. On clinical examination, if the AVM is large enough, one may detect a pulsatile sensation. On imaging, AVMs tend to have a mixed radiopaque and osteolytic appearance with well-defined borders. While many lesions are asymptomatic and do not require treatment, the most important complication of AVMs is that of uncontrolled bleeding. Low-flow lesions respond well to sclerotherapy with agents including bleomycin and ethanol. For high-flow lesions, combination

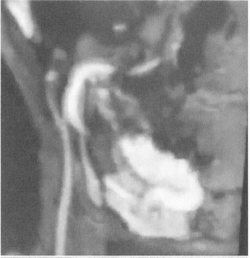

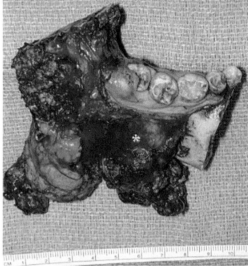

Fig. 6. Patient is a 15-year-old male with large arteriovenous malformations (AVM) of the left posterior mandible ultimately treated with resection and fibula-free flap reconstruction. (Top): Magnetic resonance angiography (MRA) shown here depicts a large cavity with contrast material filling the AVM cavity within the mandible. Clinically the patient had a palpable, pulsatile mass over the left body of the mandible. (Bottom): Resected mass showing the displacement of teeth along with large AVM cavity (depicted via *asterisk*). (Images courtesy of Dr. David Yates DMD, MD, FACS, High Desert Oral & Facial Surgery)

therapy with embolization and surgical excision is often warranted (**Fig. 6**). Excision is performed around 24 hours after embolization for bleeding control.[31]

Aneurysmal bone cyst

Aneurysmal bone cysts are benign cystic lesions of bone that are filled with blood. These lesions

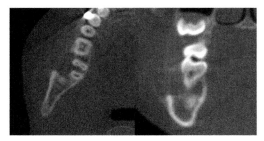

Fig. 7. Patient is a 14-year-old male who presented with a firm mass to the right lateral mandible. CT imaging showed a radiolucent lesion to the right posterolateral mandible, later proven on biopsy to represent an aneurysmal bone cyst.

are thought to be secondary to trauma, and can exhibit rapid growth, leading to a pathologic fracture.[32] Clinically, these lesions are typically asymptomatic, though can present with localized pain and swelling. On imaging, lesions are radiolucent with well-defined borders (**Fig. 7**). Treatment consists of enucleation and curettage, and the recurrence rate of these lesions is low.

Nerve Derived

Schwannoma

Schwannomas are rare benign lesions of the Schwann cells of the peripheral nervous system. The most common symptom of this lesion is swelling, though these lesions are typically otherwise asymptomatic. Radiographically, schwannomas have a radiolucent appearance, with well-defined borders, but can be seen to cause root resorption. Treatment consists of enucleation and curettage, and the involved nerve is typically preserved as the lesion arises from the surrounding cells and not the nerve itself.[33] These lesions can also be associated with neurofibromatosis type 2, as bilateral vestibular schwannomas. These patients have symptoms of tinnitus, difficulty with balance, and hearing loss, but may develop schwannomas of other nervous tissue as a progression of their disease course. If the patient is asymptomatic, conservative management through monitoring is preferred;however, if symptoms progress, surgical resection may be warranted. With rapidly growing schwannomas, bevacizumab has shown some efficacy in slowing growth prior to surgical resection.[34]

Neurofibroma

Neurofibromas are rare benign tumors of the peripheral nerve sheath. These lesions are usually seen in patients with neurofibromatosis type I (von Recklinghausen's disease).[35] Clinically, these lesions are often asymptomatic; however, as they

grow larger, can present with localized swelling. Radiographically, neurofibromas are radiolucent in appearance, with well-circumscribed borders. Treatment consists of surgical resection of the lesion along with the involved nerve. Because the lesion arises from the nerve itself, the involved nerve must be resected to prevent recurrence.

CLINICS CARE POINTS

- Benign lesions of the face and jaws can be locally aggressive. Proper diagnosis with adequate biopsy and imaging is the key to proper treatment.
- High-flow vascular malformations typically require embolization prior to surgical treatment to reduce risk of severe bleeding and the embolization should be carried out as close to the surgery date as possible to prevent revascularization of the AVM
- Fibrous dysplasia can result in stenosis of cranial nerve foramina and should be treated aggressively if cranial neuropathies are identified.
- Central giant cell lesions can appear very similar to Brown tumor of hyperparathyroidism. Work up for parathyroid abnormality should be a part of the workup for central giant cell lesions.

DISCLOSURE

There were no commercial or financial conflicts of interest from any of the authors associated with this article. Additionally, there were no funding sources for this project.

REFERENCES

1. Starch-Jensen T. Peripheral Solitary Osteoma of the Zygomatic Arch: A Case Report and Literature Review. Open Dent J 2017;11:120–5.
2. Bhatt G, Gupta S, Ghosh S, et al. Central Osteoma of Maxilla Associated with an Impacted Tooth: Report of a Rare Case with Literature Review. Head Neck Pathol 2019;13(4):554–61.
3. Singh A, Solomon MC. Osteoid osteoma of the mandible: A case report with review of the literature. J Dent Sci 2017;12(2):185–9.
4. Tepelenis K, Skandalakis GP, Papathanakos G, et al. Osteoid Osteoma: An Updated Review of Epidemiology, Pathogenesis, Clinical Presentation, Radiological Features, and Treatment Option. In Vivo 2021;35(4):1929–38.

5. Rawal YB, Angiero F, Allen CM, et al. Gnathic osteo-blastoma: clinicopathologic review of seven cases with long-term follow-up. Oral Oncol 2006;42(2): 123–30.

6. Wang L, Guo J, Tang Z. Osteoblastoma of the maxilla: A case report and review of the literature. Oral Oncol 2023;136:106268.

7. Jones AC, Prihoda TJ, Kacher JE, et al. Osteoblas-toma of the maxilla and mandible: a report of 24 cases, review of the literature, and discussion of its relationship to osteoid osteoma of the jaws. Oral Surg Oral Med Oral Pathol Oral Radiol Endod 2006;102(5):639–50.

8. Patel R, Obeid G. Osteochondroma of the Zygo-matic Arch: A Case Report and Review of the Liter-ature. J Oral Maxillofac Surg 2018;76(9):1912–6.

9. Poorna TA, Alagarsamy R, Ek J, et al. A systematic review and meta-analysis of the surgical outcomes in patients with osteochondroma of mandibular condyle. Oral Surg Oral Med Oral Pathol Oral Radiol 2023;135(6):732–45.

10. Lazow SK, Pihlstrom RT, Solomon MP, et al. Condylar chondroma: report of a case. J Oral Max-illofac Surg 1998;56(3):373–8.

11. Nehete R, Nehete A, Singla S, et al. Soft tissue chon-droma of hard palate associated with cleft palate. In-dian J Plast Surg 2012;45(3):550–2.

12. Yang X, Wang M, Gao W, et al. Chondroblastoma of mandibular condyle: Case report and literature re-view. Open Med (Wars) 2021;16(1):1372–7.

13. Bui P, Ivan D, Oliver D, et al. Chondroblastoma of the temporomandibular joint: report of a case and litera-ture review. J Oral Maxillofac Surg 2009;67(2): 405–9.

14. Bae H, Ryu DM, Kim HK, et al. A large invasive chondroblastoma on the temporomandibular joint and external auditory canal: a case report and liter-ature review. Maxillofac Plast Reconstr Surg 2021; 43(1):26.

15. Panucci BZM, Silva EV, Arévalo RHA, et al. Chondro-myxoid fibroma affecting the maxilla in a 1-year-old child: Immunohistochemical analysis and literature review. Oral Oncol 2022;124:105467.

16. Hammad HM, Hammond HL, Kurago ZB, et al. Chondromyxoid fibroma of the jaws. Case report and review of the literature. Oral Surg Oral Med Oral Pathol Oral Radiol Endod 1998;85(3):293–300.

17. Yepes JF. Dental Manifestations of Pediatric Bone Disorders. Curr Osteoporos Rep 2017;15(6):588–92.

18. Turan S, Bastepe M. GNAS Spectrum of Disorders. Curr Osteoporos Rep 2015;13(3):146–58.

19. Tsodoulos S, Ilia A, Antoniades K, et al. Cherubism: a case report of a three-generation inheritance and literature review. J Oral Maxillofac Surg 2014;72(2): 405.e1–4059.

20. Mohideen K, Balasubramaniam M, et al. Juvenile psammomatoid ossifying fibroma of the maxilla

21. Rinaggio J, Land M, Cleveland DB. Juvenile ossi-fying fibroma of the mandible. J Pediatr Surg 2003; 38(4):648–50.

22. Kaban LB, Troulis MJ, Ebb D, et al. Antiangiogenic therapy with interferon alpha for giant cell lesions of the jaws. J Oral Maxillofac Surg 2002;60(10): 1103–11.

23. Bowers LM, Cohen DM, Bhattacharyya I, et al. The non-ossifying fibroma: a case report and review of the literature. Head Neck Pathol 2013;7(2):203–10.

24. Woods TR, Cohen DM, Islam MN, et al. Desmoplas-tic fibroma of the mandible: a series of three cases and review of literature. Head Neck Pathol 2015; 9(2):196–204.

25. Jeyaraj P. Management of Central Giant Cell Granu-lomas of the Jaws: An Unusual Case Report with Critical Appraisal of Existing Literature. Ann Maxillo-fac Surg 2019;9(1):37–47.

26. Rodríguez FA, Castellón L, Moreno R, et al. Noonan syndrome with multiple Giant cell lesions, manage-ment and treatment with surgery and interferon alpha-2a therapy: Case report. Birth Defects Res 2020;112(10):732–9.

27. Schreuder WH, Lipplaa A, Cleven AHG, et al. RANKL inhibition for giant cell lesions of the jaw: A retrospective cohort analysis. Eur J Cancer 2022; 175:263–73.

28. Gokul S, Ranjini KV, Kirankumar K, et al. Congenital osteolipoma associated with cleft palate: a case report. Int J Oral Maxillofac Surg 2009;38(1):91–3.

29. Mufeed A, Hafiz A, George A, et al. Pedunculated haemangioma of the palate. BMJ Case Rep 2015; 2015. bcr2014206801.

30. Petel R, Ashkenazi M. Pediatric intraoral high-flow arteriovenous malformation: a diagnostic challenge. Pediatr Dent 2014;36(5):425–8.

31. Kolokythas A. Vascular Malformations and Their Treatment in the Growing Patient. Oral Maxillofac Surg Clin North Am 2016;28(1):91–104.

32. Richardson J, Litman E, Stanbouly D, et al. Aneu-rysmal bone cyst of the head & neck: A review of re-ported cases in the literature. J Stomatol Oral Maxillofac Surg 2022;123(1):59–63.

33. Zainab H, Kale AD, Hallikerimath S. Intraosseous schwannoma of the mandible. J Oral Maxillofac Pathol 2012;16(2):294–6.

34. Evans DG. *NF2*-Related Schwannomatosis. In: Adam MP, Mirzaa GM, Pagon RA, et al, editors. Gen-eReviews®. Seattle (WA): University of Washington, Seattle; 1998. p. 1–24.

35. Che Z, Nam W, Park WS, et al. Intraosseous nerve sheath tumors in the jaws. Yonsei Med J 2006; 47(2):264–70.

and mandible: A systematic review of published case reports. Clin Exp Dent Res 2023;9(1):186–97.

Pediatric Temporomandibular Joint Pathology

Cory M. Resnick, MD, DMD[a,b,*]

KEYWORDS

- Temporomandibular joint • Pathology • Pediatric • Costochondral graft • Hemifacial microsomia
- Treacher Collins syndrome • Juvenile idiopathic arthritis • Idiopathic condylar resorption

KEY POINTS

- Compared with adults, temporomandibular joint (TMJ) disorders in children present more commonly with dentofacial deformity and less frequently with pain.
- Progression of the TMJ deformity must be understood in development of a corrective plan.
- Stage of skeletal maturity should be considered in the timing of skeletal correction.

INTRODUCTION

Pathologic condition of the temporomandibular joint (TMJ) in children can be divided into congenital abnormalities (those present at birth) and developmental or acquired disorders. In contradistinction to TMJ dysfunction in adults, articular disc pathologic condition is not primarily implicated in most pediatric TMJ disorders. Similarly, pediatric TMJ disorders rarely present with pain, although pain may occur in later stages of the disease. More commonly, children with TMJ abnormalities are recognized because of skeletal and/or occlusal deformities, impaired mandibular mobility, masticatory dysfunction, and/or upper-airway obstruction.

Common congenital disorders affecting the TMJ include the following[1]:

- Craniofacial microsomia (CFM)
- Treacher Collins syndrome (TCS)
- Nager syndrome
- Oculoauriculovertebral syndrome (Goldenhar syndrome)
- Primary condylar aplasia
- Oculomandibulodyscephaly (Hallermann-Streiff syndrome)
- Hurler disease
- Congenital ankylosis

The 2 most common of these congenital conditions, CFM and TCS, are reviewed herein.

Prevalent developmental and acquired TMJ pathologic conditions are as follows:

- Progressive condylar resorption
  - Juvenile idiopathic arthritis (JIA)
  - Idiopathic condylar resorption (ICR)
  - Anterior disc displacement (ADD)?
- Condylar hyperplasia (CH), hemimandibular hyperplasia (HH)/elongation (HE)
- Ankylosis
- Trauma
- Neoplasms, fibro-osseous lesions, and other pathologic lesions
- Systemic steroid therapy

Of acquired diagnoses, this article focuses on the progressive resorptive and hyperplastic conditions, as these are unique to the pediatric

a Department of Oral and Maxillofacial Surgery, Harvard Medical School, Boston, MA, USA; b Department of Plastic and Oral Surgery, Boston Children's Hospital, 300 Longwood Avenue, Boston, MA 02115, USA
* Department of Plastic and Oral Surgery, Boston Children's Hospital, 300 Longwood Avenue, Boston, MA 02115.
E-mail address: Cory.Resnick@childrens.harvard.edu

Oral Maxillofacial Surg Clin N Am 36 (2024) 303–315
https://doi.org/10.1016/j.coms.2024.01.008
1042-3699/24/© 2024 Elsevier Inc. All rights reserved.

population. Cysts, tumors, and fibro-osseous lesions that may affect the TMJ are discussed elsewhere in this publication.

CONDITIONS
Craniofacial Microsomia

CFM is an asymmetric malformation of structures derived from the first and second pharyngeal arches during fetal development.[2] CFM is the second most common craniofacial anomaly after cleft lip and palate and affects approximately 1 in 5600 live births. Despite several theories, its cause remains poorly understood. CFM mostly occurs sporadically, although diagnosis of multiple members of some families has raised the possibility of a genetic underpinning.[3,4] CFM is most often unilateral, in which case it is often referred to as hemifacial microsomia, but occurs bilaterally in 10% to 15%. CFM is characterized by variable abnormalities of the orbit, mandible, external and middle ear, cranial nerves, and facial soft tissues. Macrostomia, ear tags, and epibulbar dermoids are also common, and myriad extracraniofacial manifestations may also be associated.[5] When epibulbar dermoids and extracraniofacial manifestations occur, there is overlap in terminology with the eponym Goldenhar syndrome.

The TMJ effects of CFM occur owing to hypoplasia of the mandibular ramus, condyle, and sometimes glenoid fossa on the affected side or sides. The degree of hypoplasia is typically classified as described by Pruzansky and modified by Kaban and colleagues[6] in 1988, with scores I, IIA, IIB, or III, and a higher score indicating more severe abnormality. Although some children with CFM present with masticatory dysfunction, abnormal speech development, and/or obstructive sleep apnea,[7] these manifestations are rare. Most children with CFM demonstrate a dentofacial deformity, including a multiplanar mandibular asymmetry and malocclusion. Although the maxilla typically demonstrates normal early development, canting of the maxillary dental arch occurs progressively because of dentoalveolar growth in response to the abnormal mandibular position.

Treatment is dictated by the degree of deformity, its implications on function, patient and family priorities, and growth timing. In type I and IIA deformities, the diminutive mandibular condyle can typically be spared and repositioned via osteotomy (sagittal ramus osteotomy or inverted-L osteotomy) or transport distraction osteogenesis. In type III and some type IIB mandibles, the native ramus-condyle unit is insufficient to allow stable skeletal correction and must be replaced by an autologous (costochondral graft [CCG] or free fibula flap) or alloplastic construct (**Figs. 1 and 2**). Mandibular correction usually requires simultaneous leveling of the maxilla to provide lower facial symmetry. "Early" treatment by vertical ramus distraction during the mixed dentition, while the maxilla maintains dentoalveolar growth potential and can be orthopedically directed to resolve the occlusal cant during dental eruption (**Fig. 3**), may decrease the need for a later maxillary operation,[8] but recurrence of the maxillary deformity is common in this approach.[9] A skeletal operation of the maxillomandibular complex, with or without mandibular ramus-condyle construction, can significantly improve facial symmetry, occlusion, and masticatory function and facilitate speech benefits. It is important to remember, however, that the morphologic abnormality of the mandible and lower facial structures is typically complex and composite, and ancillary procedures, such as onlay mandibular angle or body implants and soft tissue augmentation, are often necessary to optimize final symmetry.

Treacher Collins Syndrome

Mandibulofacial dysostosis, typically referred to as Treacher Collins syndrome (TCS), occurs in 1:25,000 to 1:50,000 live births. Unlike CFM, it is typically passed through families in an autosomal dominant pattern with variable penetrance. In 60% of patients, the mutation can be traced to the TCOF1 gene responsible for encoding the nucleolar phosphoprotein *treacle*. Some manifestation of TCS overlap with those of CFM, but TCS is a bilateral condition that affects the mandible symmetrically. TCS demonstrates extreme phenotypic variability, and, in addition to the mandibular deformity, may include coloboma of the lower eyelid and iris (Tessier 6, 7, 8 clefts), absence of lower eyelid lashes, downslanting palpebral fissures, hypertelorism, microtia, ear and skin tags, ossicular deformities with conductive hearing loss, macrostomia (15%), cleft palate (33%), partial or complete agenesis of the zygomatic arches, choanal atresia, and other craniofacial and extracraniofacial findings.

The mandibular deformity of TCS is typically more severe than that of CFM, and, because of the bilateral hypoplasia of the ramus-condyle units, clockwise rotation of the mandible occurs. The microretrognathia that follows frequently leads to tongue-based airway obstruction in infancy, creating a presentation of Robin sequence (micrognathia, glossoptosis, upper-airway obstruction).[10] As a result, early childhood operations, such as tracheostomy or mandibular distraction osteogenesis, are commonly used to support breathing, feeding, and growth.[11] Mandibular growth will remain

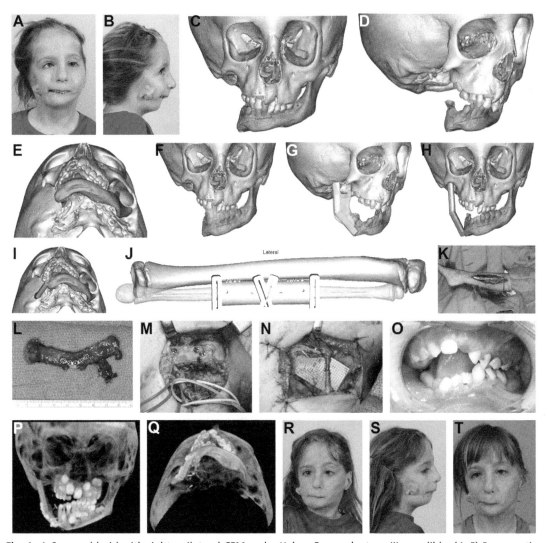

Fig. 1. A 6-year-old girl with right unilateral CFM and a Kaban-Pruzansky type III mandible. (*A–B*) Preoperative photographs show mandibular deviation to the right, retrognathia, microtia, and soft tissue insufficiency. (*C–E*) Type III mandible with minimal ramus on the right side. (*F*) Virtual repositioning of the mandible to provide occlusion on the left side and create a right posterior open bite. A surgical splint is fabricated to dictate this planned position during the operation. (*G*) A free-fibula flap is virtually positioned with one osteotomy to facilitate the planned mandibular position and mimic the contralateral mandibular contour, which has been transposed onto the affected side (*green*). (*H–I*) Planned fibula flap position. (*J*) A surgical guide is fabricated to dictate the length and internal osteotomy of the fibula flap. (*K*) Intraoperatively, the fibula flap is harvested; the internal osteotomy performed, and a miniplate is applied to provide the planned contours while the flap remains attached to the vascular pedicle. (*L*) The fibula flap is harvested, and an AlloDerm (Allergan, Inc, Parsippany, NJ, USA) cap is applied to serve as the articulating surface. (*M*) The flap is inserted, contoured, and secured to the native mandible with lag screws. (*N*) Microvascular anastomoses are performed to the facial artery and the external jugular vein. (*O*) After flap insertion and removal of the occlusal splint, the planned occlusion has been achieved. (*P–Q*) Postoperative computed tomography (CT) scan demonstrating the position of the flap. (*R–S*) One-month postoperative photographs show improved projection and symmetry of the mandible. (*T*) One-year postoperative photograph, just before beginning ear construction. (*Reproduced with permission from*: Resnick CM: TMJ reconstruction in the growing child. Oral Max Surg Clin North Am 2018; 30:109-21.)

impaired throughout development, so operations like mandibular distraction that augment the mandibular size will likely need to be repeated at or before skeletal maturity.

Classification of the mandibular deformity in TCS also uses the Pruzansky-Kaban grading system, and considerations regarding use of osteotomies, autologous, and/or alloplastic constructs for

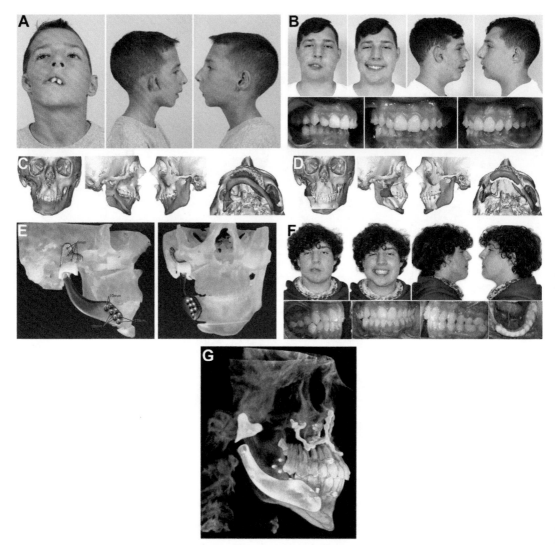

Fig. 2. An 8-year-old boy with right unilateral CFM and a Kaban-Pruzansky type III mandible. (*A*) Preoperative photographs show mandibular deviation to the right retrognathia, microtia, and soft tissue insufficiency. This patient chose delayed treatment. (*B*) Representation at age 13 years, with clear aligner orthodontic treatment in preparation for skeletal correction. (*C*) 3D CT reconstructions with type III mandible on the right side with a diminutive condylar stump. The abnormal morphology of the mandibular body is evident from below. (*D*) Virtual plan for resection (and replacement) of the right-sided condylar stump, releasing sagittal ramus osteotomy on the left, Le Fort I osteotomy, and genioplasty. (*E*) Alloplastic total TMJ prosthesis. (*F*) Two years after skeletal surgery and completion of orthodontic treatment. (*G*) Postoperative 3D CT.

mandibular correction overlap with those for CFM. For TCS, however, the deformity characteristically causes a discrepancy between the short posterior facial height owing to ramus collapse and long anterior facial height that results from the steep mandibular plane, and correction requires counterclockwise mandibular rotation. As large counterclockwise mandibular rotations may be difficult to achieve using standard osteotomies or ramus constructs owing to restriction by facial soft tissues and the pterygomasseteric muscle sling, mandibular distraction is more frequently used in TCS compared with CFM because of the ability to achieve these movements using multivector or curvilinear distraction vectors.

An anterior open bite may or may not be present, and skeletal correction usually necessitates a simultaneous or staged maxillary operation for posterior lengthening as a result of truncated posterior maxillary dentoalveolar growth from mandibular interference. In severe presentations involving tracheostomy-dependent upper-airway obstruction, a corrective approach involving construction of the bilateral rami with CCGs followed by

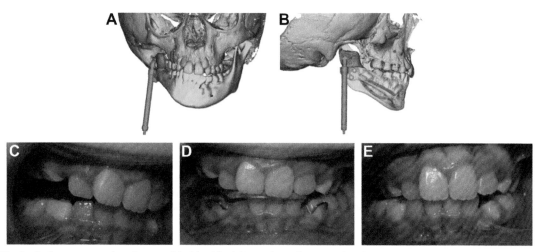

Fig. 3. Early treatment in a 9-year-old girl with right unilateral CFM and Kaban-Pruzansky type IIB mandible. (*A– B*) 3D plan for distraction osteogenesis of the right ramus using a semiburied uniderectional device. Note the proximal segment in red. (*C*) Occlusal photograph at the end of distraction, demonstrating intended right posterior open bite. (*D*) Orthodontic appliance guides the eruption of the teeth and vertical growth of the maxilla. (*E*) Occlusion after removal of dental appliance, demonstrating eruption of maxillary dentition on the affected side to close the open bite. (*Reproduced with permission from*: Resnick CM, Kaban LB, Padwa BL. Hemifacial microsomia: The disorder and its surgical management. In: Brennan PA, Schliephake H, Ghali GE, Cascarini L, editors. Maxillofacial Surgery. 3rd ed. St. Louis: Elsevier; 2017;870-93.)

simultaneous midfacial and mandibular distraction osteogenesis with hinge rotation at the nasal bones may be used.[12]

Progressive Condylar Resorption

Progressive condylar resorption may occur in patients of any age, but the likely etiopathogenesis differs significantly between children and adults. Although adult condylar resorption is most likely a manifestation of osteoarthritic remodeling and more rarely because of rheumatoid arthritis, systemic lupus erythematosus, use of systemic steroids, prior trauma, or other conditions, pediatric diagnoses are more limited. In children, progressive condylar resorption typically indicates JIA or ICR. Recent evidence suggests that ADD may also lead to progressive condylar degeneration in growing patients and may be indistinguishable from JIA with regard to acute and chronic inflammatory changes of the condyle.[13]

A is the most common chronic rheumatologic condition of childhood, affecting 1 in 1000 children worldwide. JIA represents an autoinflammatory condition with 6 subtypes that most commonly affect the hands, knees, ankles, elbows, and/or wrists. One or both TMJs are affected in 39% to 75% of patients.[14] As the TMJ affects are typically asymptomatic in early stages, diagnosis is often delayed. This condition was previously referred to as juvenile rheumatoid arthritis, but the name was changed to JIA when research demonstrated that JIA is a distinct condition from rheumatoid arthritis.

ICR is a condition of unknown cause that is characterized by progressive, bilateral, and symmetric degeneration of the mandibular condyles and condylar necks. It is seen overwhelmingly in Caucasian female patients in the second and third decades of life, prompting the eponym "cheerleaders' syndrome."[15] The female predominance has led to implication of 17B-estradiol in the pathogenesis, but the etiopathogenesis remains unclear.[16] Both JIA and ICR cause a progressive loss of posterior facial height, steepening of the mandibular plane, and loss of chin projection. Depending on the rapidity of progression, an anterior open bite may develop or dentoalveolar compensation may occur to maintain a normal occlusion.

Literature suggests that ICR can be managed effectively either by routine orthognathic surgery after observation for quiescence of the progressive degeneration for at least 2 years or by condylectomy and reconstruction with a CCG during disease activity,[17,18] and advanced JIA may be treated more effectively by extirpation of the diseased TMJ and replacement with an alloplast that is immune to further inflammatory destruction.[19] These dogmas, however, are rooted more in theory than in practice, as long-term outcomes are limited, particularly in JIA, with any reconstructive approach. Central to this theoretic management construct is the ability to reliably differentiate between these conditions.

When TMJ degeneration is observed in a child with a known rheumatologic diagnosis of JIA and/or with other affected joints suggesting JIA, the TMJ effects are presumed to result from the same disease. When a systemic diagnosis is unclear, however, JIA and ICR may be nearly indistinguishable.[20] In fact, some clinicians and researchers suggest that the 2 diagnoses actually represent variants of the same condition.

Assuming a distinction between these diagnoses, some clues may further elucidate the cause of the progressive condylar deformity. Epidemiologically, both conditions favor female over male patients, but male patients are more commonly seen in JIA compared with ICR. Also, patients with JIA often present later than those with JIA, and JIA is, by definition, diagnosed before the age of 16 years. Phenotypically, ICR is characteristically bilateral and symmetric, whereas JIA may occur in either a bilateral or a unilateral form. When JIA is bilateral, the 2 sides may be affected unequally, resulting in facial asymmetry. In both conditions, the articular disc is typically preserved in early stages of the disease, but JIA is more likely than ICR to lead to disc abnormalities in later stages. Both diseases are slowly progressive, but ICR more characteristically stabilizes and becomes quiescent eventually and/or "burns out" when the destruction reaches the sigmoid notch. In rare cases, JIA may progress to more severe condylar deformity, such as fibro-osseous ankylosis.

Imaging has historically been used to differentiate these conditions, with the assumption that nuclear medicine scans highlight metabolic turnover specific to active ICR, and gadolinium enhancement of the synovium and bone marrow in the TMJ on MRI is diagnostic of JIA (see **Fig. 3**). Recent studies, however, have called these assumptions into question and suggested that the 2 conditions may appear indistinguishable from one another and from ADD by imaging[21,22] (**Figs. 4** and **5**).

Historically, ADD observed on MRI in a young patient with progressive condylar resorption has been considered secondary to the underlying resorptive pathologic condition (typically JIA). As disc structure and position are usually normal in ICR, and in light of observation that children with ADD but without any other findings suggestive of a JIA diagnosis may demonstrate progressive condylar resorption, it is likely that ADD in a susceptible, growing TMJ can be a primary cause of condylar resorption. The role for arthroscopy to assist with diagnosis and management is emerging.[23,24]

Condylar Hyperplasia, Hemimandibular Hyperplasia/Elongation

Hyperplastic conditions that unilaterally affect one condyle, ramus, and/or mandibular body may create progressive facial asymmetry and malocclusion. Precise diagnosis, etiopathogenesis, and terminology applied to these hyperplastic conditions remain a topic of debate. Some clinicians use the term condylar hyperplasia (CH) for most mandibular hyperplastic conditions, differentiating patterns of growth by subtypes as in "CH vertical pattern" to indicate unilateral mandibular ramus and body lengthening, and "CH horizontal pattern" when a shift of the mandible toward the contralateral side occurs.[25] Another scheme for subtyping CH into types 1 to 4 has been defined by Wolford and colleagues.[26] Others subscribe to the approach of Obwegeser and Makek,[27] in which HH and HE are differentiated with similar characterization as Wolford CH types 1 and 2, respectively, emphasizing that the morphologic abnormality extends beyond the condylar head and neck. These terms speak to the understanding of the underlying etiopathogenesis of these hyperplastic conditions, in which, for example, CH vertical pattern/CH type II/HH may be caused by an osteochondroma of the condylar head, whereas other patterns of growth may differ in origin.[28]

As for progressive resorptive conditions, management of these hyperplastic diagnoses requires understanding of the pattern and trajectory of growth in combination with an assessment of the functional and social impact of the deformity. For most patients, quiescence of the morphologic abnormality will occur, but timing is variable. For some, stability coincides with cessation of skeletal growth. For others, the hyperplasia continues for some period after skeletal maturity but stabilizes eventually. Correction can be pursued during the active growth phase if desired, at which time high or proportional condylectomy is performed.[29,30] Orthognathic surgery can be performed concurrent to the condylar procedure to complete skeletal and occlusal correction.[31,32] When treatment is delayed until disease quiescence, the abnormal joint, if functional and pain-free, may be maintained. In this scenario, standard orthognathic osteotomies can be applied. Genioplasty and mandibular inferior border ostectomy and/or augmentation by autologous or alloplastic onlay implants may be necessary to complete symmetry correction due to morphologic abnormalities that extend beyond the ramus (**Fig. 6**).

TREATMENT CONSIDERATIONS

After accurate diagnosis, several unique factors deserve consideration in the management of pediatric TMJ pathologic condition.

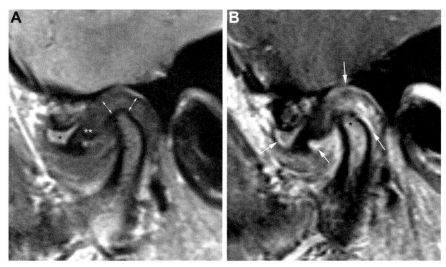

Fig. 4. ADD in an 18-year-old woman. (*A*) Sagittal oblique proton density-weighted MR image shows a large effusion (*asterisk*), an anteriorly displaced articular disc (*double asterisk*) in the anterior joint recess with thickening of the retrodiscal tissue (*double arrows*). (*B*) Corresponding contrast-enhanced T1-weighted image shows increased contrast enhancement in the TMJ space (*arrows*) and within the thickened retrodiscal tissue. Note the irregular articular surface of the condyle (*asterisk*) representing erosions. (Bradley Bousquet, Christian J. Kellenberger, Ryan M. Caprio, Snigdha Jindal, Cory M. Resnick, Does Magnetic Resonance Imaging Distinguish Juvenile Idiopathic Arthritis From Other Causes of Progressive Temporomandibular Joint Destruction?, Journal of Oral and Maxillofacial Surgery, 81 (7), 2023, 820-830, https://doi.org/10.1016/j.joms.2023.03.016.)

Timing

The 2 variables that must be critically considered in determining the timing for operative correction in a child or adolescent with TMJ pathologic condition are as follows.

Progression

Progression of the disease will influence decision making regarding operative timing. In congenital conditions, such as CFM and TCS, debate ensues about whether the disorder is progressive or if

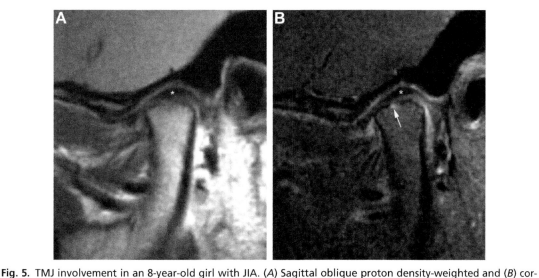

Fig. 5. TMJ involvement in an 8-year-old girl with JIA. (*A*) Sagittal oblique proton density-weighted and (*B*) corresponding contrast-enhanced T1-weighted MR images show a nondisplaced flat disc with the posterior band (*asterisk*) located at the 12 o'clock position over the condyle. There is increased contrast enhancement of the entire joint space and erosion at the condylar surface (*arrow* in *panel B*). Note severe flattening of both the condyle and the mandibular fossa. (Bradley Bousquet, Christian J. Kellenberger, Ryan M. Caprio, Snigdha Jindal, Cory M. Resnick, Does Magnetic Resonance Imaging Distinguish Juvenile Idiopathic Arthritis From Other Causes of Progressive Temporomandibular Joint Destruction?, Journal of Oral and Maxillofacial Surgery, 81 (7), 2023, 820-830, https://doi.org/10.1016/j.joms.2023.03.016.)

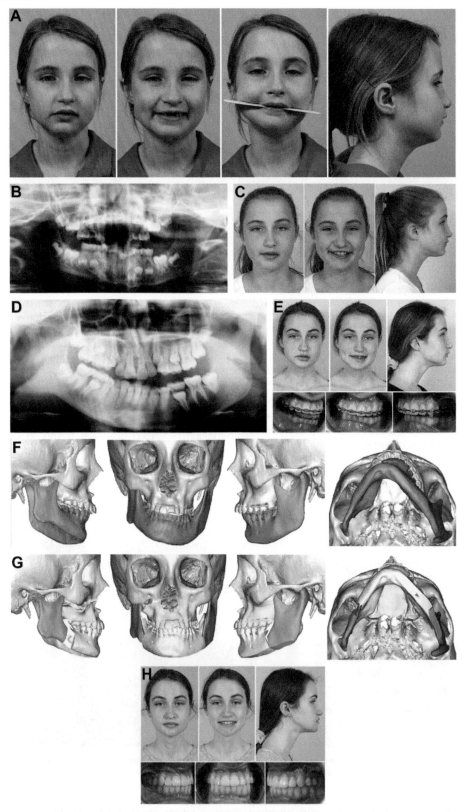

Fig. 6. An 8-year-old girl with left CH. (*A, B*) Photographs and a panoramic radiograph demonstrate lower facial asymmetry and elongated left mandibular condylar neck. The family elected to pursue delayed treatment. (*C, D*) Age 12, with progression of asymmetry. (*E, F*) Age 16, in preparation for skeletal correction. (*G*) Virtual plans for skeletal correction using bilateral sagittal ramus osteotomies, Le Fort I osteotomy, and left mandibular inferior border ostectomy. (*H*) One year after skeletal surgery and completion of orthodontic treatment.

changes that occur during growth are proportional to the original deformity. What clearly does occur during growth in these conditions is development and progression of dentoalveolar compensation. This compensation will continue until growth abates. As such, the surgeon must consider risks and benefits of normalizing the mandibular position during growth, thereby decreasing future maxillary dentoalveolar compensation and allowing correction of existing compensation by orthopedic harnessing of natural growth potential, compared with delaying skeletal correction until growth and compensation have stabilized. In the former (early treatment) approach, likelihood for recurrence of asymmetry during remaining growth is high, and the degree of return asymmetry is positively correlated with the severity of the starting deformity (Pruzansky-Kaban type I will have less return of asymmetry after early mandibular distraction compared with type IIA). As such, for patients with CFM and Pruzansky-Kaban type greater than I, operative correction during growth must be considered the first stage of a multitiered treatment plan, with patient and family expectations set to expect a second-stage skeletal operation after growth cessation. Although staged procedures, when avoidable, have several disadvantages, including increased treatment burden and higher likelihood for complications when working in scarred tissue planes, benefits of an early treatment stage include midterm improvement in facial symmetry for social and functional benefit and lessened severity of the end-stage deformity compared with delayed treatment. Conversely, when social and functional detriments can be managed nonoperatively during growth, delayed treatment until skeletal maturity with the expectation of a single-stage skeletal correction is desirable.

In acquired resorptive and overgrowth conditions, determination of the trajectory of disease progression can be accomplished by longitudinal observation, imaging, or both. When stability has been demonstrated by serial clinical examination, photographs, and/or 2-dimensional or 3-dimensional (3D) radiographs for at least 2 years, future condylar resorption or overgrowth is unlikely, and skeletal correction without TMJ replacement (in the context of a functioning and pain-free TMJ) can safely proceed.[33] Nuclear imaging studies, such as technetium-99 bone scan or single-photon emission computed tomography, can also be used to determine metabolic turnover within the mandibular condyle and ramus as a marker for growth or resorption.[34,35]

In JIA, progression of the TMJ disease is often, but not always, linked with the status of the systemic condition. TMJ signs and symptoms, such as pain and limited mouth opening, often emerge or worsen when a systemic flare affecting other joints also occurs, and, similarly, when medical control of inflammation in other joints is achieved, the TMJs also may become quiescent. Some disease-modifying medications have a better affect at the TMJs than others, however. Methotrexate, a first-line treatment for JIA, is often effective at axial and appendicular joints but is less predictable in treating TMJ disease. As such, a close collaboration between the surgeon and rheumatologist is critical in achieving optimal disease control. Gadolinium-enhanced MRIs are useful in longitudinal management of the patient with JIA-TMJ disease to determine if significant acute inflammation is present in preparation for reconstruction.

In ICR and CH/HH, skeletal correction can be pursued either during active progression of the disease or after quiescence. Treatment during active disease requires extirpation of the diseased substrate (entire condyle and condylar neck in ICR and high or proportional condylectomy in CH/HH), and simultaneous reconstruction.[31,32] After quiescence, if the stable condyle maintains good function and is pain-free, then it can be maintained, and the occlusion and asymmetry can be corrected by ramus/body osteotomies in combination with maxillary repositioning. Similar to the risk/benefit considerations in early versus delayed management in CFM, treatment during the active phase of ICR or CH/HH increases the complexity and hazard of the operation by requiring direct joint access and replacement but has the advantage of earlier correction to support social and functional goals. Some clinicians find the ultimate esthetic outcome of treatment during the active phase of CH superior to delayed management.[36]

Growth

Stage of growth and skeletal maturity are important factors in determining timing of correction. Although the side of the mandible affected by TMJ pathologic condition may have impaired growth potential with or without intervention, the contralateral side in unilateral disease and surrounding structures, such as the dentoalveolar processes and maxilla, will follow normal growth pattens in most of these conditions. Skeletal correction during growth may be more difficult due to smaller structures and presence of developing teeth, may achieve suboptimal outcomes compared with delayed treatment if final facial proportions cannot be achieved, and/or occlusal relationships cannot be optimized owing to lack of a complete adult dentition or orthodontic preparation, and stability of the result may be compromised due to unpredictable postoperative growth. As such, treatment before skeletal maturity must be carefully considered and goal oriented.

Expectation for Stability

Expectation for postoperative stability of the skeletal correction and need for future revision must be carefully considered before engaging a corrective treatment plan for a young patient with TMJ pathologic condition. Many stability considerations overlap with those discussed in the *Timing* section above. The additional variable specific to stability is the underlying pathologic condition that has created the skeletal deformity. Thorough diagnosis and understanding of the disease pathophysiology and management are necessary. For CFM and TCS, stability can be expected after skeletal maturity has been reached. Treatment during growth in TCS, however, has a high expectation for instability (lack of normal growth to maintain corrected relative mandibular position). For JIA, stability may depend on the ability to achieve and maintain medical control of the inflammatory disease, or by the potential for the disease to become naturally quiescent. This expectation varies by disease subtype. Close consultation with the treating rheumatologist and use of gadolinium-enhanced MRIs to evaluate disease activity are necessary to understand the disease trajectory. In ICR and CH/HH, quiescence can be expected in most individuals, but resorption or growth may continue beyond skeletal maturity. Stability for at least 2 years is a good rule of thumb for the expectation that the disease has become quiescent for these conditions.

Reconstructive Technique

Conceptually, joint-sparing procedures, such as ramus osteotomies, should be chosen in lieu of joint-replacing operations when a TMJ is stable, functional, and pain-free, regardless of its radiographic appearance.[37] When joint stability or function is poor or uncertain, then a joint-replacing approach should be considered.

When replacing a TMJ in a young patient, the reconstructive technique must be carefully considered, with emphasis on the expectation for durability and need for future revision. Historically, autologous tissues, such as CCGs, have been the workhorse for pediatric condyle/ramus replacement.[18] CCGs may have growth potential,[38] although also may experience overgrowth[39] and have a high rate of resorption.[40] In recent years, particularly with the increase of alloplasts, the continued use of CCGs has been called into question.[41] A free fibula flap is an autologous alternative that is more robust and predictable than the CCG owing to the larger volume of harvested bone and support by local arteriovenous anastomoses.[42] When used for unilateral construction of an asymmetric mandible without a contralateral releasing osteotomy to decrease recoil effect of the flap against the glenoid fossa, however, the free fibula flap has a high rate of postoperative ankylosis.[43]

Alloplastic TMJ replacement has emerged as a predictable alternative to autologous ramus-condyle replacement. Advantages of alloplasts include lack of donor site morbidity, decreased operative time and complexity, customizability, and dimensional stability. For systemic autoinflammatory conditions, including JIA, alloplastic TMJ reconstruction has the advantage of immunity to inflammatory degradation.[44] Furthermore, customization, precision, and lack of remodeling of alloplastic total joint replacements make them ideal for facilitating concurrent orthognathic surgical procedures.[19] Despite their myriad benefits, the use of alloplastic TMJ prosthesis in young patients must be carefully considered. Importantly, their longevity is untested for the duration a young patient will require their use. Although 20-year outcomes with custom TMJ prosthesis in adults are promising,[45] a young patient will require their use for much longer. Borrowing from the experience of our orthopedic colleagues, total hip replacements have an approximately 58% survival rate at 25 years after insertion.[46] Furthermore, although alloplasts avoid some of the pitfalls of autologous tissues, they introduce others, such as a higher likelihood of biofilm and infection, and the potential for heterotopic bone formation.[47] Notably, although the theoretic potential for resorption of autologous grafts in the context of future arthritic flares in autoinflammatory disease exists, limited experience with routine orthognathic osteotomies in patients with quiescent JIA has not demonstrated significant postoperative relapse.[48,49]

Occlusal Relationships

Management of malocclusion is commonly a component of surgical correction for pediatric TMJ pathologic conditions. In younger patients, collaboration with a pediatric or family dentist to manage dental eruption may be prudent. For patients in the late-mixed and permanent dentitions, partnership with an orthodontist for dental decompensation in conjunction with skeletal correction is paramount. Location of unerupted dentition should be considered when planning osteotomies and fixation.

Morphologic Abnormalities not Addressed by Skeletal Correction

Many pathologic conditions of the pediatric TMJ create morphologic abnormalities of the mandible and surrounding structures that are not fully corrected by skeletal surgery of the maxillomandibular complex. To achieve holistic correction of symmetry and profile, ancillary procedures are often necessary. Some of these procedures can be performed concurrently with skeletal correction, whereas others may be staged and/or incremental. Genioplasty and inferior border ostectomy are examples of procedures that are commonly performed concurrent to orthognathic procedures. Alloplastic onlay implants of the mandibular angle and/or body may be best staged to reduce infection risk. Soft tissue augmentation with techniques such as autologous fat injection can be performed at any time and are often incremental.

All of the conditions reviewed in this article typically require additional procedures beyond maxillomandibular skeletal correction to optimize facial symmetry. Examples of common ancillary procedures include the following:

- CFM: Macrostomia correction, skin tag removal, microtia construction, onlay mandibular angle/body onlay implants, genioplasty, soft tissue augmentation, facial nerve reanimation
- TCS: All procedures noted for CFM, plus coloboma repair, zygomatic arch construction
- JIA and ICR: Genioplasty, mandibular angle onlay implants
- CH: Inferior border ostectomy, mandibular angle/body onlay implants

SUMMARY

Pediatric TMJ pathologic conditions represent a broad range of disorders that frequently cause facial asymmetry and/or retrognathism and malocclusion. Masticatory dysfunction, limited joint mobility, and pain variably occur. When the pathologic condition is nonneoplastic, is stable, and is not associated with functional disturbance or pain, joint-sparing procedures are preferred for correction. When TMJ replacement is necessary, careful consideration should be given to the risks, benefits, and uncertainty of various reconstructive options.

CLINICS CARE POINTS

- Accurate diagnosis is paramount in managing pediatric temporomandibular joint pathologic condition.

- Progression versus stability of the temporomandibular joint abnormality must be determined to inform the treatment plan.
- A functional mandibular condyle that is pain-free and has demonstrated stability for greater than 2 years or via imaging can be maintained during skeletal correction.
- Careful consideration should be given to likelihood of future revision procedures when choosing a reconstructive approach.

DISCLOSURE

C.M. Resnick is a consultant for AbbVie Pharmaceuticals without a relevant relationship to the subject matter contained within this article.

REFERENCES

1. Kaneyama K, Segami N, Hatta T. Congenital deformities and developmental abnormalities of the mandibular condyle in the temporomandibular joint. Congenit Anom (Kyoto) 2008;48(3):118–25.
2. Resnick CM, Kaban LB, Padwa BL. Hemifacial microsomia: the disorder and its surgical management. Maxillofacial Surgery. Churchill Livingstone; 2017. p. 870–93.
3. Boles DJ, Bodurtha J, Nance WE. Goldenhar complex in discordant monozygotic twins: a case report and review of the literature. Am J Med Genet 1987; 28(1):103–9.
4. Zielinski D, Markus B, Sheikh M, et al. OTX2 duplication is implicated in hemifacial microsomia. PLoS One 2014;9(5):e96788.
5. Horgan JE, Padwa BL, LaBrie RA, et al. OMENS-Plus: analysis of craniofacial and extracraniofacial anomalies in hemifacial microsomia. Cleft Palate Craniofac J 1995;32(5):405–12.
6. Kaban LB, Moses MH, Mulliken JB. Surgical correction of hemifacial microsomia in the growing child. Plast Reconstr Surg 1988;82(1):9–19.
7. Caron C, Pluijmers BI, Maas B, et al. Obstructive sleep apnoea in craniofacial microsomia: analysis of 755 patients. Int J Oral Maxillofac Surg 2017; 46(10):1330–7.
8. Kaban LB, Padwa BL, Mulliken JB. Surgical correction of mandibular hypoplasia in hemifacial microsomia: the case for treatment in early childhood. J Oral Maxillofac Surg 1998;56(5):628–38.
9. Pluijmers BI, Caron CJ, Dunaway DJ, et al. Mandibular reconstruction in the growing patient with unilateral craniofacial microsomia: a systematic review. Int J Oral Maxillofac Surg 2014;43(3):286–95.
10. Resnick CM, Calabrese CE. Is Obstructive Apnea More Severe in Syndromic Than Nonsyndromic

Patients With Robin Sequence? J Oral Maxillofac Surg 2019;77(12):2529–33.

11. Resnick CM, LeVine J, Calabrese CE, et al. Early Management of Infants With Robin Sequence: An International Survey and Algorithm. J Oral Maxillofac Surg 2019;77(1):136–56.

12. Hopper RA, Kapadia H, Susarla S, et al. Counterclockwise Craniofacial Distraction Osteogenesis for Tracheostomy-Dependent Children with Treacher Collins Syndrome. Plast Reconstr Surg 2018;142(2):447–57.

13. Bousquet B, Kellenberger CJ, Caprio RM, et al. Does Magnetic Resonance Imaging Distinguish Juvenile Idiopathic Arthritis From Other Causes of Progressive Temporomandibular Joint Destruction? J Oral Maxillofac Surg 2023;81(7):820–30.

14. Resnick CM. Temporomandibular Joint Reconstruction in the Growing Child. Oral Maxillofac Surg Clin North Am 2018;30(1):109–21.

15. Wolford LM. Idiopathic condylar resorption of the temporomandibular joint in teenage girls (cheerleaders syndrome). SAVE Proc 2001;14(3):246–52.

16. Nicolielo LFP, Jacobs R, Ali Albdour E, et al. Is oestrogen associated with mandibular condylar resorption? A systematic review. Int J Oral Maxillofac Surg 2017;46(11):1394–402.

17. Ji YD, Resnick CM, Peacock ZS. Idiopathic condylar resorption: A systematic review of etiology and management. Oral Surg Oral Med Oral Pathol Oral Radiol 2020;130(6):632–9.

18. Peacock ZS, Lee CCY, Troulis MJ, et al. Long-Term Stability of Condylectomy and Costochondral Graft Reconstruction for Treatment of Idiopathic Condylar Resorption. J Oral Maxillofac Surg 2019;77(4):792–802.

19. Wolford LM, Kesterke MJ. Does Combined Temporomandibular Joint Reconstruction With Patient-Fitted Total Joint Prosthesis and Orthognathic Surgery Provide Stable Skeletal and Occlusal Outcomes in Juvenile Idiopathic Arthritis Patients? J Oral Maxillofac Surg 2022;80(1):138–50.

20. Hugle B, Spiegel L, Hotte J, et al. Isolated Arthritis of the Temporomandibular Joint as the Initial Manifestation of Juvenile Idiopathic Arthritis. J Rheumatol 2017;44(11):1632–5.

21. Kellenberger CJ, Bucheli J, Schroeder-Kohler S, et al. Temporomandibular joint magnetic resonance imaging findings in adolescents with anterior disk displacement compared to those with juvenile idiopathic arthritis. J Oral Rehabil 2019;46(1):14–22.

22. Pedersen TK, Stoustrup P. How to diagnose idiopathic condylar resorptions in the absence of consensus-based criteria? J Oral Maxillofac Surg 2021;79(9):1810–1.

23. Kinard BE, Bouloux GF, Prahalad S, et al. Arthroscopy of the Temporomandibular Joint in Patients With Juvenile Idiopathic Arthritis. J Oral Maxillofac Surg 2016;74(7):1330–5.

24. Leschied JR, Smith EA, Baker S, et al. Contrast-enhanced MRI compared to direct joint visualization at arthroscopy in pediatric patients with suspected temporomandibular joint synovitis. Pediatr Radiol 2019;49(2):196–202.

25. Chouinard AF, Kaban LB, Peacock ZS. Acquired Abnormalities of the Temporomandibular Joint. Oral Maxillofac Surg Clin North Am 2018;30(1):83–96.

26. Wolford LM, Movahed R, Perez DE. A classification system for conditions causing condylar hyperplasia. J Oral Maxillofac Surg 2014;72(3):567–95.

27. Obwegeser HL, Makek MS. Hemimandibular hyperplasia–hemimandibular elongation. J Maxillofac Surg 1986;14(4):183–208.

28. Sun R, Sun L, Sun Z, et al. A three-dimensional study of hemimandibular hyperplasia, hemimandibular elongation, solitary condylar hyperplasia, simple mandibular asymmetry and condylar osteoma or osteochondroma. J Cranio-Maxillo-Fac Surg 2019;47(11):1665–75.

29. Ghawsi S, Aagaard E, Thygesen TH. High condylectomy for the treatment of mandibular condylar hyperplasia: a systematic review of the literature. Int J Oral Maxillofac Surg 2016;45(1):60–71.

30. Nino-Sandoval TC, Maia FPA, Vasconcelos BCE. Efficacy of proportional versus high condylectomy in active condylar hyperplasia - A systematic review. J Cranio-Maxillo-Fac Surg 2019;47(8):1222–32.

31. Maniskas SA, Ly CL, Pourtaheri N, et al. Concurrent High Condylectomy and Orthognathic Surgery for Treatment of Patients With Unilateral Condylar Hyperplasia. J Craniofac Surg 2020;31(8):2217–21.

32. Turvey TA, Hannan E, Brader T, et al. Active Unilateral Condylar Hyperplasia Treated With Simultaneous Condylectomy and Orthognathic Surgery: A Clinical Report. J Oral Maxillofac Surg 2022;80(10):1593–612.

33. Posnick JC, Fantuzzo JJ. Idiopathic condylar resorption: current clinical perspectives. J Oral Maxillofac Surg 2007;65(8):1617–23.

34. Kaban LB, Cisneros GJ, Heyman S, et al. Assessment of mandibular growth by skeletal scintigraphy. J Oral Maxillofac Surg 1982;40(1):18–22.

35. Pogrel MA, Kopf J, Dodson TB, et al. A comparison of single-photon emission computed tomography and planar imaging for quantitative skeletal scintigraphy of the mandibular condyle. Oral Surg Oral Med Oral Pathol Oral Radiol Endod 1995;80(2):226–31.

36. Maniskas S, Ly CL, Parsaei Y, et al. Facial Asymmetry in Unilateral Condylar Hyperplasia: Comparing Treatment for Active versus Burnt-Out Disease. Plast Reconstr Surg 2020;146(4):439e–45e.

37. Posnick JC, Kaban LB. A conceptual framework for treating jaw deformities in patients with abnormal condyles: preservation versus replacement of the glenoid fossa-disc-condyle-ramus. Int J Oral Maxillofac Surg 2022;51(1):98–103.

38. Kumar P, Rattan V, Rai S. Do costochondral grafts have any growth potential in temporomandibular joint surgery? A systematic review. J Oral Biol Craniofac Res 2015;5(3):198–202.

39. Yang S, Fan H, Du W, et al. Overgrowth of costochondral grafts in craniomaxillofacial reconstruction: Rare complication and literature review. J Cranio-Maxillo-Fac Surg 2015;43(6):803–12.

40. Medra AM. Follow up of mandibular costochondral grafts after release of ankylosis of the temporomandibular joints. Br J Oral Maxillofac Surg 2005;43(2):118–22.

41. Hawkins A, Mercuri LG, Miloro M. Are Rib Grafts Still Used for Temporomandibular Joint Reconstruction? J Oral Maxillofac Surg 2020;78(2):195–202.

42. Dowgierd K, Pokrowiecki R, Mysliwiec A, et al. Use of a Fibula Free Flap for Mandibular Reconstruction in Severe Craniofacial Microsomia in Children with Obstructive Sleep Apnea. J Clin Med 31 2023;12(3).

43. Resnick CM, Genuth J, Calabrese CE, et al. Temporomandibular Joint Ankylosis After Ramus Construction With Free Fibula Flaps in Children With Hemifacial Microsomia. J Oral Maxillofac Surg 2018;76(9):2001 e1–e2001 e15.

44. Brown Z, Rushing DC, Perez DE. Alloplastic Temporomandibular Joint Reconstruction for Patients With Juvenile Idiopathic Arthritis. J Oral Maxillofac Surg 2020;78(9):1492–8.

45. Wolford LM, Mercuri LG, Schneiderman ED, et al. Twenty-year follow-up study on a patient-fitted temporomandibular joint prosthesis: the Techmedica/TMJ Concepts device. J Oral Maxillofac Surg 2015;73(5):952–60.

46. Evans JT, Evans JP, Walker RW, et al. How long does a hip replacement last? A systematic review and meta-analysis of case series and national registry reports with more than 15 years of follow-up. Lancet 2019;393(10172):647–54.

47. Bach E, Sigaux N, Fauvernier M, et al. Reasons for failure of total temporomandibular joint replacement: a systematic review and meta-analysis. Int J Oral Maxillofac Surg 2022;51(8):1059–68.

48. Kinard BE, Behlen VH, Kau CH, et al. Is Orthognathic Correction with TMJ Preservation A Stable Treatment Option for Patients with Juvenile Idiopathic Arthritis? J Maxillofac Oral Surg 2022;21(4):1286–90.

49. Raffaini M, Arcuri F. Orthognathic surgery for juvenile idiopathic arthritis of the temporomandibular joint: a critical reappraisal based on surgical experience. Int J Oral Maxillofac Surg 2022;51(6):799–805.

Pediatric Salivary Gland Pathology

Shaunak N. Amin, MD[a], Kristopher T. Patterson, BS[b], David J. Cvancara, BS[b],
John P. Dahl, MD, PhD, MBA[c,d],*

KEYWORDS

- Parotid gland • Submandibular gland • Sublingual gland • Saliva • Salivary duct

KEY POINTS

- Benign and malignant salivary gland disorders are uncommon overall in the pediatric population but can be frequently seen in pediatric otolaryngology or oral and maxillofacial surgery practices.
- Ultrasound and cross-sectional imaging with computed tomography or MRI can be very useful in the diagnosis of most pediatric salivary gland masses or inflammatory conditions.
- Sialorrhea is a frequently seen symptom in patients with chronic neuromuscular disease, and treatment can include rehabilitation, medical management, and surgery.
- Salivary gland neoplasms are more likely to be malignant in children than in adults, and the clinician should have a low threshold for fine-needle aspiration or excisional biopsy.

INTRODUCTION

Benign and malignant salivary gland disorders are uncommon in the pediatric population; however, these can be frequently seen in pediatric otolaryngology or oral and maxillofacial surgery practices. The astute clinician should be aware of the clinical presentation, diagnosis, and management options for common inflammatory, infectious, benign, and malignant disorders of salivary glands.

PHYSIOLOGY

Salivary glands are ectodermally derived and develop from oral epithelium outgrowths expanding into the surrounding mesenchyme. These cores arborize, enlarge, and canalize before terminating into acini. Acinar cells are responsible for the production of saliva, which then passes through intercalated, intralobular, and excretory ducts before collecting in the main excretory duct of the gland. Ductal cells are responsible for further modifications of saliva until its secretion into the oral cavity.

Saliva is a complex solution which is primarily composed of water (99%), but additionally contains enzymes such as amylase and lipase, proteins including secretory IgA, mucins, and lactoferrin, and electrolytes. These elements are paramount in oral cavity physiology and assist with lubrication of food, digestion, inhibition of bacterial overgrowth, and maintenance of a neutral pH.[1] In children, the daily secretion of saliva ranges between 0.5 and 1.5 L.[2,3] There are 3 pairs of major salivary glands which contribute to 90% of total salivary secretions: the parotid, submandibular, and sublingual glands. Additionally, there are thousands of minor salivary glands lining the upper aerodigestive tract primarily occurring in the buccal, lingual, labial, and palatal regions which produce the remaining 10%. Resting salivary secretions are produced primarily by the submandibular glands (60%–75% of total saliva production), while the parotid is the major producer of stimulated saliva.[3]

[a] Department of Otolaryngology-Head and Neck Surgery, University of Washington, Box 356515 Health Sciences Building, Suite BB1165, Seattle, WA 98195-65, USA; [b] School of Medicine, University of Washington, Box 356515 Health Sciences Building, Suite BB1165, Seattle, WA 98195-65, USA; [c] Department of Otolaryngology-Head and Neck Surgery, University of Washington, Seattle, WA, USA; [d] Division of Pediatric Otolaryngology-Head and Neck Surgery, Seattle Children's Hospital, Seattle, WA, USA
* Corresponding author. M/S OA.9.220, PO Box 5371, Seattle, WA 98105-5005.
E-mail address: jake.dahl@seattlechildrens.org

Oral Maxillofacial Surg Clin N Am 36 (2024) 317–332
https://doi.org/10.1016/j.coms.2024.02.001
1042-3699/24/© 2024 Elsevier Inc. All rights reserved.

Salivary flow is mediated by the autonomic nervous system. Parasympathetic outflow is the primary modulator of saliva production through the release of acetylcholine onto M_3 muscarinic receptors, which results in increased blood flow to salivary glands, increased salivary secretion from acinar cells, and higher flow of watery saliva. Conversely, sympathetic innervation plays a relatively minor role in regulation of salivary production and flow. Through the effects of norepinephrine on alpha- and beta-adrenergic receptors, sympathetic outflow causes reduced the salivary secretion and production of viscous saliva.

ANATOMY

The parotid glands are the largest major salivary glands and are the first to develop embryologically. The parotid glands exist as paired glands which lie between the external auditory canal, mandibular ramus, and mastoid tip. The extratemporal facial nerve courses and arborizes within the parenchyma of the parotid gland and divides the gland into superficial and deep lobes. The parotid gland is enveloped by the superficial portion of the deep cervical fascia and is separated from the submandibular gland by the stylomandibular ligament. The parotid acinar system drains into a terminal excretory duct known as Stensen's duct. Stensen's duct is 4 to 7 cm in length and courses anteriorly over the masseter muscle, pierces the buccinator muscle, and empties into the oral cavity via an opening in the buccal mucosa opposite from the maxillary second molar. The narrowest component of Stensen's duct is at the ostium with an average diameter of approximately 0.5 mm.[4,5] In approximately 20% of the population, accessory parotid glands exist along, and empty into, Stensen's duct.[6] The primary parasympathetic innervation to the parotid glands is via the glossopharyngeal nerve with preganglionic fibers synapsing in the otic ganglion and postganglionic fibers traveling to the gland via the auriculotemporal nerve. Sympathetic innervation to the parotid gland occurs via the superior sympathetic ganglion.[5]

The next largest salivary glands are the submandibular glands, which experience rapid growth in the first 2 years of life. These exist as paired glands located in the floor of the mouth between the anterior and posterior digastric tendons and just inferior to the body of the mandible. The posterior free-edge of the mylohyoid abuts the submandibular gland and divides it into a large superficial portion and small deep lobe. Similar to the parotid gland, the submandibular gland is enveloped by the superficial layer of deep cervical fascia.

Importantly, the submandibular gland maintains a close anatomic relationship with the marginal mandibular branch of the facial nerve, the facial vein and artery, the lingual nerve, and the hypoglossal nerve. Acinar units and ductal systems from the submandibular gland drain into a final secretory duct known as Wharton's duct. Wharton's duct is approximately 5 cm in length and courses anteriorly between the mylohyoid, hyoglossus, and genioglossus muscles before opening into the oral cavity through a papilla lateral to the lingual frenulum. The ostium of Wharton's duct is the narrowest portion of the final ductal system with a diameter of approximately 0.5 mm.[4] The primary parasympathetic innervation of the submandibular glands is via the chorda tympani nerve, a branch of the intratemporal facial nerve, with preganglionic fibers synapsing with postganglionic fibers at the submandibular ganglion. Sympathetic innervation occurs via fibers from the superior sympathetic ganglion.[7]

Sublingual glands are the smallest of the 3 major salivary glands and, similarly to the submandibular glands, exhibit rapid growth in the first 2 years of life. The sublingual glands are unencapsulated and are located in the floor of the mouth, superficial to the mylohyoid muscle, and just deep to the oral mucosa. In young children, these glands are often contiguous with the submandibular glands. Unlike the other major salivary glands, the sublingual glands typically drain directly into the floor of the mouth via several small ducts known as ducts of Rivinus; however, occasionally some of the ducts of Rivinus drain into a common terminal duct known as the Bartholin duct. The parasympathetic and sympathetic innervations of the sublingual glands are similar to those of the submandibular glands.[8]

HISTORY AND PHYSICAL EXAMINATION

In children with suspected salivary gland disorders, detailed history and physical examinations are critical in determining a differential diagnosis. A thorough history should include the location, onset, duration, severity, and frequency of symptoms as well as any alleviating and exacerbating factors. A careful review of medications is also useful as a significant number of medications can affect salivary production and secretion. Physical examination should include a comprehensive head and neck evaluation to assess for concomitant pathologies with a detailed examination of all salivary glands. When assessing salivary glands, it is important to note the size, mobility, symmetry, tenderness, and consistency of the glands as well as assess the overlying skin for edema, erythema, fistulas, or dermal involvement. The floor of mouth and buccal mucosa should be palpated and each main ductal orifice should be examined while manually massaging the associated gland to assess for secretion of saliva or purulence. The mucosa surrounding ductal orifices should additionally be examined to looks for signs of inflammation. In the case of a suspected salivary mass or malignancy, a comprehensive facial nerve examination should be performed.

A list of common history and examination findings which are associated with specific salivary gland pathologies, is summarized in **Table 1**.

DIAGNOSTIC MODALITIES
Laboratory Evaluation

Although laboratory evaluations generally have limited diagnostic utility in the evaluation of salivary gland pathologies in children, they are helpful in narrowing the differential diagnosis and can aid in diagnosis of select diseases. If concerned for an infectious process, white blood cell count or C-reactive protein may be helpful to confirm suspicions and can be used to monitor response to treatment.[9,10] In the case of bacterial sialadenitis, cultures of any purulent secretions can be very useful in identifying the causative organisms and determining antibiotic sensitivities. In select cases, specific tests can be ordered to confirm or rule out diagnoses. Examples include obtaining a purified protein derivative skin test in the case of suspected mycobacterial infection, human immunodeficiency virus (HIV) viral load in patients with bilateral cystic swelling and positive family history,

and mumps serology in an unvaccinated patient with orchitis.

Diagnostic Imaging

Imaging plays an essential role in the diagnostic workup of many pediatric patients with salivary gland pathologies with some patients requiring multiple modalities or serial examinations to confirm and monitor diagnoses.

Plain radiography has limited utility in the workup of salivary gland pathologies but may be useful in low-resource settings to confirm sialolithiasis. However, the sensitivity of sialoliths on plain radiographs is low, particularly with parotid calculi (radiolucent in 80% of cases); thus, there is a high false-negative rate.[11] Furthermore, extrasalivary diseases such as phleboliths, lingual artery atherosclerosis, and calcified lymphadenopathy can all lead to false positives.[12]

Ultrasonography, on the other hand, is the preferred initial imaging modality in children with salivary gland disorders. It allows for excellent superficial visualization of the major salivary glands and their associated structures and has additional benefits of being noninvasive, cost-effective, does not involve radiation, and generally does not require sedation or anesthesia. Despite its advantages, ultrasonography is limited as it is an operator-dependent test and is inadequate for evaluation of deeper pathology, particularly with regard to neoplasms which often require additional advanced imaging. Nonetheless, ultrasound is used in many surgical practices as part of routine examination and assessments. Ultrasonography excels at detection of sialoliths with sensitivity of up to 90%

Table 1
History and physical examination findings which are commonly associated with salivary gland pathologies

Pathology	Associated History or Examination Finding(s)
Neoplasm	Painless growth, facial nerve weakness
Vascular anomaly	Perinatal swelling
Infectious/inflammatory	Acute onset of pain or swelling, erythema or purulence at ductal orifice
Obstructive	Postprandial pain and swelling, reduced salivary flow at ductal orifice, recent facial trauma
Atypical mycobacterial	Overlying violaceous discoloration
Bartonella	Recent cat exposure/scratch
Autoimmune	Other systemic conditions
Mumps	Tender bilateral swelling, unvaccinated, concomitant orchitis
HIV-associated BLECs	Bilateral painless cystic swelling, paternal/maternal history of HIV
Sjogren's syndrome	Xerostomia and dry eyes, positive family history

in stones greater than 2 mm.[13] Additionally, ultrasound has comparable precision to computed tomography (CT) and MRI in the diagnosis of superficial parotid or submandibular gland lesions. Furthermore, ultrasound is excellent in the diagnosis of vascular lesions and can be used to assist in needle aspirations of abscesses and fine-needle aspiration (FNA) of superficial neoplasms.[12]

Despite the utility of ultrasound, cross-sectional imaging via CT or MRI is still often required in evaluation of suspected malignancies, severe infectious processes, and inflammatory and obstructive processes. Contrasted CT is often the preferred imaging modality for suspected inflammatory or obstructive conditions including sialadenitis, sialolithiasis, ranulas, and abscesses, and pathologies which spread to the deep neck spaces or adjacent lymph nodes. Particular advantages of CT over MRI include time of procedure, lack of need for sedation for pediatric patients, and low costs. MRI, on the other hand, is the preferred modality for evaluation of masses of the parotid and parapharyngeal spaces due to excellent soft tissue detail, which allow for fine delineation of tumor extent in relation to critical neurovascular structures such as the facial nerve or internal carotid artery. Fat-suppressed and gadolinium-enhanced images are useful in identification of perineural spread. MRI additionally is useful for the evaluation of high-flow (eg, hemangiomas, arteriovenous malformations) versus low-flow (eg, lymphatic malformations) vascular anomalies through assessment of flow voids. The benefits of MRI include the aforementioned excellent soft tissue detail as well as the lack of radiation exposure; however, the drawbacks include cost, lack of availability, and need for sedation in young patients.[14,15]

Additional, more advanced, imaging modalities exist for evaluation of select salivary gland disorders. Sialography utilizes injected contrast material that is injected into affected salivary ducts to detect obstruction including stricture, stenosis, or sialolith; however, this is often unfeasible in uncooperative pediatric patients.[16,17] Scintigraphy has select usefulness in the evaluation of residual excretory function in inflammatory conditions such as Sjogren's syndrome (SS) and postradiation xerostomia. In this technique, technetium-99m pertechnetate is injected intravenously, and the uptake, concentration, and excretion of tracer by salivary glands are measured.[18] Further discussion of these techniques is beyond the scope of this article.

SIALORRHEA

Sialorrhea is defined as an excessive salivary flow in the oral cavity. Sialorrhea can be classified as anterior or posterior sialorrhea. Anterior sialorrhea, or drooling, refers to the spillage of saliva beyond the border of the lower lip, while posterior sialorrhea is the flow of saliva into the pharynx.[19] Sialorrhea can be further classified as primary (excess production of saliva or hypersalivation) or secondary (decreased frequency of swallowing saliva), with the latter form being much more common among patients. Swallowing requires a complex mechanism of coordinated orofacial sensory and motor systems. Drooling is common in normally developing babies up to the first 18 to 24 months of life at which point these complex neuromuscular swallowing mechanisms mature and they achieve salivary continence.[20] Neurologic dysfunction is often implicated in pathologic sialorrhea in children. In fact, the most common etiologies of sialorrhea in children are cerebral palsy with an estimated prevalence of 10% to 38% of individuals affected by the condition.[21]

Sialorrhea poses a significant burden on children through its physical and psychosocial impacts. Drooling can result in perioral maceration of the skin and secondary infections, foul odor, feeding difficulty, speech problems, and soiled clothing.[22] In addition, posterior sialorrhea can cause coughing, gagging, vomiting, and aspiration, with aspiration pneumonia being a potentially life-threatening complication.

Treatment

Treatment for sialorrhea is usually administered in a stepwise approach beginning with conservative treatments before advancing to more invasive measures (Sialorrhea in Cerebral Palsy: https://www.aacpdm.org/publications/care-pathways/sialorrhea-in-cerebral-palsy). If present, anatomical causes for sialorrhea should first be corrected. This may include orthodontic appliances for dental malocclusion or incomplete lip closure as well as proper wheelchair or braces fitting to correct postural issues that may be contributing to a patient's sialorrhea.[23] Once any anatomic anomalies are addressed, a variety of rehabilitative therapies can be employed. Positioning exercises, speech and oral motor therapy, oral sensory awareness training, and behavioral therapy are several noninvasive treatments that have shown long-lasting and effective results.[24]

The cornerstone of pharmacologic therapy in sialorrhea is utilization of the anticholinergic class of medications as salivary gland function is mediated by parasympathetic innervation.[25] Glycopyrrolate and scopolamine are the most widely used anticholinergics used in the treatment of sialorrhea.[26] While all anticholinergics have been shown to be efficacious in the treatment of sialorrhea, the use of this medication is often limited due to a relatively high incidence of unfavorable side effects, including dry mouth, constipation, urinary retention, blurred vision, irritability, and behavioral changes. To mitigate the risk of systemic absorption of anticholinergic agents, sublingual atropine has shown to be effective in the short-term treatment of sialorrhea with minimal side effects; however, its efficacy in the pediatric population is less clear and optimal dosing regimen has yet to be established.[27,28]

Botulinum toxin A (BoNT-A) injections have been a widely popular treatment option for sialorrhea for over 2 decades in part due to its minimally invasive nature, proven efficacy, and relatively mild side-effect profile.[22,29] BoNT-A exerts its therapeutic effects through blocking synaptic transmission of acetylcholine via cleavage of SNAP-25 at presynaptic nerve terminals, inducing chemical denervation of the parasympathetic fibers supplying the salivary glands.[30] The effects of BoNT-A last 3 to 6 months; therefore, redosing is required at this frequency for sustained treatment response. The parotid and submandibular glands are usually the target of the BoNT-A therapy, and injections are performed under ultrasound guidance or through manual palpation of the glands with identification of anatomic landmarks[31] The main complication of BoNT-A injections appears to be due to local diffusion of the toxin into surrounding neck musculature and with reported dysphagia, dysphonia and, rarely, aspiration pneumonia. Special dental care should be given to children receiving salivary gland BoNT-A injections as an increased risk of dental carries have been described in these patients.[32]

In patients with refractory sialorrhea despite rehabilitative and medical treatments, radiation and surgical therapy may be considered. Targeted radiotherapy to the submandibular and parotid glands has been shown to produce long-lasting improvement in sialorrhea; however, potential for malignancy later in life largely precludes this treatment modality in the pediatric population.[33] Surgical treatment usually involves a combination of salivary gland excision, duct ligation, and duct diversion. A meta-analysis revealed that overall, slightly more than 80% of pediatric patients experienced significant relief from sialorrhea when any type of salivary gland surgery was performed.[34] The most effective surgical intervention was found to be bilateral submandibular gland excision with bilateral parotid duct diversion which had a reported success rate of nearly 88%. The major complications associated with surgical treatment are xerostomia and increased incidence of dental caries. Novel procedures to treat sialorrhea, such as endoscopic submandibular ganglion neurectomy, have emerged; however, long-term data are not available to compare this method to more established techniques.[35]

BENIGN DISORDERS
Infectious

Acute bacterial sialadenitis is an uncommon infection in the pediatric population that most often involves the parotid gland (**Table 2**). Acute parotitis commonly presents with sudden onset of fever, pain, edema, and erythema of the affected parotid gland. Unilateral involvement and purulent drainage from the associated duct are common. Complications associated with bacterial parotitis include abscess formation, facial palsy, and phlegmons that may lead to airway obstruction if significant.[36] Sialadenitis originating from the submandibular gland can also occur and is often associated with an obstructing sialolith. Pathogens associated with acute bacterial sialadenitis include *Staphylococcus aureus*, *Haemophilus influenzae*, *Peptostreptococcus*, *Streptococcus pneumoniae*, *Moraxella catarrhalis*, *Escherichia coli*, and *Bacteroides* species. Treatment is aimed at directed antibiotic therapy and supportive measures. Supportive therapy includes hydration, sialagogues, analgesics, and warm compress.[37]

Viral sialadenitis is caused by a number of viruses with one of the most important viral pathogens being Paramyxovirus. Paramyxovirus, the virus responsible for mumps, is historically the most common cause of sialadenitis in children, although the incidence of mumps has decreased significantly since the introduction of the measles-mumps-rubella vaccine.[38] Unlike bacterial causes, sialadenitis from mumps nearly always involves bilateral parotid gland swelling without purulence. While most diagnoses of mumps parotitis are made clinically, serum IgM antibodies can be used to confirm infection from the mumps virus. The Epstein–Barr virus and cytomegalovirus, both part of the herpes virus family, are also implicated in cases of viral sialadenitis. In children with HIV, sialadenitis is one of the most common presenting symptoms, with involvement of the parotid gland more common than the submandibular or sublingual glands. The clinical picture for HIV-associated parotitis is often bilateral, painless swelling of the glands. Additionally, neoplasm should be considered in cases of HIV-associated sialadenitis where there is rapid growth of salivary lesions or abnormal appearance on physical examination.[39] With all forms of uncomplicated viral sialadenitis, the mainstay of treatment is supportive therapy.

Table 2
Benign conditions of the salivary glands and their clinical features, diagnosis, and treatment

Disorder	Etiology	Presentation	Diagnosis	Treatment
Infectious				
Acute bacterial sialadenitis	*S aureus* most common	Acute pain and swelling	Clinical, bacterial cultures	Antibiotics and supportive care
Mumps	Paramyxovirus	Bilateral swelling, ± tenderness	IgM serology testing, PCR	Supportive care
Epstein–Barr virus	Human herpesvirus 4	Often asymptomatic, triad of fever, sore throat, and posterior cervical adenopathy	Serology testing, monospot test	Supportive care
Human immunodeficiency virus (HIV)	HIV	Bilateral cystic enlargement, painless	ELISA, CT or MRI, ± biopsy	Antiretrovirals, supportive care
Granulomatous				
Mycobacterial	*M avium* complex (MAC), *M tuberculosis*	Cervicofacial lymphadenopathy, skin changes (violaceous hue, fistula formation)	Clinical, FNA, PCR	Antimycobacterial therapy, surgery for advanced stages
Actinomycosis	Gram-positive anaerobic bacilli (*Actinomyces israelii*)	Nontender mass with sinus tracts, or acute painful swelling with fever	Histology showing sulfur granules	Prolonged antibiotics (penicillin), ± surgery
Cat-scratch disease	*B henselae*	Regional lymphadenopathy, ± fever, self-limited	Antibody titers, histology showing positive Warthin–Starry stain	Supportive care, antibiotics for complicated infections
Sarcoidosis	Noncaseating granulomas	Parotid gland enlargement with other systemic symptoms (ie, bilateral hilar adenopathy, cutaneous, joint, ocular lesions)	Chest radiograph, angiotensin-converting enzyme level, histology	Corticosteroids

Inflammatory/Autoimmune/Cystic

Juvenile recurrent parotitis (JRP)	Nonobstructive, nonsuppurative inflammation	Recurrent tenderness and swelling of parotid gland(s)	Doppler ultrasound or MR sialography	Supportive care
Necrotizing sialometaplasia	Ischemic changes or minor salivary gland acini	Painless ulceration, commonly on hard or soft palate	Biopsy	Conservative as lesion heals over course of months
Sialolithiasis	Calculi formation from salivary stasis	Tenderness and swelling of affected gland	Dental radiograph, ultrasound, or CT	Sialendoscopy, lithotripsy, sialolithotomy, rarely gland excision
Sjogren's syndrome	CD4 lymphocyte-mediated infiltration of salivary gland parenchyma	Recurrent salivary gland swelling, xerostomia, Keratoconjunctivitis sicca	Clinical, autoantibodies (SS-A/SS-B), salivary gland biopsy	Mostly symptomatic management, ± systemic pharmacotherapy
Mucocele/Ranula	Injury or obstruction of salivary duct	Fluctuant swelling, often in floor of mouth	Clinical, ultrasound, FNA	Observation, incision, and drainage

Granulomatous

Unlike acute bacterial or viral sialadenitis that involves the salivary gland parenchyma, granulomatous diseases of the salivary glands result in inflammation of the periglandular lymph nodes. In immunocompetent children, *Mycobacterium tuberculosis* is extremely rare and should be considered in cases where the patient is from endemic regions with a slow-growing firm nodular mass involving a unilateral parotid gland.[40] Nontuberculous mycobacterium (NTM), such as *Mycobacterium avium* complex, is found ubiquitously in the environment and represents a more clinically significant etiology of caseating granulomatous sialadenitis in children, particularly in the 1 to 3 age range.[41,42] NTM most commonly presents with cervicofacial lymphadenopathy which usually involves the parotid and submandibular regions. The skin overlying the infection can develop a classic violaceous hue, and advance progression can lead to cutaneous fistulas or sinus tracts formation. Treatment for NTM infections can include antibiotic (combination of macrolide with rifamycin or ethambutol) or surgical therapy.

Other causes of granulomatous salivary gland disease in children include actinomycosis and cat-scratch disease (CSD). *Actinomyces* are gram-positive anaerobes that normally colonize the human mouth; as a result, sialadenitis due to these pathogens is often seen in the setting of dental procedures or oral trauma.[43] Actinomycosis' presentation is usually described as either a slow-growing, nontender mass with multiple sinus tracts or as an acute painful swelling associated with fever. Diagnosis is made by histologic analysis demonstrating hallmark sulfur granules. Treatment consists of prolonged penicillin-based antibiotic therapy with surgery reserved for advanced cases complicated by chronic abscesses or persistent sinus tracts. CSD is caused by the intracellular bacteria *Bartonella henselae*. Transmission is often due to cat scratches or bites, and clinically, the infection classically presents with regional lymphadenopathy with fever absent in about half of patients.[44] Antibody titers, histologic appearance, and PCR analysis can all aid in the correct diagnosis. In contrast to other bacterial infections of the salivary glands, treatment is supported as the infection is self-limiting. However, antibiotic therapy and surgery may be indicated for some patients with complicated infections.

While sarcoidosis is rarely seen in pediatric populations, it can cause noncaseating granulomatous sialadenitis. Sarcoidosis should be suspected in cases of parotid gland enlargement with other systemic findings including bilateral hilar adenopathy and cutaneous, joint, and eye lesions. Chest radiograph and serum angiotensin-converting enzyme level may aid in the diagnosis, but pathologic specimens demonstrating noncaseating granulomas are highly suggestive of sarcoid.[45] Treatment is not required in cases of asymptomatic involvement of the salivary glands in the absence of other systemic disease. However, systemic involvement usually warrants corticosteroid therapy.

Inflammatory/Autoimmune/Cystic

Juvenile recurrent parotitis (JRP) is the second most common salivary disease in children after mumps. Onset of JRP occurs between the ages of 3 and 6 years with a predilection for males.[46] The pathogenesis of JRP is unclear, with many experts hypothesizing multiple factors may be involved in disease development including congenital ductal malformation, hereditary genetic factors, infections, allergy, and autoimmune components.[47] JRP manifests as recurrent episodes of parotid gland inflammation with symptom-free intervals lasting from days to years. Clinically, these children present with tender and edematous jaws, often accompanied by fever and malaise. Swelling is more commonly unilateral and it can be differentiated from other infections etiologies by the absence of purulent secretion when the gland is expressed.[48] Treatment is aimed at managing symptoms with most patients demonstrating spontaneous resolution of the disease by early adulthood.

Necrotizing sialometaplasia is a self-limited inflammatory condition of the salivary glands that rarely affects children and adolescents. The disease may occur in all locations where there is salivary gland tissue; however, lesions often affect the minor salivary glands on the hard and soft palate.[49] Most cases present as painless ulcerations that may resemble malignant neoplasms. Biopsy is often performed to rule out malignancy and treatment is conservative as the lesions heal without any interventions over the course of several months.

SS is a chronic inflammatory autoimmune disease of the salivary and lacrimal glands. SS is exceedingly rare in pediatric populations and usually presents as chronic sialadenitis with the classic constellation of ocular and oral dryness occurring less frequently compared to adult patients.[50] Extraglandular manifestations can also be seen such as arthralgias and neurologic and renal diseases.[51] Diagnosis of SS in pediatric patients is complicated as many children do not meet the criteria published for adult diagnosis of

SS. Therefore, diagnostic criteria in children should be tailored to this specific population and may utilize a combination of subjective ocular or oral dryness, laboratory evidence of autoantibodies (SS-A and SS-B), and biopsy of the minor salivary gland or tail of the parotid gland.[52] Currently, no pediatric-specific treatment recommendations exist for SS, and management is mostly symptomatic. Some of the most commonly prescribed systemic therapies for SS in children are hydroxychloroquine, corticosteroids, methotrexate, azathioprine, and rituximab; however, evidence of the efficacy of these pharmacotherapies are not clear.

Salivary cysts can develop in the setting of trauma or obstruction of the excretory duct of the salivary glands. Mucoceles are common oral lesions found in children and represent mucous extravasation in the surrounding gland parenchyma. Ranulas are a form of mucocele that are found on the floor of the mouth, usually originating from the sublingual glands (**Fig. 1**).[53] Mucoceles and ranulas are pseudocysts as they lack an epithelial lining. In contrast, mucous retention cysts are true cysts of the minor salivary glands that result from direct ductal obstruction. Salivary cysts can often be observed up to 6 months before definitive surgical excision of the cyst or involved gland is pursued (**Fig. 2**).[54,55]

Sialolithiasis

Salivary gland stones, or sialolithiasis, are exceedingly rare in the pediatric population but should be considered in cases of recurrent or chronic sialadenitis, especially of the submandibular gland where approximately 85% of sialoliths originate. Salivary calculi typically present with tenderness and swelling of the gland involved and imaging with dental radiographs, ultrasound, or CT scan

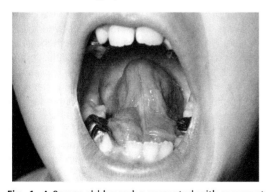

Fig. 1. A 9 year old boy who presented with recurrent cystic swelling of the floor of mouth following prior marsupialization at an outside facility. The patient subsequently underwent right submandibular gland excision with final pathologic diagnosis of a plunging ranula.

confirmed the diagnosis. Stones that are refractory to conservative management can be further treated with a variety of modern surgical approaches including sialendoscopy with stone removal, intraductal lithotripsy, sialolithotomy with sialodochoplasty, and, as an option of last resort, excision of the symptomatic gland.[56–58]

Vascular Anomalies

Vascular anomalies represent a wide range of pathology commonly seen involving the salivary glands in pediatric populations and are characterized as either vascular tumors or vascular malformations. Hemangiomas are the most common parotid tumor of childhood and exhibit a female predominance.[59] Diagnosis is typically clinical, with the characteristic appearance of a soft mass often with overlying bluish cutaneous discoloration exhibiting a natural history of rapid proliferation within the first months of life followed by another growth spurt occurring in the 4th to 6th months of life, ultimately resolving after a slow involution phase. MRI can be used to define the lesion's extension into surrounding tissues. Propranolol has been shown to be an effective first-line treatment for complicated pediatric hemangiomas.[60] Of the vascular malformations to involve the salivary glands lymphatic malformations are the most common. Most lymphatic malformations are diagnosed by age 2 years, and these lesions often present abruptly as a palpable mass, sometimes in the setting of a recent infection or trauma. Imaging with MRI will reveal well-circumscribed, multicystic masses. Lymphatic malformations can be described radiographically as either macrocystic or microcystic. Both surgery and sclerotherapy have been shown to be effective treatments for lymphatic malformations, with macrocystic lesions demonstrating a greater likelihood of eradication compared to microcystic disease.[61] Pharmacologic therapies including sirolimus and alpelisib, that target the PIK3CA pathway, are being used with increasing frequency in the treatment of lymphatic malformations.

SALIVARY GLAND NEOPLASMS

Salivary gland tumors are relatively rare within pediatric populations and comprise only 8% of all pediatric head and neck tumors.[62] While salivary gland tumors exhibit comparable histologic patterns and locations in both pediatric and adult populations, pediatric populations tend to have a higher preponderance of malignant pathology (50% vs 15%–25%).[62–64] Fortunately, pediatric salivary gland tumors tend to be lower grade and have more favorable outcomes if caught and

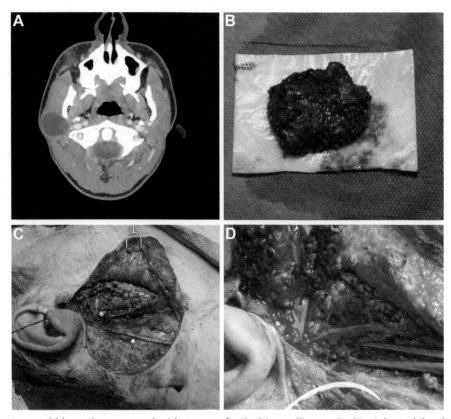

Fig. 2. A 14 year old boy who presented with 1 year of palpable swelling under his right earlobe. (*A*) CT neck demonstrating well-demarcated 3 × 3 cm cystic mass of the right superficial parotid gland extending into the deep lobe. (*B*) Gross surgical specimen following superficial parotidectomy and removal of mass. Final pathology was consistent with a salivary cyst. (*C*) Intraoperative photograph following mass removal with demonstration of branching of the facial nerve (*asterisk*) and the greater auricular nerve (*arrow*). (*D*) Close-up photograph demonstrating branching of the facial nerve just deep to the superficial lobe of the parotid gland.

managed early.[65] History and physical examination should be comprehensive with special attention placed on pain as it relates to the mass, family history of head and neck salivary gland malignancy, cervical adenopathy or direct mass extension, and cranial nerve examination. If malignancy is a possibility, imaging modalities such as ultrasound or MRI have become standard techniques for characterizing the tumor as well as surgical planning.[66] The primary diagnostic approach for assessing a salivary gland mass involves utilizing the FNA biopsy, while intraoperative excisional biopsy serves as an alternative option. Incisional biopsy or core biopsy is typically contraindicated for salivary gland masses given the increased risk of seeding and recurrence.

Benign Neoplasms

Pleomorphic (mixed) adenoma is the most common epithelial salivary gland tumor in the pediatric population and is composed of cell lines that stem from both mesenchymal and epithelial origins.[64] Clinically, this tumor is identified in pediatric patients around puberty as a slow-growing, freely moving, asymptomatic mass typically located within the tail of the parotid gland or on the hard palate.[64] Although characterized as a benign neoplasm, there is a 1.5% to 9.5% chance of conversion to a malignant neoplasm if left untreated with increasing risk over time.[67,68] Because of this, management of a pleomorphic adenoma, regardless of size, is complete surgical excision. Enucleation, incomplete resection, or tumor spillage is not appropriate given the 40% recurrence rate associated with seeding the resection bed.[69,70] Despite this, pleomorphic adenoma is associated with recurrence rates that are higher in the pediatric population relative to adult patients (20% vs 1%).

Warthin tumors (papillary cystadenoma lymphomatosum) comprise 2% of benign salivary gland tumors in the pediatric population. Clinically, these tumors reside almost exclusively in the parotid gland.[71] Common manifestations include a painless and slow-growing mass, typically unilateral presentation (although 10% are bilateral), and cystic composition (however, both homogenous cystic or solid components can be present on imaging).[71] While benign, Warthin tumors are quite rare and can easily be mistaken for malignant processes, therefore complete surgical excision is the recommended treatment.[72,73]

First branchial anomalies or other ductal cysts are congenital malformations of ductal anatomy. Given the embryonic and anatomic origin of these ducts, they are almost exclusively found in the parotid gland and often present in neonates as unilateral parotid gland swelling. First branchial anomalies generally require surgical management including a superficial parotidectomy, in order to identify and preserve the facial nerve.

Plexiform neurofibroma is a rare, benign nerve sheath tumor more commonly seen in patients with neurofibromatosis type 1.[74–76] Presentation is highly reliant on the location and size of the tumor. Full or partial surgical excision is a treatment to consider in some patients, in order to eliminate the risk of malignant transformation and optimize quality of life. Newer medical therapies, including trametinib, are also being used for the treatment of plexiform neurofibromas including those involving the salivary glands.

Other benign salivary gland tumors that are uncommonly encountered in the pediatric population, include embryoma, monomorphic adenoma, lymphoepithelial tumor, cystadenoma, xanthoma, neurilemmoma, lipoma, and teratoma.

Malignant Neoplasms

The most common malignant salivary gland tumor, mucoepidermoid carcinoma (MEC), accounts for roughly 50% of salivary gland tumors in the pediatric population. The major risk factor for MEC is prior exposure to radiation. The average age of onset for these tumors ranges from 10 to 16 years with earlier onset associated with worse prognosis.[77] MEC typically presents as a firm, fixed, slow-growing mass that can be painful to palpation. MRI can show a wide breadth of features ranging from tumors with well-circumscribed borders to those with extrafacial or nodal extension; however, signs of necrosis or high cellularity on T2 imaging are suspicious of more aggressive tumors and warrants biopsy.[66] Histologically, low-grade tumors often display a cystic architecture with mucinous differentiation as well as cytologic atypia and low mitotic activity and have good overall prognosis.[63,78] Alternatively, high-grade MEC displays a more squamous differentiation and is sometimes difficult to differentiate from squamous cell carcinoma on histologic analysis. These tumors display marked cytologic atypia and a high rate of mitotic activity and are much more aggressive with lower survival rates.[63,78] Therapeutic options include wide local excision of the tumor. Neck dissection should be considered if preoperative imaging or operative findings are concerning for cervical metastasis. Chemotherapy using methotrexate and doxorubicin has been shown to have some efficacy in MEC; however, there is not a consensus.[62] Postoperative radiation therapy should additionally be considered for all lesions, especially in patients with high-grade tumors, pending patient goals of care and multidisciplinary tumor board discussion.[79–81]

Acinic cell carcinoma represents the second most common malignant neoplasm of the salivary glands in the pediatric population.[63,82,83] Clinically, this tumor occurs during the second decade of life and presents as a slowly enlarging mass that can be painful. Derived from serous acinar cells, approximately 80% of acinic cell carcinomas arise within the parotid gland. Histologically, there is a diverse set of patterns including solid/lobular, microcystic, papillary-cystic, and follicular; however, most subtypes are considered low grade. Treatment involves wide local excision of the lesion, typically through superficial parotidectomy with negative margins. While nodal metastasis is occasionally present, there is continued debate regarding the role that neck dissection and adjuvant radiation therapy may play.[84,85] Regardless, prognosis following wide local excision is generally favorable in patients with low-grade, well-differentiated tumors. Of note, acinic cell carcinoma is associated with an approximately 35% rate of locoregional recurrence, often occurring many years after initial diagnosis, and therefore follow-up screening should be considered.[86,87]

Adenoid cystic carcinoma is classically known for neurotrophic behavior and perineural invasion and extension as opposed to spread via cervical lymphatic system. Clinical presentation depends on the location of the lesion which is more commonly seen in minor salivary glands. Histologically, there are 3 distinct growth patterns including tubular, cribriform, and solid; however, a single tumor can be composed of all 3 patterns in varying proportions. A greater proportion of the solid pattern in an individual tumor is associated with a poorer prognosis. Gold standard therapeutic options include wide local excision, whereas neck dissection and postoperative radiation therapy should be considered following a multidisciplinary tumor board.[88,89] Of note, chemotherapy using cisplatin, doxorubicin, and 5-fluorouracil has had favorable outcomes in

Table 3
American Joint Committee on Cancer major salivary glands cancer staging

T Category	T Criteria
TX	Primary tumor cannot be assessed
T0	No evidence of primary tumor
Tis	Carcinoma in situ
T1	Tumor ≤2 cm in greatest dimension without extraparenchymal extension
T2	Tumor >2 cm but <4 cm in greatest dimension without extraparenchymal extension
T3	Tumor >4 cm and/or tumor having extraparenchymal extension
T4[a]	
T4a	Tumor invades the skin, mandible, ear canal, and/or facial nerve
T4b	Tumor invades skull base and/or pterygoid plates and/or encases carotid artery

cN Category	cN Criteria
NX	Regional nodes cannot be assessed
N0	No regional lymph node metastasis
N1	Single ipsilateral lymph node ≤3 cm in greatest dimension and ENE (−)
N2[a]	
N2a	Single ipsilateral lymph node >3 cm but <6 cm in greatest dimension and ENE (−)
N2b	Multiple ipsilateral lymph nodes, none >6 cm in greatest dimension and ENE (−)
N2c	Bilateral or contralateral lymph nodes, none >6 cm in dimension and ENE (−)
N3[a]	
N3a	Metastasis in a lymph node >6 cm in greatest dimension and ENE (−)
N3b	Metastasis in any node(s) with clinically overt ENE (+)

pN Category	pN Criteria
NX	Regional lymph nodes cannot be assessed
N0	No regional lymph node metastasis
N1	Single ipsilateral lymph node ≤3 cm in greatest dimension and ENE (−)
N2[a]	
N2a[b]	1. Single ipsilateral lymph node ≤3 cm in greatest dimension and ENE (+) 2. Single ipsilateral lymph node >3 cm but <6 cm in dimension and ENE (−)
N2b	Multiple ipsilateral lymph nodes <6 cm in greatest dimension and ENE (−)
N2c	Bilateral or contralateral lymph node(s) <6 cm in greatest dimension and ENE (−)
N3[a]	
N3a	Metastasis in a lymph node >6 cm in greatest dimension and ENE (−)
N3b[b]	1. Metastasis in a single ipsilateral node >3 cm in greatest dimension and ENE (+) 2. Multiple ipsilateral, contralateral, or bilateral nodes, any with ENE (+) 3. Single contralateral node of any size and ENE (+)

M Category	M Criteria
cM0	No distant metastasis
cM1	Distant metastasis

Abbreviations: cN, clinical N; ENE, extranodal extension; M, metastasis; N, nodal; pN, pathologic N; T, primary tumor.
[a] = Subclassification present.
[b] = More than one criterion can be met to meet staging category.

select patients with adenoid cystic carcinoma.[62] Similar to acinic cell carcinoma, adenoid cystic carcinoma is associated with delayed recurrence highlighting the importance of long-term follow-up.[64,90]

The American Joint Committee on Cancer staging system for major salivary gland carcinomas is summarized in **Table 3**.

CLINICS CARE POINTS

- There is a wide range of salivary gland pathology in children.
- A thorough understanding of the differential diagnoses will allow clinicians to pursue an appropriate diagnostic evaluation that includes physical examination, laboratory studies, and imaging.
- The majority of benign salivary conditions can be treated medically prior to considering surgical interventions.
- Malignant salivary lesions require a multidisciplinary team-based approach and complete surgical excision is a primary treatment modality.

DISCLOSURE

Dr SN Amin and Mr KT Patterson were supported by the T32DC000018 from the National Institute on Deafness and Other Communication Disorders during their work on this article. The authors have no conflicts of interest to disclose.

REFERENCES

1. Carpenter GH. The secretion, components, and properties of saliva. Annu Rev Food Sci Technol 2013;4(1):267–76.
2. Hughes A, Lambert EM. Drooling and Aspiration of Saliva. Otolaryngol Clin North Am 2022;55(6):1181–94.
3. Navazesh M, Kumar SKS. Measuring salivary flow: challenges and opportunities. J Am Dent Assoc 2008;139(Suppl):35S–40S.
4. Zenk J, Hosemann WG, Iro H. Diameters of the main excretory ducts of the adult human submandibular and parotid gland: a histologic study. Oral Surg Oral Med Oral Pathol Oral Radiol Endod 1998;85(5):576–80.
5. Kochhar A, Larian B, Azizzadeh B. Facial Nerve and Parotid Gland Anatomy. Otolaryngol Clin North Am 2016;49(2):273–84.
6. Newberry TR, Kaufmann CR, Miller FR. Review of accessory parotid gland tumors: Pathologic incidence and surgical management. American Journal of Otolaryngology - Head and Neck Medicine and Surgery 2014;35(1):48–52.
7. Silvers AR, Som PM. Salivary glands. Radiol Clin North Am 1998;36(5):941–66.
8. Grewal JS, Ryan J. Anatomy, Head and Neck, Submandibular Gland. StatPearls. 2020. Available at: http://www.ncbi.nlm.nih.gov/pubmed/31194412. [Accessed 25 November 2023].
9. Chafin JB, Bayazid L. Pediatric Salivary Gland Disease. Pediatr Clin North Am 2022;69(2):363–80.
10. Wei W, Parvin MN, Tsumura K, et al. Induction of C-reactive protein, serum amyloid P component, and kininogens in the submandibular and lacrimal glands of rats with experimentally induced inflammation. Life Sci 2001;69(3):359–68.
11. Burke CJ, Thomas RH, Howlett D. Imaging the major salivary glands. Br J Oral Maxillofac Surg 2011;49(4):261–9.
12. Chen T, Szwimer R, Daniel SJ. The changing landscape of pediatric salivary gland stones: A half-century systematic review. Int J Pediatr Otorhinolaryngol 2022;159. https://doi.org/10.1016/J.IJPORL.2022.111216.
13. Jager L, Menauer F, Holzknecht N, et al. Sialolithiasis: MR sialography of the submandibular duct–an alternative to conventional sialography and US? Radiology 2000;216(3):665–71.
14. Afzelius P, Nielsen MY, Ewertsen C, et al. Imaging of the major salivary glands. Clin Physiol Funct Imaging 2016;36(1):1–10.
15. Thoeny HC. Imaging of salivary gland tumours. Cancer Imag 2007;7(1):52–62.
16. Gadodia A, Seith A, Sharma R, et al. Magnetic resonance sialography using CISS and HASTE sequences in inflammatory salivary gland diseases: comparison with digital sialography. Acta Radiol 2010;51(2):156–63.
17. Gadodia A, Bhalla AS, Sharma R, et al. MR sialography of iatrogenic sialocele: comparison with

conventional sialography. Dentomaxillofac Radiol 2011;40(3):147–53.

18. Henriksen AM, Nossent HC. Quantitative salivary gland scintigraphy can distinguish patients with primary Sjøgren's syndrome during the evaluation of sicca symptoms. Clin Rheumatol 2007;26(11): 1837–41.

19. Adadan Güvenç I. Sialorrhea: A Guide to Etiology, Assessment, and Management. In: Salivary glands - New approaches in diagnostics and treatment. IntechOpen; 2019. https://doi.org/10.5772/intechopen. 82619.

20. Isaacson J, Patel S, Torres-Yaghi Y, et al. Sialorrhea in Parkinson's Disease. Toxins 2020;12(11). https:// doi.org/10.3390/TOXINS12110691.

21. Dias BLS, Fernandes AR, Maia Filho H de S. Sialorrhea in children with cerebral palsy. J Pediatr 2016; 92(6):549–58.

22. Lakraj A, Moghimi N, Jabbari B. Sialorrhea: Anatomy, Pathophysiology and Treatment with Emphasis on the Role of Botulinum Toxins. Toxins 2013;5(5): 1010–31.

23. Thomas-Stonell N, Greenberg J. Three treatment approaches and clinical factors in the reduction of drooling. Dysphagia 1988;3(2):73–8.

24. James E, Ellis C, Brassington R, et al. Treatment for sialorrhea (excessive saliva) in people with motor neuron disease/amyotrophic lateral sclerosis. Cochrane Database Syst Rev 2022;2022(5). https:// doi.org/10.1002/14651858.CD006981.PUB3.

25. You P, Strychowsky J, Gandhi K, et al. Anticholinergic treatment for sialorrhea in children: A systematic review. Paediatr Child Health 2022;27(2):82.

26. Lovardi E, De Ioris MA, Lettori D, et al. Glycopyrrolate for drooling in children with medical complexity under three years of age. Ital J Pediatr 2022;48(1). https://doi.org/10.1186/S13052-021-01195-1.

27. Azapağası E, Kendirli T, Perk O, et al. Sublingual Atropine Sulfate Use for Sialorrhea in Pediatric Patients. J Pediatr Intensive Care 2020;9(3):196.

28. Petkus KD, Noritz G, Glader L. Examining the Role of Sublingual Atropine for the Treatment of Sialorrhea in Patients with Neurodevelopmental Disabilities: A Retrospective Review. J Clin Med 2023; 12(16):5238.

29. Türe E, Yazar A, Dündar MA, et al. Treatment of sialorrhea with botulinum toxin A injection in children. Niger J Clin Pract 2021;24(6):847–52.

30. Nigam P, Nigam A. BOTULINUM TOXIN. Indian J Dermatol 2010;55(1):8.

31. Gerlinger I, Szalai G, Hollódy K, et al. Ultrasound-guided, intraglandular injection of botulinum toxin A in children suffering from excessive salivation. J Laryngol Otol 2007;121(10):947–51.

32. Ferraz dos Santos B, Dabbagh B, Daniel SJ, et al. Association of onabotulinum toxin A treatment with salivary pH and dental caries of neurologically impaired children with sialorrhea. Int J Paediatr Dent 2016;26(1):45–51.

33. Bittmann S, Luchter E, Bittmann L, et al. Current Aspects of Treatment Options of Chronic Sialorrhea in Children. J Clin Med Res 2022;14(6):246.

34. Reed J, Mans CK, Brietzke SE. Surgical Management of Drooling: A Meta-analysis. Arch Otolaryngol Head Neck Surg 2009;135(9):924–31.

35. Ozturk K, Erdur O, Gul O, et al. Feasibility of endoscopic submandibular ganglion neurectomy for drooling. Laryngoscope 2017;127(7):1604–7.

36. Whitley MK, Zur KB. Salivary gland diseases in children. GMS Curr Top Otorhinolaryngol, Head Neck Surg 2014;13:1467–78.

37. Stong BC, Sipp JA, Sobol SE. Pediatric parotitis: A 5-year review at a tertiary care pediatric institution. Int J Pediatr Otorhinolaryngol 2006;70(3): 541–4.

38. Francis CL, Larsen CG. Pediatric sialadenitis. Otolaryngol Clin North Am 2014;47(5):763–78.

39. Michelow P, Meyers T, Dubb M, et al. The utility of fine needle aspiration in HIV positive children. Cytopathology 2008;19(2):86–93.

40. Patankar SS, Chandorkar SS, Garg A. Parotid Gland Tuberculosis: A Case Report. Indian J Surg 2012; 74(2):179.

41. Pham-Huy A, Robinson JL, Tapiéro B, et al. Current trends in nontuberculous mycobacteria infections in Canadian children: A pediatric investigators collaborative network on infections in Canada (PICNIC) study. Paediatr Child Health 2010;15(5):276–82.

42. Wolinsky E. Mycobacterial lymphadenitis in children: a prospective study of 105 nontuberculous cases with long-term follow-up. Clin Infect Dis 1995;20(4):954–63.

43. Valour F, Sénéchal A, Dupieux C, et al. Actinomycosis: etiology, clinical features, diagnosis, treatment, and management. Infect Drug Resist 2014;7:183–97.

44. Scherl C. Referateband: Rare Diseases of the Salivary Glands and of Facial Nerve. Laryngo-Rhino-Otol 2021;100(Suppl 1):S1.

45. Shah KK, Pritt BS, Alexander MP. Histopathologic review of granulomatous inflammation. J Clin Tuberc Other Mycobact Dis 2017;7:1.

46. Capaccio P, Sigismund PE, Luca N, et al. Modern management of juvenile recurrent parotitis. J Laryngol Otol 2012;126(12):1254–60.

47. Tomar RPS, Vasudevan R, Kumar M, et al. Juvenile recurrent parotitis. Med J Armed Forces India 2014;70(1):83.

48. Wood J, Toll EC, Hall F, et al. Juvenile recurrent parotitis: Review and proposed management algorithm. Int J Pediatr Otorhinolaryngol 2021;142:110617.

49. Raquel de Souto Medeiros M, César da Silva Barros C, Cristina da Costa Miguel M, et al. Necrotizing sialometaplasia: A report of two cases and review of the literature. Stomatologija, Baltic Dental and Maxillofacial Journal. 2022;24(2).

50. Randell RL, Lieberman SM. Unique Aspects of Pediatric Sjögren Disease. Rheum Dis Clin North Am 2021;47(4):707–23.

51. Wright TB. Updates in childhood Sjogren's syndrome. Curr Opin Pediatr 2022;34(2):217–22.

52. Schiffer BL, Stern SM, Park AH. Sjögren's syndrome in children with recurrent parotitis. Int J Pediatr Otorhinolaryngol 2020;129:109768.

53. Bowers EMR, Schaitkin B. Management of Mucoceles, Sialoceles, and Ranulas. Otolaryngol Clin North Am 2021;54(3):543–51.

54. Nguyen BN, Malone BN, Sidman JD, et al. Excision of sublingual gland as treatment for ranulas in pediatric patients. Int J Pediatr Otorhinolaryngol 2017;97:154–6. https://doi.org/10.1016/J.IJPORL.2017.04.003.

55. Harrison JD. Modern management and pathophysiology of ranula: literature review. Head Neck 2010; 32(10):1310–20.

56. Kraaij S, Karagozoglu KH, Forouzanfar T, et al. Salivary stones: symptoms, aetiology, biochemical composition and treatment. Br Dent J 2014; 217(11):E23.

57. Ogden MA, Rosbe KW, Chang JL. Pediatric sialendoscopy indications and outcomes. Curr Opin Otolaryngol Head Neck Surg 2016;24(6):529–35.

58. Koch M, Zenk J, Iro H. Algorithms for Treatment of Salivary Gland Obstructions. Otolaryngol Clin North Am 2009;42(6):1173–92.

59. Kessler AT, Bhatt AA. Review of the Major and Minor Salivary Glands, Part 2: Neoplasms and Tumor-like Lesions. J Clin Imaging Sci 2018;8:48.

60. Mantadakis E, Tsouvala E, Deftereos S, et al. Involution of a large parotid hemangioma with oral propranolol: an illustrative report and review of the literature. Case Rep Pediatr 2012;2012:1–5.

61. Balakrishnan K, Menezes MD, Chen BS, et al. Primary surgery vs primary sclerotherapy for head and neck lymphatic malformations. JAMA Otolaryngol Head Neck Surg 2014;140(1):41–5.

62. De Ribeiro KCB, Kowalski LP, Saba LMB, et al. Epithelial salivary glands neoplasms in children and adolescents: a forty-four-year experience. Med Pediatr Oncol 2002;39(6):594–600.

63. Xu B, Aneja A, Ghossein R, et al. Salivary gland epithelial neoplasms in pediatric population: a single-institute experience with a focus on the histologic spectrum and clinical outcome. Hum Pathol 2017;67:37–44.

64. Orvidas LJ, Kasperbauer JL, Lewis JE, et al. Pediatric parotid masses. Arch Otolaryngol Head Neck Surg 2000;126(2):177–84.

65. Sultan I, Rodriguez-Galindo C, Al-Sharabati S, et al. Salivary gland carcinomas in children and adolescents: a population-based study, with comparison to adult cases. Head Neck 2011;33(10):1476–81.

66. D'Arco F, Ugga L. Computed tomography and magnetic resonance imaging in pediatric salivary gland diseases: a guide to the differential diagnosis. Pediatr Radiol 2020;50(9):1293–307.

67. Bokhari MR, Greene J. Pleomorphic Adenoma. StatPearls. 2023. Available at: https://www.ncbi.nlm.nih.gov/books/NBK430829/. [Accessed 28 November 2023].

68. Ohtaké S, Cheng J, Ida H, et al. Precancerous foci in pleomorphic adenoma of the salivary gland: recognition of focal carcinoma and atypical tumor cells by P53 immunohistochemistry. J Oral Pathol Med 2002;31(10):590–7.

69. Bradley PJ. The recurrent pleomorphic adenoma conundrum. Curr Opin Otolaryngol Head Neck Surg 2018;26(2):134–41.

70. Witt RL, Eisele DW, Morton RP, et al. Etiology and management of recurrent parotid pleomorphic adenoma. Laryngoscope 2015;125(4):888–93.

71. Lowe LH, Stokes LS, Johnson JE, et al. Swelling at the angle of the mandible: imaging of the pediatric parotid gland and periparotid region. Radiographics 2001;21(5):1211–27.

72. Daoud EV, McLean-Holden AC, Pfeifer CM, et al. Pediatric Warthin-like Mucoepidermoid Carcinoma: Report of Two Cases with One Persistent/Recurrent as Conventional Mucoepidermoid Carcinoma. Head Neck Pathol 2020;14(4):923–8.

73. Heatley N, Harrington KJ, Thway K. Warthin Tumor-Like Mucoepidermoid Carcinoma. Int J Surg Pathol 2018;26(1):31–3.

74. Kotch C, Dombi E, Shah AC, et al. Retrospective Cohort Analysis of the Impact of Puberty on Plexiform Neurofibroma Growth in Patients with Neurofibromatosis Type 1. J Pediatr 2023. https://doi.org/10.1016/j.jpeds.2023.113513.

75. Lai JS, Jensen SE, Patel ZS, et al. Using a qualitative approach to conceptualize concerns of patients with neurofibromatosis type 1 associated plexiform neurofibromas (pNF) across the lifespan. Am J Med Genet 2017;173(1):79–87.

76. Prada CE, Rangwala FA, Martin LJ, et al. Pediatric Plexiform Neurofibromas: Impact on Morbidity and Mortality in Neurofibromatosis Type 1. J Pediatr 2012;160(3):461–7.

77. Verma J, Teh BS, Paulino AC. Characteristics and outcome of radiation and chemotherapy-related mucoepidermoid carcinoma of the salivary glands. Pediatr Blood Cancer 2011;57(7):1137–41.

78. Katabi N, Ghossein R, Ali S, et al. Prognostic features in mucoepidermoid carcinoma of major salivary glands with emphasis on tumour histologic grading. Histopathology 2014;65(6): 793–804.

79. Dombrowski ND, Wolter NE, Irace AL, et al. Mucoepidermoid carcinoma of the head and neck in children. Int J Pediatr Otorhinolaryngol 2019;120:93–9.

80. Janz TA, Camilon PR, Nguyen SA, et al. Has the management of pediatric mucoepidermoid

carcinoma of the parotid gland changed? Laryngoscope 2018;128(10):2408–14.

81. Ryan JT, El-Naggar AK, Huh W, et al. Primacy of surgery in the management of mucoepidermoid carcinoma in children. Head Neck 2011;33(12):1769–73.

82. Galer C, Santillan AA, Chelius D, et al. Minor salivary gland malignancies in the pediatric population. Head Neck 2012;34(11):1648–51.

83. Cockerill CC, Gross BC, Contag S, et al. Pediatric malignant salivary gland tumors: 60 year follow up. Int J Pediatr Otorhinolaryngol 2016;88:1–6.

84. Moon P, Tusty M, Divi V, et al. Significance of Nodal Metastasis in Parotid Gland Acinar Cell Carcinoma. Laryngoscope 2021;131(4):E1125–9.

85. Andreoli MT, Andreoli SM, Shrime MG, et al. Radiotherapy in parotid acinic cell carcinoma: does it have an impact on survival? Arch Otolaryngol Head Neck Surg 2012;138(5):463–6.

86. Neskey DM, Klein JD, Hicks S, et al. Prognostic factors associated with decreased survival in patients with acinic cell carcinoma. JAMA Otolaryngol Head Neck Surg 2013;139(11):1195–202.

87. Gomez DR, Katabi N, Zhung J, et al. Clinical and pathologic prognostic features in acinic cell carcinoma of the parotid gland. Cancer 2009;115(10):2128–37.

88. Cassidy RJ, Switchenko JM, El-Deiry MW, et al. Disparities in Postoperative Therapy for Salivary Gland Adenoid Cystic Carcinomas. Laryngoscope 2019;129(2):377–86.

89. Chen Y, Zheng ZQ, Chen FP, et al. Role of Postoperative Radiotherapy in Nonmetastatic Head and Neck Adenoid Cystic Carcinoma. J Natl Compr Cancer Netw 2020;18(11):1476–84.

90. Yoshida EJ, García J, Eisele DW, et al. Salivary gland malignancies in children. Int J Pediatr Otorhinolaryngol 2014;78(2):174–8.

Pediatric Orbital and Skull Base Pathology

Dominic Nistal, MD[a], Amy Lee, MD[a,b], Jacob Ruzevick, MD[a,b],*

KEYWORDS

- Pediatric skull base tumor • Orbital lesions • Transcranial approach
- Endoscopic endonasal approach • Transorbital approach

KEY POINTS

- The wide breadth of pediatric skull base and orbital pathologies benefit from multidisciplinary evaluation and treatment.
- Endoscopic approaches are evolving to represent the primary approach to many skull base and orbital approaches, though open transcranial approaches must remain in the arsenal of treating surgeons.
- A thorough understanding of the natural history of skull base and orbital pathologies helps to inform recommendations for treatment and long-term surveillance.

INTRODUCTION

Pediatric orbital and skull base pathologies comprise a spectrum of benign and aggressive soft tissue and bony lesions. A complex and thorough understanding of the anatomy and surgical approaches to the orbit, anterior, middle, and posterior skull base is paramount for the safe preservation of critical neurologic function.

MULTIDISCIPLINARY WORKUP OF SKULL BASE AND ORBITAL LESIONS

The clinical presentation of orbital and skull base lesions in the pediatric population can vary widely. Though the exact epidemiology is limited, the majority of patients present with some combination of proptosis, restricted extraocular movements, nasal obstruction, epistaxis, rhinorrhea, endocrinopathies, headaches, visual changes, cranial neuropathies, seizures, developmental delay, or cognitive decline with the anatomic location dictating the individual clinical presentation. Cranial and maxillofacial imaging is the corner stone for the diagnosis of pediatric skull base and orbital pathology. A combination of CT, CTA, MRI, and catheter angiography is used for the evaluation of bony, soft tissue, and vascular anatomy and pathology.

APPROACHES
Transcranial Approaches

Despite the growing popularity of endoscopic endonasal and transorbital approaches, transcranial approaches to the orbit and skull base must remain in the technical repertoire of the modern skull base surgeon. The frontotemporal, or pterional craniotomy remains the workhorse of open surgical approaches to the parasellar region and anterior skull base, allowing access to similar bony and soft tissue structures. Extending beyond standard bifrontal or frontotemporal craniotomies does improve access to skull base structures but is associated with their own challenges and potential complications. Unilateral orbital rim osteotomies provide access to the orbit and orbital apex as well as increased dural retraction for approaches to the parasellar region or even ventral brainstem. An orbital osteotomy can be combined with a zygomatic osteotomy to improve access to the basal temporal lobe or for subtemporal approaches,

[a] Department of Neurological Surgery, University of Washington, 1959 Northeast Pacific Street, Box 356470, Seattle, WA 98195, USA; [b] Seattle Children's Hospital, 4800 Sandpoint Way NE, Seattle, WA 98105, USA
* Corresponding author. 1959 Northeast Pacific Street, Box 356470, Seattle, WA 98195.
E-mail address: ruzevick@uw.edu

Oral Maxillofacial Surg Clin N Am 36 (2024) 333–342
https://doi.org/10.1016/j.coms.2024.02.003
1042-3699/24/© 2024 Elsevier Inc. All rights reserved.

though care should be taken in appropriate patient selection as craniofacial growth is only 80% complete by age 4, and at least one group has reported altered facial growth patterns following a zygomatic osteotomy.[1] For large tumors of the midline anterior skull base, a bilateral naso-orbital osteotomy minimizes the need for brain retraction as the osteotomy is flush with the floor of the anterior cranial fossa. While helpful in select cases, extensive reconstructions are needed and are often met with significant morbidity (**Fig. 1**).

Endoscopic Endonasal Approaches and Their Variants

The endoscopic endonasal approach has continued to gain in popularity over the past decade as surgeon experience has grown and surgical instruments and optics have improved. The aeration of pediatric sinuses is variable but in general does not reach mature levels until approximately 14 years.[2] This makes access to the midline anterior cranial skull base challenging in young patients as bone must be aggressively removed to provide safe access to midline skull base structures.

The direct endoscopic approach to the sella remains the foundational approach on which extended approaches are based. While a detailed, stepwise approach is described in detail elsewhere, the primary goal remains the visualization of the sella via a wide sphenoidotomy. While this approach is helpful for the treatment of primary sellar pathology such as pituitary neuroendocrine tumors or Rathke's Cleft cysts, the extension of the direct transsphenoidal approach through the tuberculum is necessary for pathology extending into the suprasellar space (**Figs. 2** and **3**). Similarly,

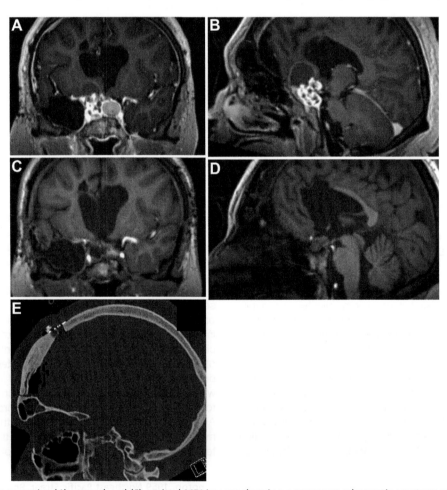

Fig. 1. Preoperative (*A*) coronal and (*B*) sagittal MRI images showing a recurrent adamantinomatous craniopharyngioma in a 16-year-old child who had previously undergone multiple endoscopic endonasal and open transcranial approaches. The lesion was approached via a bifrontal, transcranial approach. A gross total resection of tumor was achieved as shown in postoperative (*C*) coronal and (*D*) sagittal MRI images. (*E*) Postoperative sagittal CT showing cranial reconstruction.

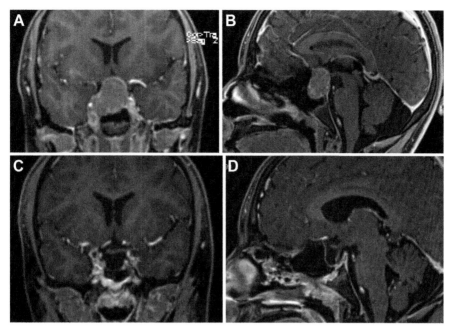

Fig. 2. Preoperative (*A*) coronal and (*B*) sagittal images showing a nonfunctional pituitary neuroendocrine tumor in a 14-year-old patient presenting with bitemporal hemianopsia. The patient underwent an endoscopic endonasal transsphenoidal approach for gross total resection (panels *C* and *D*) of tumor with preservation of pituitary function and normalization of visual fields.

for clival skull base lesions, such as chordoma, resection of the clivus and posterior clinoid processes, often with the skeletonization of the paraclival carotid arteries, are needed.

Multiple retrospective series have shown that direct endoscopic approaches to the midline skull base are safe when performed by an experienced multidisciplinary team. CSF leak remains the most common postoperative complication with an estimated rate of 10% though other potential complications include meningitis (3.8%), endocrinologic morbidity, transient (3.8%) and permanent (2.3%) cranial neuropathies, among others.[3–5] Outcomes

and evolution of endoscopic skull base reconstruction in the pediatric population remains limited, though techniques are largely borrowed from a wider experience in the adult population and include local reconstruction with surgical adjuncts to free or pedicled nasoseptal flaps.

Transorbital Approach

The transorbital neuroendoscopic (TONES) approach is a relatively new surgical approach, though it is gaining worldwide popularity due to its ability to visualize deep skull base locations

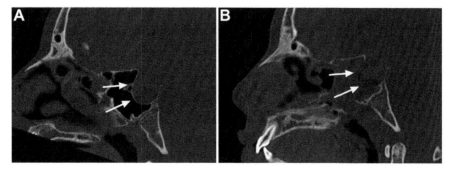

Fig. 3. (*A*) preoperative sagittal CT scan showing the expanded sella (*white arrows*) due to a nonfunctional pituitary neuroendocrine tumor in a 14-year-old patient presenting with bitemporal hemianopsia. Preoperative imaging is shown in **Fig. 2**. (*B*) postoperative sagittal CT scan showing the degree of bony removal (*white arrows*) for access to the sellar and suprasellar tumor. The floor of the sella is left intact to assist in sellar reconstruction.

without the need for craniotomy and with minimal morbidity.[6] While it can be used in isolation, its benefit often comes when used in a multi-portal strategy so as to potential avoid morbid and disfiguring transfacial approaches. Similar to the endoscopic endonasal approach, one concern limiting the application of TONES in the pediatric population remains the size and subsequent development of the orbit.[7] While the majority of reported TONES cases have been performed in adults, available pediatric series' show this approach is safe and not associated with alterations in normal orbital development (**Fig. 4**).[8,9]

CONGENITAL SKULL BASE LESIONS

Congenital skull base lesions are commonly a result of embryologic abnormalities due to a failure of closure of the anterior neuropore, resulting in dermoid cysts and encephaloceles.[10] Their incidence is rare, only occurring 1 in every 20,000 to 40,000 births, and often present secondary to a CSF leak or infection.[11,12]

1. Dermoid cysts

Dermoid cysts develop secondary to a failure of dural involution and closure resulting in the entrapment of ectodermal elements along the lines of embryonic closure.[13] These lesions are benign and result in stratified squamous epithelium lined cysts filled with keratin debris and hair. They are typically slow growing with less than 35% of these lesions extending into the bone or epidural

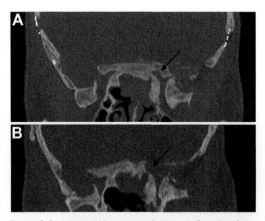

Fig. 4. (*A*) preoperative coronal CT scan showing bony growth and stenosis of the left optic canal (*black arrow*) with subsequent vision decline in a 15-year-old patient with neurofibromatosis type 2. A transorbital neuroendoscopic approach was performed for optic nerve decompression with (*B*) coronal CT showing 180-degree decompression of the optic nerve within the optic canal (*black arrow*). Postoperatively, the patient had improvement in vision.

space.[14] Approximately 40% of cases are identified at birth with up to approximately 60% of cases identified by 5 years of age.[15] They typically present as a midline firm subcutaneous dome-shaped lesion that is frequently asymptomatic and nonpulsatile, and can secrete sebaceous material that can result in inflammation and/or infection.[13,16] Treatment is directed toward those lesions extending into the intracranial space to prevent potential meningitis or abscess formation.

2. Skull base dehiscence/encephalocele

Skull base encephaloceles are a heterogenous group of skull defects resulting in the herniation of any combination of brain, cerebrospinal fluid, or dura through the skull. They can be a result of a congenital defect of the anterior neuropore whereby there is failure of closure of the skull resulting in skull base dehiscence and protrusion of neural elements or a result of trauma, prior craniotomy, or erosion secondary to a mass lesion or elevated intracranial pressure.[17]

While not considered a surgical emergency, anterior skull base encephaloceles carry the risk of cerebrospinal fluid leak and resultant meningitis. For defects in the anterior skull base including the sphenoid and ethmoid regions, the endoscopic endonasal approach is the favored approach as it allows a direct trajectory view of the defect with the opportunity for multiple reconstructive options without a disfiguring scar or morbid transcranial approach.[18] For nonskull base anterior craniofacial encephaloceles, the goal of surgery remains the reduction/resection of the herniated brain tissue, repair of the dural defect, reconstruction of the skull defect, and resection of excess skin.

SKULL BASE NEOPLASMS

1. Juvenile Nasopharyngeal Angiofibroma (JNA)

Juvenile nasopharyngeal angiofibroma is a rare, benign, angiofibromatous hamartoma originating from the sphenopalatine foramen.[19] While histologically benign, it characteristically invades throughout the nasal cavity and paranasal sinuses including the pterygopalatine fossa causing the obstruction of mucous and airflow as well as painless epistaxis. Larger lesions can extend throughout the sphenoid and maxillary sinuses and extend into the infratemporal fossa, orbit, or middle cranial fossa.[19,20] They almost exclusively develop in adolescent boys with many tumors showing limited growth beyond young adulthood.[21]

Surgical resection is the mainstay treatment. Preoperative endovascular embolization is especially helpful so as to avoid potentially catastrophic hemorrhage during resection. In cases of advanced disease with significant residual tumor, radiation therapy is a potential adjuvant therapy with multiple series showing tumor control rates between 80% and 90%.[20,22] Medical therapy including hormone or cytotoxic therapy remains limited and their use rarely results in meaningful tumor response.[23]

2. Rhabdomyosarcoma

Rhabdomyosarcoma is a rare soft tissue sarcoma arising from primitive mesenchymal origin and is the most common childhood soft tissue sarcoma compromising approximately 50% of pediatric soft tissue sarcomas and 3% of childhood tumors.[24] It arises from skeletal muscle and typically presents as an enlarging, painless subcutaneous mass.[25] The embryonal subtype occurs more frequently in the head and neck with initial treatment being surgical resection, especially for those patients with localized disease.[26] Patients with a skull base or intracranial extension of disease tend to be diagnosed later in their disease course, leading to poorer prognosis and likely requirement for additional radiation and chemotherapy.[27]

3. Midline skull base lesions

Midline skull base lesions include sellar and parasellar lesions involving the pituitary gland, infundibulum, or parasellar skull base structures as well as clival and petroclival lesions. The most common pathologies in the midline skull base in children include pituitary or infundibular neoplastic lesions, such as pituitary neuroendocrine tumors or craniopharyngioma as well as benign cystic lesions, such as Rathke's cleft cysts. Midline clival lesions include chordoma or aneurysmal bone cysts, among others.

a. Pituitary neuroendocrine tumors

Pituitary neuroendocrine tumors in children comprise approximately 3% of intracranial tumors in the pediatric population.[28,29] Management of pediatric pituitary neuroendocrine tumors benefits from multidisciplinary evaluation by neurosurgeons, skull base rhinologists/otolaryngologists, endocrinologists, and ophthalmologists. Surgical resection of nonfunctional pituitary neuroendocrine tumors is primarily guided by neurologic or endocrine deficits associated with a mass effect on the optic chiasm or pituitary gland. Functional tumors, such as ACTH- or GH -secreting tumors are best treated with upfront surgery for attempted biochemical remission. Prolactin-secreting pituitary neuroendocrine tumors generally are best treated with

dopamine agonists as a first line therapy. In cases of treatment refractory disease or intolerance to medical therapy, surgery can be considered, though long-term biochemical remission is uncommon.[30] The need for adjuvant therapy or repeat surgical resection for secretory tumors has been reported as high as 30% to 50%.[28]

b. Rathke's Cleft Cyst

Rathke's cleft cysts (RCC) are rare lesions in children which arise from Rathke's pouch remnants due to a failure of obliteration of the craniopharyngeal duct, resulting in an expansile midline pituitary cystic lesion.[31] They are most commonly discovered in imaging workup for associated endocrine (frequently growth hormone deficit due to compression of the pituitary gland), visual deficits (due to compression of the optic chiasm), or headaches.[32,33] Treatment includes observation for those patients without symptoms secondary to mass effect on the pituitary gland or optic chiasm or fenestration via the endoscopic endonasal approach for symptomatic patients. Surgical morbidity related to these lesions is comparable to the adult population including diabetes insipidus and cerebrospinal fluid leak, occurring in approximately 20% and 25% of patients, respectively.[31–33]

c. Craniopharyngioma

Pediatric craniopharyngioma is a complex pathology requiring multidisciplinary collaboration as it leads to significant morbidity including endocrinologic dysfunction, visual changes, and potential hypothalamic dysfunction. Adamantinomatous craniopharyngioma is predominantly seen in children and young adults and is thought to arise from remnants of ectodermal cells during embryogenesis due to failure of obliteration of the craniopharyngeal duct.[34] Initial management of pediatric craniopharyngioma remains controversial with options including attempt at surgical gross total resection versus surgical biopsy with subsequent radiation therapy. Benefits of surgical resection include immediate decompression of the optic chiasm and resection of tumor that may invade the third ventricle as well as decompression of the hypothalamus. Risks of a purely surgical approach include sinonasal morbidity, risk of vascular injury, likely panhypopituitarism including diabetes insipidus, devascularization of the undersurface of the optic chiasm causing visual decline, iatrogenic injury to the hypothalamus and adjacent brain structures, and complications associated with complex skull base reconstruction. Alternatively, the risk of radiation therapy includes delayed panhypopituitarism, growth of tumor-associated cysts, neurocognitive changes, delayed vascular changes, or potential radiation induced neoplasms in the future, among others.[35] Following initial treatment, tumor and/or cyst recurrence is common. Surgical resection or fenestration is often recommended once previously treated with radiation. Catheter-based approaches with the injection of local chemotherapy for the treatment of expanding cysts can also be considered though open approaches are preferred to stereotactic approaches given the risk of injury to adjacent structures due to a firm cyst wall causing an errant course of a catheter.[36]

d. Chordoma

Clival chordoma is an invasive, slow growing, and frequently recurring subtype of sarcoma. They arise from remnants of the notochord and are pathologically defined by the presence of brachyury. Patients often present with cranial neuropathies, most frequently a 6th nerve palsy, or after incidental discovery in workup of other pathology (headaches, tonsillar evaluation, or sinusitis).[37] The first line therapy for skull base chordoma is surgical resection for an attempt at gross total resection.[37] However, complete surgical resection of the skull base chordoma is challenging given the small working corridors and risk to critical neurovascular structures adjacent to the clivus. Given its location, the extended endoscopic endonasal approach is preferred given the trajectory view to the clivus. Extensive bony resection is frequently required, including the skeletonization of the paraclival carotid arteries as well as the resection of the posterior clinoid processes with subsequent complex skull base reconstruction via pedicled naso-septal flaps.

SKULL BASE FIBROOSSEOUS LESIONS

Fibroosseous lesions of the skull base are both erosive and expansile lesions whereby normal bone is replaced by the variable growth of fibroblasts. They are generally benign, though they can devolve into neoplastic lesions requiring more aggressive treatment.[38]

1. Fibrous dysplasia

Fibrous dysplasia is a benign lesion that characterized by the replacement of normal bone and marrow with fibrous tissue intermixed with irregular mixed woven bone.[39] The majority of cases occur spontaneously in affected regions of the head and neck resulting in craniofacial abnormalities or stenosis of the cranial foramina and subsequent cranial neuropathies.[38,40] The majority of head and neck or skull base fibrous dysplasia is incidentally discovered or asymptomatic and requires only periodic imaging evaluation. In cases affecting cranial foramina, simple decompression can save or restore neurologic function either through transcranial, transorbital, or endoscopic endonasal approaches.[38]

2. Osteoma

Osteoid osteoma is the most common benign bony lesion of the anterior skull base in children.[41] They are often asymptomatic and frequently discovered incidentally. They are benign lesions without the risk of malignant transformation. The most common location for osteoma in the anterior skull base is the paranasal sinuses and frontal sinus.[42] While many are asymptomatic, the most common symptomatic presentation is pain localized to the osteoma. Conservative treatment with nonsteroidal antiinflammatory medications is the recommended first line therapy. Surgical management is directed toward the management of symptoms such as pain that is not responsive to medical therapy, cosmetic disruption, or cranial neuropathies.[43,44]

3. Aneurysmal Bone Cyst

Aneurysmal bone cyst is a rare benign vascular lesion that can grow aggressively in any bone causing local destruction and structural weakening.[45] When present within the skull base or facial bones, patients typically present with an insidious onset of pain or headaches. Treatment is recommended as there have been case reports of malignant transformation of these lesions, which involves curettage of the affected bone.[46]

4. Juvenile Ossifying fibroma

Juvenile ossifying fibroma is a benign but highly destructive lesion typically presenting as a rapidly growing craniofacial lesion, often leading to skull base and facial deformity.[38] There are two categories of juvenile ossifying fibroma; psammomatoid and trabecular, with the trabecular subtype typically affecting the mandible whereas psammomatoid lesions more frequently affecting the anterior skull base, nasal sinuses, and orbits.[47] Treatment is directed to limit bony deformity, decompression of critical structures, and preservation of adjacent neurovascular structures. Aggressive lesional resection with adjacent bone is required as juvenile ossifying fibromas have high rates of recurrence.[48]

ORBITAL LESIONS

1. Neuroblastoma

Neuroblastoma is the most common extracranial tumor in children, originating from neural crest progenitor cells.[49] The most common site of origin is the adrenal glands with orbital neuroblastoma being a rare presentation.[50] Orbital neuroblastoma is most commonly a metastatic lesion, but it has also been described as a primary lesion.[51] Typically, patients will present with periorbital ecchymoses, proptosis, or visual symptoms. Delay in diagnosis can lead to compromise of orbital structures and development of intracranial extension. Treatment is dependent on tumor location, grade, stage, and risk to adjacent neurologic structures. Multidisciplinary evaluation can help guide decision making regarding surgical resection via craniotomy or TONES as well as chemo/immunotherapy, radiation therapy, or stem cell transplantation.[51]

2. Optic pathway glioma

Optic pathway glioma describes primary lesions of the optic apparatus (nerve and chiasm), optic tracts, optic radiations, or hypothalamus. They are histologically grade 1 pilocytic astrocytoma that originate anatomically along the optic pathway and can arise sporadically or be associated with the tumor predisposition syndrome, neurofibromatosis type 1.[52] Presentation is dependent upon tumor location and includes vision loss, proptosis, headaches, and hydrocephalus. Following the diagnosis of optic pathway glioma, observation is frequently used with a stable lesional appearance and visual examination. Surgical resection or debulking is reserved for cases causing compression or extension to other critical structures along the optic pathway that may not have tumor involvement, including contralateral optic structures or periorbital structures. Surgical resection or tumor debulking has not been shown to improve survival or morbidity and therefore has grown out of favor as a primary therapy for these lesions.[53]

3. Plexiform neurofibroma

Neurofibromas are common benign nerve sheath tumors that can occur anywhere along the neural or cutaneous axis. Plexiform neurofibromas (PN) are pathognomonic for neurofibromatosis type 1 and have a higher risk of malignant transformation than localized or diffuse neurofibromas.[54] Surgical resection is the mainstay of treatment as these tumors typically do not respond to radiation or chemotherapy.[55] Lesions involving the skull base commonly show widening of the exiting cranial nerve foramina as well as spread into adjacent soft tissue spaces.[56] The recurrence rate for large skull base PN's is high, with the mean time to recurrence being between 2 and 3 years after surgical resection.[56]

4. Leukemia, Lymphoproliferative disease, and Orbital inflammatory syndrome

Ocular involvement of leukemia or other lymphoproliferative diseases is rare and can be primary or secondary upon presentation.[57] Infiltration of disease into the cranial nerves can lead to papilledema, visual deficits, or cranial neuropathies with restrictions on extraocular movements. Current treatment for ocular leukemia is nonsurgical including systemic therapy, radiotherapy, or intravitreal steroids or chemotherapy agents.[58]

Orbital inflammatory syndrome (OIS) is a rare, benign, noninfectious inflammatory process typically presenting with edema, a mass-like periorbital lesion, and other systemic signs of inflammation including headache, fatigue, nausea, and vomiting.[59] Medical intervention is the most effective treatment with corticosteroid administration resulting in 75% symptomatic improvement and a nearly 40% cure rate.[60] Surgery is reserved for severe cases that are nonresponsive to medical therapy or those requiring biopsy due to diagnostic uncertainty.[61]

5. Langerhans Cell Histiocytosis

Langerhans cell histiocytosis (LCH) is a reactive and potentially neoplastic process whereby there is an abnormal proliferation of antigen presenting immune cells (Langerhans cells). Similar to OIS, these lesions respond well to medical therapies including chemotherapy and radiation.[62] A biopsy for the confirmation of diagnosis followed by surgical excision is the mainstay of treatment given that orbital LCH is typically an isolated process and preservation of the orbital and periorbital structures is best achieved with targeted resection.[63]

6. Vascular lesions

Vascular lesions of the orbit consist of vascular proliferative tumors, vascular malformations, and their subtypes. These include hemangiomas, venous malformations, arteriovenous malformations, arteriovenous fistulas, and cavernous malformations.[64]

Orbital hemangioma can present as either an infantile or congenital subtype. Infantile hemangioma is more common, usually discovered at birth or soon after due to a proliferative phase in the first 6 to 12 months of life.[65] Medical therapy with beta-blockers is the first line and most effective form of therapy.[66] Congenital hemangiomas present at birth without a proliferative phase and do not typically regress spontaneously. No medical therapy has demonstrated clinical benefit for congenital hemangiomas, which are thus more frequently considered for surgical resection in conjunction with preoperative embolization.[67]

Vascular malformations of the orbit can present either spontaneously or as a result of syndromic disease such as Sturge-Weber, Klippel-Trenaunay, or Parks Weber syndromes. Typically, vascular lesions of the orbit are found incidentally, and observation is often first line management. However, surgical or interventional therapies are indicated in cases of symptomatic progression.[68]

SUMMARY

Pediatric orbital and skull base pathologies encompass a breadth of inflammatory, sporadic, syndromic, and neoplastic processes which require a broad and complex clinical approach for both medical and surgical treatment of these diverse lesions. The intricate anatomy of the anterior skull base and orbit make the clinical presentation and natural history of these disease processes extremely challenging to diagnose and manage. However, a multidisciplinary approach in both the diagnostic and treatment phases of care allows for a significant positive clinical impact and a high chance of cure. Advances in minimally invasive surgical approaches, including endoscopic endonasal and transorbital approaches allows for more targeted surgical approaches through smaller corridors without sacrificing working angles and allowing for shorter hospital stays with low rates of surgical morbidity.

CLINICS CARE POINTS

- Pediatric skull base and orbital pathologies represent a diverse spectrum of disease with potential catastrophic clinical outcomes.
- Endoscopic approaches are evolving to allow for more minimally invasive approaches to the skull base and orbit without sacrificing visualization or working angles.
- A more thorough understanding of the molecular drivers of pediatric skull base and orbital disease will allow for targeted therapies, potentially preventing the morbidity associated with maximally and minimally invasive surgical approaches.

DISCLOSURE

All authors confirm there are no commercial or financial conflicts of interest.

REFERENCES

1. Hanbali F, Tabrizi P, Lang FF, et al. Tumors of the skull base in children and adolescents. J Neurosurg 2004;100(2 Suppl Pediatrics):169–78.
2. Scuderi AJ, Harnsberger HR, Boyer RS. Pneumatization of the paranasal sinuses: normal features of importance to the accurate interpretation of CT scans and MR images. AJR Am J Roentgenol 1993;160(5):1101–4.
3. Lopez EM, Farzal Z, Dean KM, et al. Outcomes in Pediatric Endoscopic Skull Base Surgery: A Systematic Review. J Neurol Surg B Skull Base 2023;84(1):24–37.
4. Chivukula S, Koutourousiou M, Snyderman CH, et al. Endoscopic endonasal skull base surgery in the pediatric population. J Neurosurg Pediatr 2013;11(3):227–41.
5. McDowell MM, Zwagerman NT, Wang EW, et al. Long-term outcomes in the treatment of pediatric skull base chordomas in the endoscopic endonasal era. J Neurosurg Pediatr 20 2020;27(2):170–9.
6. Moe KS, Bergeron CM, Ellenbogen RG. Transorbital neuroendoscopic surgery. Neurosurgery 2010;67(3 Suppl Operative):ons16–28.
7. Escaravage GK Jr, Dutton JJ. Age-related changes in the pediatric human orbit on CT. Ophthalmic Plast Reconstr Surg 2013;29(3):150–6.
8. Balakrishnan K, Moe KS. Applications and outcomes of orbital and transorbital endoscopic surgery. Otolaryngol Head Neck Surg 2011;144(5):815–20.
9. Dallan I, Cristofani-Mencacci L, Fiacchini G, et al. Endoscopic-assisted transorbital surgery: Where do we stand on the scott's parabola? personal considerations after a 10-year experience. Front Oncol 2022;12:937818.
10. Adil E, Robson C, Perez-Atayde A, et al. Congenital nasal neuroglial heterotopia and encephaloceles: an update on current evaluation and management. Laryngoscope 2016;126(9):2161–7.
11. Hughes GB, Sharpino G, Hunt W, et al. Management of the congenital midline nasal mass: a review. Head Neck Surg 1980;2(3):222–33.
12. Riley CA, Soneru CP, Overdevest JB, et al. Pediatric sinonasal and skull base lesions. World J Otorhinolaryngol Head Neck Surg 2020;6(2):118–24.
13. Julapalli MR, Cohen BA, Hollier LH, et al. Congenital, ill-defined, yellowish plaque: the nasal dermoid. Pediatr Dermatol 2006;23(6):556–9.
14. Prior A, Anania P, Pacetti M, et al. Dermoid and Epidermoid Cysts of Scalp: Case Series of 234 Consecutive Patients. World Neurosurg 2018;120:119–24.
15. Orozco-Covarrubias L, Lara-Carpio R, Saez-De-Ocariz M, et al. Dermoid cysts: a report of 75 pediatric patients. Pediatr Dermatol 2013;30(6):706–11.

16. Nakajima K, Korekawa A, Nakano H, et al. Subcutaneous dermoid cysts on the eyebrow and neck. Pediatr Dermatol 2019;36(6):999–1001.

17. Gump WC. Endoscopic Endonasal Repair of Congenital Defects of the Anterior Skull Base: Developmental Considerations and Surgical Outcomes. J Neurol Surg B Skull Base 2015;76(4):291–5.

18. Komotar RJ, Starke RM, Raper DM, et al. Endoscopic endonasal versus open repair of anterior skull base CSF leak, meningocele, and encephalocele: a systematic review of outcomes. J Neurol Surg A Cent Eur Neurosurg 2013;74(4):239–50.

19. Alshaikh NA, Eleftheriadou A. Juvenile nasopharyngeal angiofibroma staging: An overview. Ear Nose Throat J 2015;94(6):E12–22.

20. Mallick S, Benson R, Bhasker S, et al. Long-term treatment outcomes of juvenile nasopharyngeal angiofibroma treated with radiotherapy. Acta Otorhinolaryngol Ital 2015;35(2):75–9.

21. Guertl B, Beham A, Zechner R, et al. Nasopharyngeal angiofibroma: an APC-gene-associated tumor? Hum Pathol 2000;31(11):1411–3.

22. Min HJ, Chung HJ, Kim CH. Delayed cerebrospinal fluid rhinorrhea four years after gamma knife surgery for juvenile angiofibroma. J Craniofac Surg 2014; 25(6):e565–7.

23. Scholfield DW, Brundler MA, McDermott AL, et al. Adjunctive Treatment in Juvenile Nasopharyngeal Angiofibroma: How Should We Approach Recurrence? J Pediatr Hematol Oncol 2016;38(3):235–9.

24. Sultan I, Qaddoumi I, Yaser S, et al. Comparing adult and pediatric rhabdomyosarcoma in the surveillance, epidemiology and end results program, 1973 to 2005: an analysis of 2,600 patients. J Clin Oncol 2009;27(20):3391–7.

25. Dagher R, Helman L. Rhabdomyosarcoma: an overview. Oncol 1999;4(1):34–44.

26. Daya H, Chan HS, Sirkin W, et al. Pediatric rhabdomyosarcoma of the head and neck: is there a place for surgical management? Arch Otolaryngol Head Neck Surg 2000;126(4):468–72.

27. Radzikowska J, Kukwa W, Kukwa A, et al. Management of pediatric head and neck rhabdomyosarcoma: A case-series of 36 patients. Oncol Lett 2016;12(5):3555–62.

28. Perry A, Graffeo CS, Marcellino C, et al. Pediatric Pituitary Adenoma: Case Series, Review of the Literature, and a Skull Base Treatment Paradigm. J Neurol Surg B Skull Base 2018;79(1):91–114.

29. Chen J, Schmidt RE, Dahiya S. Pituitary Adenoma in Pediatric and Adolescent Populations. J Neuropathol Exp Neurol 2019;78(7):626–32.

30. Petersenn S, Fleseriu M, Casanueva FF, et al. Diagnosis and management of prolactin-secreting pituitary adenomas: a Pituitary Society international Consensus Statement. Nat Rev Endocrinol 2023; 19(12):722–40.

31. Trifanescu R, Ansorge O, Wass JA, et al. Rathke's cleft cysts. Clin Endocrinol (Oxf) 2012;76(2):151–60.

32. Jahangiri A, Molinaro AM, Tarapore PE, et al. Rathke cleft cysts in pediatric patients: presentation, surgical management, and postoperative outcomes. Neurosurg Focus 2011;31(1):E3.

33. Higuchi Y, Hasegawa K, Kubo T, et al. The clinical course of Rathke's cleft cysts in pediatric patients: impact on growth and pubertal development. Clin Pediatr Endocrinol 2022;31(1):38–43.

34. Miller DC. Pathology of craniopharyngiomas: clinical import of pathological findings. Pediatr Neurosurg 1994;21(Suppl 1):11–7.

35. Edmonston DY, Wu S, Li Y, et al. Limited surgery and conformal photon radiation therapy for pediatric craniopharyngioma: long-term results from the RT1 protocol. Neuro Oncol 2022;24(12):2200–9.

36. Zhang S, Fang Y, Cai BW, et al. Intracystic bleomycin for cystic craniopharyngiomas in children. Cochrane Database Syst Rev 2016;7(7):Cd008890.

37. Rassi MS, Hulou MM, Almefty K, et al. Pediatric Clival Chordoma: A Curable Disease that Conforms to Collins' Law. Neurosurgery 2018;82(5): 652–60.

38. Wilson M, Snyderman C. Fibro-Osseous Lesions of the Skull Base in the Pediatric Population. J Neurol Surg B Skull Base 2018;79(1):31–6.

39. Ma J, Liang L, Gu B, et al. A retrospective study on craniofacial fibrous dysplasia: preoperative serum alkaline phosphatase as a prognostic marker? J Cranio-Maxillo-Fac Surg 2013;41(7):644–7.

40. Robinson C, Collins MT, Boyce AM. Fibrous Dysplasia/McCune-Albright Syndrome: Clinical and Translational Perspectives. Curr Osteoporos Rep 2016;14(5):178–86.

41. Ren X, Yang L, Duan XJ. Three-dimensional printing in the surgical treatment of osteoid osteoma of the calcaneus: A case report. J Int Med Res 2017; 45(1):372–80.

42. Sofokleous V, Maragoudakis P, Kyrodimos E, et al. Management of paranasal sinus osteomas: a comprehensive narrative review of the literature and an up-to-date grading system. Am J Otolaryngol 2021;42(5):102644.

43. Langlie JA, Hullfish H, Jabori SK, et al. Diagnosis and Management of Craniofacial Osteomas. J Craniofac Surg 2023;34(5):1515–21.

44. Boffano P, Roccia F, Campisi P, et al. Review of 43 osteomas of the craniomaxillofacial region. J Oral Maxillofac Surg 2012;70(5):1093–5.

45. Schreuder HW, Veth RP, Pruszczynski M, et al. Aneurysmal bone cysts treated by curettage, cryotherapy and bone grafting. J Bone Joint Surg Br 1997;79(1):20–5.

46. Brindley GW, Greene JF Jr, Frankel LS. Case reports: malignant transformation of aneurysmal bone cysts. Clin Orthop Relat Res 2005;438:282–7.

47. Thompson L. World Health Organization classification of tumours: pathology and genetics of head and neck tumours. Ear Nose Throat J 2006;85(2):74.

48. Aggarwal S, Garg A, Aggarwal A, et al. Juvenile ossifying fibroma: Psammamatoid variant. Contemp Clin Dent 2012;3:330–3.

49. Matthay KK, Maris JM, Schleiermacher G, et al. Neuroblastoma. Nat Rev Dis Primers 2016;2:16078.

50. Yang WJ, Zhou YY, Zhao F, et al. Orbital neuroblastoma metastasis: A case report and literature review. Medicine (Baltimore) 2019;98(36):e17038.

51. Vallinayagam M, Rao VA, Pandian DG, et al. Primary orbital neuroblastoma with intraocular extension. Indian J Ophthalmol 2015;63(8):684–6.

52. Robert-Boire V, Rosca L, Samson Y, et al. Clinical Presentation and Outcome of Patients With Optic Pathway Glioma. Pediatr Neurol 2017;75:55–60.

53. Farazdaghi MK, Katowitz WR, Avery RA. Current treatment of optic nerve gliomas. Curr Opin Ophthalmol 2019;30(5):356–63.

54. Hernández-Martín A, Duat-Rodríguez A. An Update on Neurofibromatosis Type 1: Not Just Café-au-Lait Spots, Freckling, and Neurofibromas. An Update. Part I. Dermatological Clinical Criteria Diagnostic of the Disease. Actas Dermosifiliogr 2016;107(6):454–64. Neurofibromatosis tipo 1: más que manchas café con leche, efélides y neurofibromas. Parte I. Actualización sobre los criterios dermatológicos diagnósticos de la enfermedad. doi:10.1016/j.ad.2016.01.004.

55. Kebudi R, Cakir FB, Gorgun O. Interferon-α for unresectable progressive and symptomatic plexiform neurofibromas. J Pediatr Hematol Oncol 2013;35(3):e115–7.

56. Wise JB, Cryer JE, Belasco JB, et al. Management of head and neck plexiform neurofibromas in pediatric patients with neurofibromatosis type 1. Arch Otolaryngol Head Neck Surg 2005;131(8):712–8.

57. de Queiroz Mendonca C, Freire MV, Viana SS, et al. Ocular manifestations in acute lymphoblastic leukemia: A five-year cohort study of pediatric patients. Leuk Res 2019;76:24–8.

58. Vishnevskia-Dai V, Sella King S, Lekach R, et al. Ocular Manifestations of Leukemia and Results of Treatment with Intravitreal Methotrexate. Sci Rep 2020;10(1). 1994.

59. Espinoza GM. Orbital inflammatory pseudotumors: etiology, differential diagnosis, and management. Curr Rheumatol Rep 2010;12(6):443–7.

60. Reggie S, Neimkin M, Holds J. Intralesional corticosteroid injections as treatment for non-infectious orbital inflammation. Orbit 2018;37(1):41–7.

61. Yeşiltaş YS, Gündüz AK. Idiopathic Orbital Inflammation: Review of Literature and New Advances. Middle East Afr J Ophthalmol 2018;25(2):71–80.

62. DiCaprio MR, Roberts TT. Diagnosis and management of langerhans cell histiocytosis. J Am Acad Orthop Surg 2014;22(10):643–52.

63. Herwig MC, Wojno T, Zhang Q, et al. Langerhans cell histiocytosis of the orbit: five clinicopathologic cases and review of the literature. Surv Ophthalmol 2013;58(4):330–40.

64. Colafati GS, Piccirilli E, Marrazzo A, et al. Vascular lesions of the pediatric orbit: A radiological walk-through. Front Pediatr 2022;10:734286.

65. Sullivan TJ. Vascular Anomalies of the Orbit–A Reappraisal. Asia Pac J Ophthalmol (Phila). 2018; 7(5):356–63.

66. Sethuraman G, Yenamandra VK, Gupta V. Management of infantile hemangiomas: current trends. J Cutan Aesthet Surg 2014;7(2):75–85.

67. Leung AKC, Lam JM, Leong KF, et al. Infantile Hemangioma: An Updated Review. Curr Pediatr Rev 2021;17(1):55–69.

68. Wu ZY, Yan JH, Han J, et al. Diagnosis and surgical management of 209 cases of orbital cavernous hemangioma. Zhonghua Yan Ke Za Zhi 2006;42(4):323–5.

Pediatric Cranial Vault Pathology

Andrew D. Linkugel, MD[a,b], Erin E. Anstadt, MD[a,b], Jason Hauptman, MD, PhD[b,c], Russell E. Ettinger, MD[a,b],*

KEYWORDS

• Pediatric • Skull • Reconstruction • Bone tumor

KEY POINTS

- Pathology of the pediatric cranial vault is best approached in a multidisciplinary manner.
- Extent of planned resection, need for adjuvant therapy, soft tissue coverage, and remaining growth of the skull are all critical considerations in pediatric cranial vault pathology.
- In general, reconstruction with autologous bone of calvarial defects is preferred.

INTRODUCTION

Bone and soft tissue tumors originating from the calvarium are extremely rare, comprising approximately 2% of all musculoskeletal tumors.[1] Fortunately, the majority of primary skull masses are surgically curable and have favorable outcomes with low recurrence rates.[2,3] Here, we aim to describe their distribution and characteristics, approach to diagnosis, and briefly discuss treatment options.

Scalp and skull lesions are defined as abnormal masses of the calvarium from the external occipital protuberance to the supraorbital margin. They may involve skin, subcutaneous tissue, galea, pericranium, and calvarial bone.[4] Many pediatric scalp and skull masses are congenital or developmental tumors. Cranial bone tumors can be divided into benign, malignant, and undefined neoplasms. Benign congenital tumors, such as dermoid cysts, are more common in neonates, while malignant and aggressive lesions are more likely to present in older children.[5] Calvarial tumors can extend from the bone toward the scalp or can extend intracranially; intracranial extension occurs at a reported rate of 37% to 57%.[5,6] Intraosseous

calvarial lesions are often slowly progressive. They may be asymptomatic or characterized by swelling, local pain, or sensitivity.[5,7] In general, clinical management varies depending on the diagnosis: most benign lesions require complete excision only, while malignant lesions potentially require resection plus adjuvant therapies.[7]

CRANIOSYNOSTOSIS

Craniosynostosis represents a clinically significant entity and is among the most common cranial vault pathologies seen in infants and children. Craniosynostosis refers to the premature fusion of one or more cranial sutures and has associated characteristic phenotypes related to the suture(s) involved (**Fig. 1**).[8] It has an incidence estimated to be 1 in every 2500 births.[9,10] It can be seen as part of a syndrome or as an isolated finding; more than 80% of cases seen are considered isolated or nonsyndromic.[10] Single-suture craniosynostosis restricts skull growth perpendicular to the affected suture, and compensatory growth is often seen in the unaffected regions of the skull. Sagittal synostosis remains the most common type of single-suture synostosis, with an incidence of 1 in 2000 to 5000

a Division of Plastic Surgery, Seattle Children's Hospital, University of Washington School of Medicine, Seattle, WA, USA; b Craniofacial Center, Seattle Children's Hospital, 4800 Sand Point Way Northeast, Seattle, WA 98105, USA; c Department of Neurosurgery, Seattle Children's Hospital, University of Washington School of Medicine, Seattle, WA, USA
* Corresponding author. Seattle Children's Hospital, 4800 Sand Point Way NE, M/S OB.9.520, Seattle, WA 98105.
E-mail address: russell.ettinger@seattlechildrens.org

Oral Maxillofacial Surg Clin N Am 36 (2024) 343–353
https://doi.org/10.1016/j.coms.2024.03.003
1042-3699/24/© 2024 Elsevier Inc. All rights are reserved, including those for text and data mining, AI training, and similar technologies.

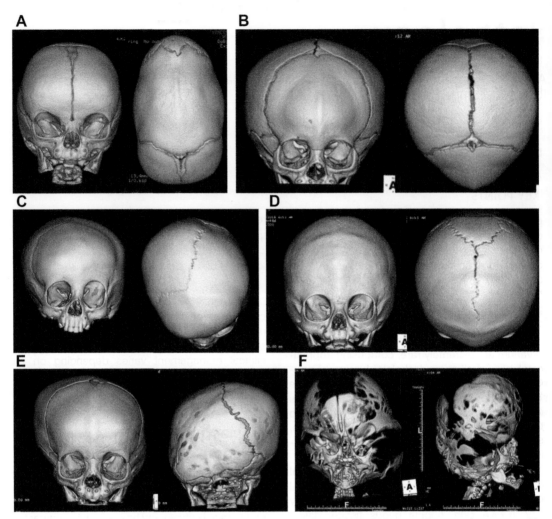

Fig. 1. Patterns of calvarial vault dysmorphology in craniosynostosis. Sagittal craniosynostosis is characterized by scaphocephaly with frontal bossing and occipital bulleting (*A*). Metopic craniosynostosis is characterized by trigonocephaly with angulation of the zygomaticofrontal sutures (*B*). Unicoronal craniosynostosis is characterized by flattening of the ipsilateral frontoparietal area with elevation and retrusion of the ipsilateral superior orbit (*C*). Bicoronal craniosynostosis is characterized by turribrachycephaly (*D*). Lambdoid craniosynostosis is characterized by occipital bossing and skull base tilt (*E*). Multisuture craniosynostosis, such as in this case of Pfeiffer syndrome (*F*), can result in a kleeblattschadel (cloverleaf) skull deformity with increased intracranial pressure resulting in a "copper-beaten" pattern of the calvarial bone.

live births.[8,11] Etiology and pathogenesis for this condition are not completely understood.[9,10] Several genetic mutations have been implicated in the development of syndromic and nonsyndromic craniosynostosis, including mutations in fibroblast growth factor receptor genes (FGFR1, FGFR2, FGFR3; multisuture), the BBS9 gene (isolated sagittal), and FREM1 and SMAD6 genes (metopic). Other hypotheses, including intrauterine constraint and environmental exposures (such as smoking, antacids, nutritional deficiencies), have also been considered but remain undersupported by the literature.[10]

Surgical intervention for craniosynostosis can improve head shape and prevent neurologic sequelae of intracranial hypertension due to limited skull growth.[10,11] Thus, the primary operative goals are to release the involved sutures and expand the calvarial vault to address cephalocranial disproportion and normalize the head shape. Although single-suture synostosis can be typically corrected in a single operation, multisuture and syndromic synostosis may require staged reconstruction, with posterior vault expansion as the first stage followed by anterior vault expansion.[10] The main categories of surgical approaches include endoscopic suturectomy followed by postoperative helmet therapy, open calvarial vault expansion, distraction osteogenesis, and spring-mediated cranioplasty. Specific patient needs, such as multisutural involvement, age, severity of deformity, and overall health status, will influence decisions regarding the surgical approach, and individual surgeon preferences vary widely.

DIAGNOSTIC EVALUATION

A comprehensive approach to patients with calvarial vault lesions includes medical history, physical examination, radiologic evaluation, and multidisciplinary management planning. A well-rounded craniofacial team should include plastic surgery, neurosurgery, otolaryngology, ophthalmology, oral/maxillofacial surgery, social work, neuropsychology, genetics, pediatrics and pediatric anesthesiology/critical care, respiratory/occupational/physical therapy, audiology, and speech pathology.

Clinical presentation of these lesions can vary depending on the location, etiology, and extent. Asymptomatic lesions may be incidental findings on imaging studies. Patients with involvement of the scalp, outer table, periosteum, or dura may have localized pain with a palpable mass. Inner table involvement can result in neurologic symptoms such as headaches, neurologic deficits, meningeal irritation, and seizures. Skull base involvement may manifest as cranial nerve deficits.[12] Understanding the patient's medical and familial history can provide critical insight into the diagnosis.

Physical examination with documentation of the size, location, texture of the lesion as well as any associated symptoms, soft tissue abnormalities, or neurologic deficits is critical. Thorough evaluation for additional lesions should also be performed.

Accurate diagnosis can involve multiple imaging modalities as well as tissue biopsy. Imaging features often suggest either benign or malignant etiologies, but histologic tissue examination after biopsy is confirmatory. Imaging can also provide guidance for tissue sampling and avoid interventions for nonaggressive lesions.[13] While computed tomography (CT) with a bone window is critical, MRI is helpful for evaluating soft tissue extension and brain metastases. Bone scan has poor diagnostic utility in osteolytic bone metastases.[12] In infants with primarily hematopoietic bone marrow, the skull has low signal intensity on T1-weighted images. The diploic space becomes T1 hyperintense by age 15 years in most individuals. Thus, bone marrow disease can be suggested by uniform low signal intensity at T1-weighted MRI after

7 years of age.[13] Imaging should be analyzed for extent (focal vs diffuse), location, suture crossing, multiplicity, attenuation (lytic, sclerotic, mixed), internal structure, presence of bone expansion and periosteal reaction, relationship with dura and diploic veins, and soft tissue involvement.[13] One can infer the speed of growth of a lesion by its edges: smooth edges and homogenous internal structure are often consistent with slowly progressive processes, while irregular edges with heterogenous internal structure suggest more aggressive and potentially malignant lesions.[7,13] Care should be taken to observe any extension of the lesion, involvement of adjacent critical structures and vasculature. Benign lesions are often limited to bone, while more aggressive lesions may infiltrate adjacent tissue. Contrast agents can be helpful to characterize inflammation or scarring in the dura (manifested as linear homogenous contrast enhancement, whereas tumor infiltration is often associated with irregular heterogenous enhancement). If the epidural space is preserved, dural infiltration is less likely.[7]

Following targeted imaging, biopsy is necessary to confirm diagnosis. Complete excision of the lesion and reconstruction is often recommended if feasible.[12] In pediatric patients, minimizing blood loss is critical. Timing for this procedure is considered in the context of the patient's medical history, clinical complaints, and the differential diagnosis.

RECONSTRUCTION

Defects of the pediatric skull require consideration of the age of the patient and need for lifetime durability.[14] Spontaneous ossification of skull defects, driven by the dura,[15] is possible in young children (generally <2 years old) and is the foundational principle of cranial vault expansion for craniosynostosis. Acquired defects in older children require autologous or alloplastic cranioplasty for brain protection and restoration of the calvarial contour. Reconstruction with autologous bone is the gold standard, and split bone from elsewhere on the skull (even in young children[16]), rib, and iliac crest are all potential donor sites. For cases where autologous reconstruction is not feasible, synthetic alloplasts including porous polyethylene[17] and polyetheretherketone can be customized preoperatively with virtual planning and are generally preferable to titanium cranioplasty in children.[14] When adjuvant radiation is required for cranial vault malignancies, alloplastic reconstruction should be avoided whenever possible. To protect bony reconstruction and fixation hardware, the pericranial flap is a versatile source of vascularized tissue that can be raised in various orientations on its circumferential blood supply.[18]

CASE EXAMPLES
Case 1: Encephalocele

This newborn was diagnosed prenatally with a large occipital encephalocele and delivered via elective C-section. He had no other significant abnormalities noted on examination and did not require cardiorespiratory support after birth. The encephalocele measured about 7 cm in diameter and was covered with skin without leakage of cerebral spinal fluid (CSF) (**Fig. 2**A, B). Magnetic resonance angiogram and venogram (MRA/V) performed shortly after birth showed a largely fluid-filled encephalocele with meninges and a small amount of brain matter present (**Fig. 2**C). Imaging also showed a Chiari I malformation and small CSF spaces. The patient underwent reconstruction in early infancy with switch cranioplasty to address the bony defect, posterior and middle cranial vault expansion with barrel stave osteotomies, and reconstruction with local scalp flaps to address the soft tissue defect. There was no alopecia or contour irregularity postoperatively (**Fig. 2**D, E).

Case 2: Dermoid Cyst

A 15-month-old girl was evaluated for a mass on the vertex of her scalp measuring about 4 cm in diameter (**Fig. 3**A). The mass had slowly increased in size since birth. She was asymptomatic and growing and developing normally. CT bone windows showed a patent anterior fontanelle with depression of the surrounding calvarium in the setting of compression from the mass (**Fig. 3**B). T2-weighted MRI showed an extradural homogenously enhancing mass (**Fig. 3**C). MRV confirmed a patent sagittal sinus deep to the mass (**Fig. 3**D). During resection, the mass was identified in the subgaleal plane and removed en bloc from the dura of the anterior fontanelle. Interrogation of the contents of the mass revealed both clear fluid and soft tissue including keratinous debris and hair (**Fig. 3**E).

Case 3: Intraosseous Vascular Malformation

A 2-year-old boy presented with a slowly enlarging asymptomatic calvarial mass. CT was significant for a mass in the right parietal bone involving both inner and outer table measuring approximately 3.5 cm in diameter leading to asymmetry of the lambdoid sutures and occiput (**Fig. 4**A). MRI provided key information for preoperative diagnosis. While the mass was isointense to muscle on T1-weighted images, T2-weighted images

(**Fig. 4**B) showed a strikingly hyperintense mass with avid postcontrast enhancement. While the dura showed some reactive changes and there was mass effect on the underlying gyri, there was no edema or invasion of the brain parenchyma. CT angiography excluded any significant arterial feeding vessel, so preoperative embolization was not performed. Whole-body PET was performed to exclude malignancy and was significant for mild fluorodeoxyglucose uptake in the skull lesion and some reactive cervical lymph nodes with no other areas of suspicious uptake. Taken together, the imaging workup was most consistent with calvarial intraosseous vascular malformation. Resection and reconstruction were planned with a multidisciplinary approach. A posterior scalp (modified pterional) surgical approach (**Fig. 4**C) was designed to allow coverage with an anteriorly based pericranial flap. Dissection proceeded in the subgaleal plane until the mass was fully exposed, and a planned resection with approximately 1 cm margins and including the pericranium was marked (**Fig. 4**D). The lesion was excised en bloc using a single burr hole (**Fig. 4**E). The mass was fed by several parasitized dural vessels that were coagulated to facilitate removal. The excision resulted in a right parietal skull defect approximately 6 cm diameter. A second craniotomy corresponding to the size of the defect was performed further anterior on the parietal bone. The autologous bone graft was split, with the outer table used to reconstruct the resection defect and the inner table used to reconstruct the donor site. Fixation was achieved with resorbable plates and screws, and bone gaps were filled with particulate bone autograft (**Fig. 4**F). An anteriorly based pericranial flap was elevated from the underlying bone and preserved for coverage of the reconstruction (**Fig. 4**G). Final pathology, again consistent with calvarial intraosseous vascular malformation, showed infiltration of variably sized vessels into mature bone with some cortical destruction. There were no features, such as atypia or mitoses, suggestive of malignancy. Immunohistochemistry staining for glucose transporter 1 (GLUT-1) was negative, as expected in this type of lesion.[19] The patient went on to recover uneventfully.

Case 4: Langerhans Cell Histiocytosis

A 4-year-old boy presented with about 1 month of painless swelling in the right lateral forehead, initially thought to be secondary to minor trauma. CT was performed and showed a mixed attenuation mass measuring about 6 cm in the largest dimension in the frontal and parietal bones with

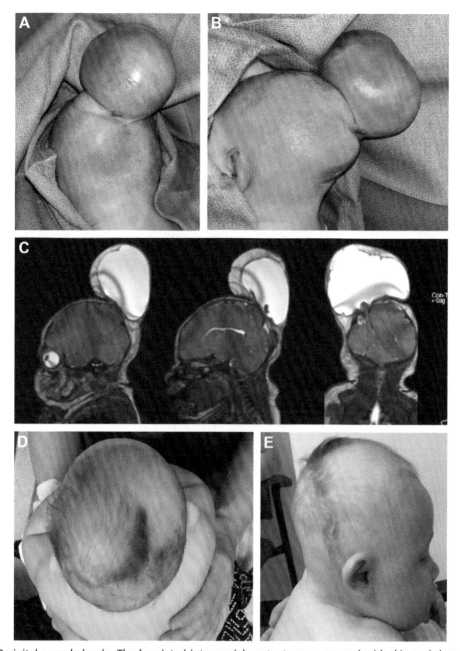

Fig. 2. Occipital encephalocele. The herniated intracranial contents were covered with skin and there was no leakage of CSF. No other significant congenital abnormalities were present (*A, B*). MRA/V was significant for a largely fluid-filled encephalocele with duplicated falcine dural venous sinuses draining the area (*C*). Postoperative soft tissue healing was unremarkable (*D, E*).

thinning of the inner table and obliteration of the outer table (**Fig. 5**A). MRI showed invasion of the pericranium, reactivity but no invasion of the dura, and mild mass effect on the underlying brain. The mass included septations and fluid–fluid levels (**Fig. 5**B). Biopsy of the lesion was performed and showed proliferation of histiocytic cells with immunostaining positive for langerin, consistent with

Langerhans cell histiocytosis. The lesion was surrounded by inflammatory cells and non-neoplastic reactive bone. PET was performed for staging and showed low uptake in the frontoparietal mass and no regional or distant metastasis in bone or other tissue. With no involvement anywhere except the calvarium, this case fit unifocal-monosystem subgroup of Langerhans cell histiocytosis.[20] He was

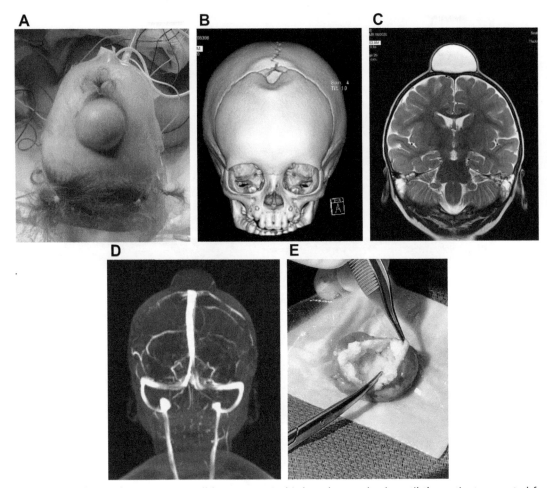

Fig. 3. Dermoid cyst. The mass was small but present at birth and grew slowly until the patient presented for resection at 15 months of age (*A*). CT showed a patent anterior fontanelle with intact but depressed calvarium deep to the mass (*B*). MRI, including venogram, showed a homogeneously enhancing extradural mass on T2 images (*C*) overlying a patent sagittal sinus (*D*). Excision of the mass revealed a cyst with clear fluid, keratinous debris, and hair (*E*).

discussed at tumor board and since the location in the calvarium (frontoparietal rather than temporal bone) did not represent a central nervous system metastasis risk, resection alone without adjuvant chemotherapy was recommended. The patient has recovered unremarkably, has not required adjuvant chemotherapy or radiation, and is undergoing serial surveillance with head CT and skeletal survey plain films to query recurrence or development of additional skeletal lesions.

Case 5: Osteoma

A 15-year-old boy presented with a painless right skull mass recently noted during a haircut. CT was performed and showed a pedunculated extracranial sclerotic bone lesion measuring about 3 cm in the largest dimension with preserved architecture of the inner table (**Fig. 6**). MRI showed hyperostosis

of the involved area without soft tissue invasion. In a similar manner to the prior cases, the patient underwent resection including pericranium and immediate autologous reconstruction with split calvarial bone graft from nearby parietal bone. Exposed mastoid air cells after resection were occluded with bone wax, and the reconstruction was covered with an anteriorly based pericranial flap. Final pathology of the lesion showed sessile lamellar bone with Haversian canals and no atypia, consistent with osteoma. The patient went on to recover unremarkably without further treatment.

Case 6: Cemento-Ossifying Fibroma

A 15-year-old boy presented with a unilateral sinonasal mass and associated right eye proptosis, slightly decreased sense of smell, and nasal congestion. There were no vision changes,

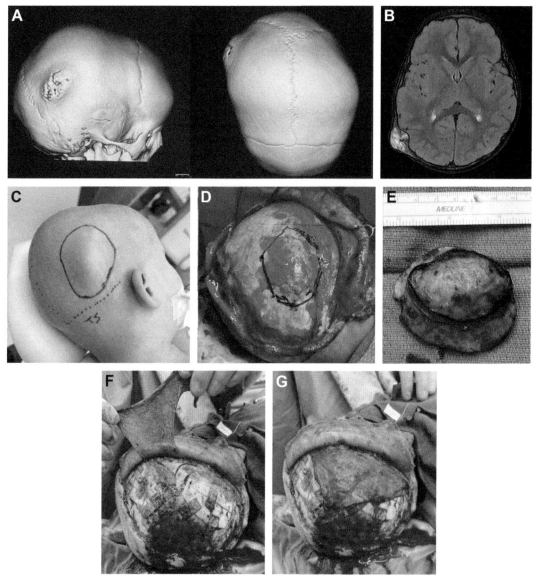

Fig. 4. Intraosseous vascular malformation. The patient presented with a slowly growing painless mass of the right parietal bone causing slight deformation of the occiput (*A*). The mass was hyperintense on T2-weighted MR images with postcontrast enhancement (*B*). A posterior scalp approach (*C*) was designed to allow coverage of the resection and reconstruction with an anteriorly based pericranial flap. Initial dissection was performed in the subgaleal plane to allow full-thickness resection including associated pericranium, and approximately 1 cm of visibly normal tissue was included in the planned resection (*D*). The en bloc resection measured 6 cm in the largest dimension (*E*), and reconstruction was accomplished with autologous split calvarial bone graft and resorbable fixation (*F*). The bone graft and hardware were covered with a pericranial flap (*G*).

headaches, paresthesias, or weakness. On examination, he had proptosis and hypoglobus of the right eye with intact visual acuity and nasal obstruction (**Fig. 7**A). CT and MRI demonstrated an expansile osseous lesion (4.6 × 3.2 × 6.1 cm) in the right ethmoid paranasal sinus with superior extension into the right frontal sinus, abutting the anterior skull base, and laterally into the right maxillary sinus and medial orbit with compression of the orbital contents (**Fig. 7**B, C). The mass was multiloculated with fluid–fluid levels of layered proteinaceous and blood products. Bony margins were thinned, suggesting a lytic lesion. Differential diagnosis included aneurysmal bone cyst, telangiectatic osteosarcoma, and ossifying fibroma. Cerebral angiogram showed no occlusion or

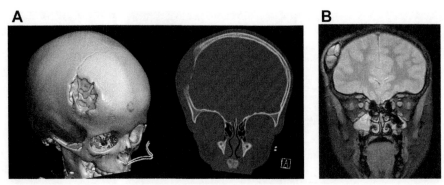

Fig. 5. Langerhans cell histiocytosis. A 4 year old patient presented with painless swelling of the right forehead. CT imaging showed a 6 cm mass along the coronal suture with invasion of the inner table and obliteration of the outer table (*A*). On T2-weighted MR images, an expansile lesion in the diploic space with septations and fluid–fluid levels is seen. There is invasion of the overlying pericranium with reactivity but no invasion of the dura. No postcontrast enhancement is present (*B*). Definitive management included en bloc resection with autologous split cranioplasty.

aneurysm about the circle of Willis and patent circulation. He underwent preoperative embolization of feeder vessels from the right internal maxillary artery, right middle meningeal artery, and right ophthalmic internal carotid artery branches prior to surgical resection of the mass. Resection required combined approaches by craniofacial surgery, otolaryngology, and neurosurgery and involved bifrontal craniotomy with orbital osteotomies to access the anterior skull base and orbits, as well as transnasal/transantral endoscopic approaches to complete the resection involving nasal tissues. The lesion was extradural and associated with significant remodeling of the anterior cranial fossa causing displacement of the brain and orbital contents. Following tumor resection (**Fig. 7**D), the medial orbital wall, roof, and anterior cranial base were reconstructed with calvarial bone graft, and the frontal sinus was cranialized including inset of a pericranial flap (**Fig. 7**E, F). The bandeau and frontal bone were replaced (**Fig. 7**G), and redraping of the scalp demonstrated

immediate improvement in the right proptosis (**Fig. 7**H). Postoperative MRI demonstrated slight kinking of the right optic nerve instead of smooth compression as seen in preoperative imaging. Ophthalmologic examinations over 2 years postoperatively were notable for right optic nerve atrophy with preserved visual acuity (20/20 bilaterally) and color vision, albeit with a corresponding visual field defect in the right eye; no follow-up interventions were required for this. Pathology showed an aneurysmal bone cyst with an associated cemento-ossifying fibroma. At 1 year follow-up imaging, recurrent expansile masses involving the orbital floor/roof/medial walls and right ethmoid sinus were seen. Given the benign pathology, lack of symptoms, and satisfactory esthetic result (**Fig. 7**I, J), no surgical intervention has been pursued.

Case 7: Fibrous Dysplasia

A 7-year-old girl presented with slight asymmetry of the right forehead and temporal region and

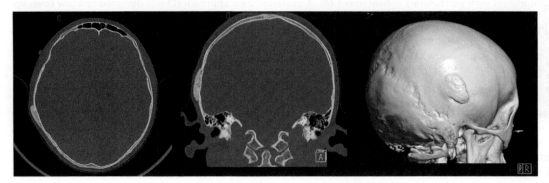

Fig. 6. Osteoma. A teenage boy presented with a small mass noted during a haircut. CT showed a pedunculated lesion protruding from the outer table of the right parietal bone. MRI was unremarkable, and he underwent resection with autologous cranioplasty for definitive management.

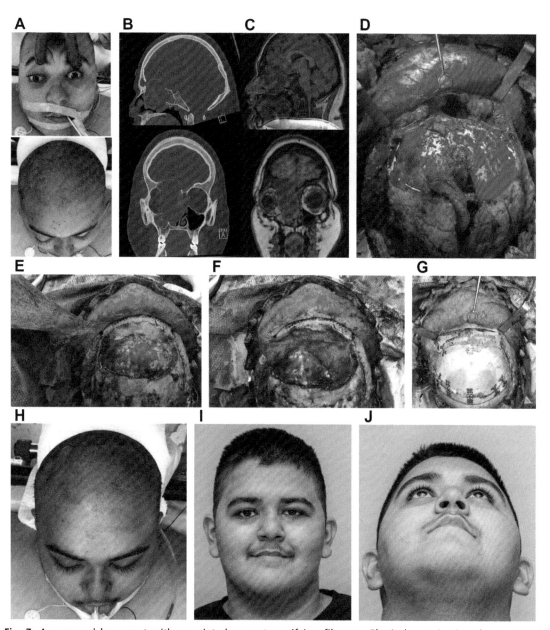

Fig. 7. Aneurysmal bone cyst with associated cemento-ossifying fibroma. Physical examination demonstrated right proptosis and hypoglobus (*A*). On CT above, the right-sided mass can be seen involving the entirety of the right ethmoid/paranasal sinuses with deformity of the orbit, anterior skull base, and nasal cavity (*B*). Bony margins are ballooned and thin, but intact. On MRI, the mass demonstrated contrast enhancement and no diffusion restriction (*C*). Resection was accomplished with a bifrontal craniotomy and removal of the orbital bandeau and resulted in defects of the right orbital roof and medial wall as well as the anterior cranial base (*D*). The missing bone was reconstructed with split calvarial graft (*E*), and the frontal sinus was cranialized with inset of a pericranial flap (*F*). The frontal bone was replaced (*G*), and there was immediate improvement in the right proptosis (*H*). The improvement in globe position was maintained in follow-up (*I*, *J*).

intermittent headaches. On examination, she had a symmetric face with mild fullness over the right temple as compared to the left, but no tenderness and symmetric brows and orbits. CT demonstrated an expansile ground-glass bone lesion involving the greater wing of the sphenoid, right orbital roof, and lateral orbital wall in addition to the inferior frontal bone, suggestive of fibrous dysplasia (**Fig. 8**). Given her lack of symptoms and benign characteristics of the lesion, she was

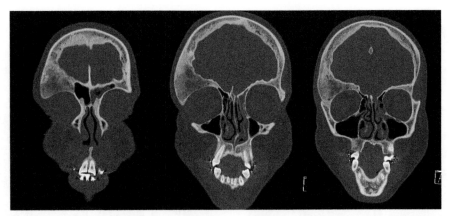

Fig. 8. Fibrous dysplasia. CT demonstrates a ground-glass expansile lesion involving the right frontal and sphenoid bones on CT scan. While there is demonstrated bony asymmetry of the orbit, this did not translate to significant facial asymmetry on clinical examination.

followed with serial CT imaging. Follow-up imaging at 1 month demonstrated stable osseous changes. Two years later, there was mild interval increase involving the right frontal calvarium and possible dysplasia involving the left orbital roof. At both 3 and 7 years from initial diagnosis, no significant changes in the character or extent of the lesion were seen. She had intermittent sharp headaches that resolved spontaneously but otherwise no significant symptoms associated with the lesion. She was happy with her appearance and did well academically in school. As such, surgical debulking of the dysplastic bone was deferred.

SUMMARY

Calvarial vault pathologies are tremendously varied. A systematic approach to diagnosis, extirpation, and reconstruction of these defects in a multidisciplinary setting provides a framework to address this variety. Reconstructive goals generally include (1) brain protection and (2) re-establishment of calvarial contour with stable soft tissue coverage. For many lesions, extirpation and reconstruction can be curative in a single stage. However, some lesions cannot be entirely resected and require surveillance through skeletal maturity and beyond.

CLINICS CARE POINTS

- Cranial vault pathologies can be broadly classified into congenital, benign, and malignant lesions.
- Imaging workup generally consists of CT (bone/bony invasion) and/or MRI (soft tissue/soft tissue invasion).

- Preliminary diagnosis can often be achieved by imaging criteria alone, but tissue sampling can be used to determine the necessary extent of resection.
- Depth and margin of excision vary depending on the subtype of cranial vault pathology.
- Reconstruction should be autologous when feasible in children. Alloplasts must be used judiciously in the context of remaining skull growth.

DISCLOSURE

The authors have nothing to disclose.

REFERENCES

1. Liu H, Zhang X, Zhang M, et al. Skull bone tumor: a review of clinicopathological and neuroimaging characteristics of 426 cases at a single center. Cancer Commun 2019;39:8.
2. Gibson SE, Prayson RA. Primary skull lesions in the pediatric population: a 25-year experience. Arch Pathol Lab Med 2007;131(5):761–6.
3. Hayden Gephart MG, Colglazier E, Paulk KL, et al. Primary pediatric skull tumors. Pediatr Neurosurg 2012;47(3):198–203.
4. Yang L, Yang MC, Qu PR, et al. A retrospective study comprising 228 cases of pediatric scalp and skull lesions. BMC Pediatr 2023;23:478.
5. Sahinoglu M, Gundogdu DK, Karabagli P, et al. Pediatric calvarial tumors: 10 years of clinical experience and differences from the literature. J Craniofac Surg 2021;32(5):1668.
6. Yoon SH, Park SH. A study of 77 cases of surgically excised scalp and skull masses in pediatric patients. Childs Nerv Syst 2008;24(4):459–65.

7. Nasi-Kordhishti I, Hempel JM, Ebner FH, et al. Calvarial lesions: overview of imaging features and neurosurgical management. Neurosurg Rev 2021; 44(6):3459–69.

8. Alperovich M, Runyan CM, Gabrick KS, et al. Long-term neurocognitive outcomes of spring-assisted surgery versus cranial vault remodeling for sagittal synostosis. Plast Reconstr Surg 2021;147(3): 661–71.

9. Persing JA. MOC-PS(SM) CME article: management considerations in the treatment of craniosynostosis. Plast Reconstr Surg 2008;121(4 Suppl):1–11.

10. Xue AS, Buchanan EP, Hollier LH. Update in Management of Craniosynostosis. Plast Reconstr Surg 2022;149(6):1209e–23e.

11. Ruane EJ, Garland CB, Camison L, et al. A treatment algorithm for patients presenting with sagittal craniosynostosis after the age of 1 year. Plast Reconstr Surg 2017;140(3):582–90.

12. Gupta S, Sharma G, Sajeevan S, et al. Varied clinical presentation and management of calvarial metastases. Asian J Neurosurg 2022;17(4):631–4.

13. Khodarahmi I, Alizai H, Chalian M, et al. Imaging spectrum of calvarial abnormalities. Radiographics 2021;41(4):1144–63.

14. Bykowski MR, Goldstein JA, Losee JE. Pediatric cranioplasty. Clin Plast Surg 2019;46(2):173–83.

15. Hobar PC, Schreiber JS, McCarthy JG, et al. The role of the dura in cranial bone regeneration in the immature animal. Plast Reconstr Surg 1993;92(3): 405–10.

16. Vercler CJ, Sugg KB, Buchman SR. Split cranial bone grafting in children younger than 3 years old: debunking a surgical myth. Plast Reconstr Surg 2014;133(6):822e–7e.

17. Lin AY, Kinsella CRJ, Rottgers SA, et al. Custom porous polyethylene implants for large-scale pediatric skull reconstruction: early outcomes. J Craniofac Surg 2012;23(1):67.

18. Argenta LC, Friedman RJ, Dingman RO, et al. The versatility of pericranial flaps. Plast Reconstr Surg 1985;76(5):695.

19. Prasad GL, Pai K. Pediatric cranial intraosseous hemangiomas: a review. Neurosurg Rev 2018; 41(1):109–17.

20. Zhang XH, Zhang J, Chen ZH, et al. Langerhans cell histiocytosis of skull: a retrospective study of 18 cases. Ann Palliat Med 2017;6(2):15164–964.

Head and Neck Vascular Anomalies in Children

Jeremy S. Ruthberg, MD[a,*], Srinivas M. Susarla, DMD, MD, MPH[b], Randall A. Bly, MD[a,c]

KEYWORDS

- Vascular anomaly • Vascular tumor • Vascular malformation • Hemangioma
- Lymphatic malformation • Propranolol • Sclerotherapy • Facial nerve mapping

KEY POINTS

- Vascular lesions are subdivided into 2 categories: vascular tumors and vascular malformations under the current classification system of the International Society for the Study of Vascular Anomalies.
- Due to complexity and potential for high morbidity and functional impairment, vascular anomaly management requires a multidisciplinary approach, with a combination of medical, laser, chemical, orthognathic, and surgical therapies available.
- Ultrasound can be used as an in-clinic screening tool to evaluate the flow characteristics of vascular anomalies in pediatric patients while limiting ionizing radiation or sedation.
- The standard imaging technique for studying vascular anomalies is magnetic resonance imaging with gadolinium enhancement.

INTRODUCTION

Vascular anomalies represent a diverse and complex set of conditions that can significantly impact the health and well-being of patients. Oral and maxillofacial surgeons are commonly consulted for evaluation of patients with vascular anomalies; vascular anomalies may affect the head and neck in nearly 60% of cases.[1] Vascular anomalies can have significant functional and esthetic concerns for patients. Depending on growth patterns, size, and location, a patient's symptoms may include dysphagia, airway compromise, obstructive sleep apnea, dysfunctional mastication, abnormal speech, and others.

Our understanding of the pathogenesis of vascular lesions has dramatically shifted over the past 40 years. However, the management of facial vascular anomalies remains a challenge, demanding a multidisciplinary approach. Part of the confusion around management is due to persistence of inconsistent, sometimes inaccurate, largely descriptive nomenclature used by clinicians and researchers. Historically, vascular lesions were classified by descriptors and associations with foods (eg, "cherry", "strawberry," and "port-wine stain"). Others have used the word hemangioma to describe both acquired and congenital lesions.

Mulliken and Glowacki comprised a biologic classification system after analyzing the clinical behavior and endothelial cell characteristics of vascular anomalies in 1982, subdividing vascular lesions into 2 primary categories: hemangiomas and malformations.[2] Hemangiomas were defined as tumors with abnormal endothelial cell cycles and vascular malformations as structural abnormalities of blood vessels with normal endothelial cells.[3]

[a] Department of Otolaryngology-Head and Neck Surgery, University of Washington Medical Center, 1959 Northeast Pacific Street, UW Box 356515, Seattle, WA 98195, USA; [b] Division of Craniofacial Plastic Surgery, Seattle Children's Hospital, 4800 Sand Point Way NE, OB.9.520, Seattle, WA 98105, USA; [c] Division of Pediatric Otolaryngology-Head and Neck Surgery, University of Washington Medical Center, 1959 Northeast Pacific Street, UW Box 356515, Seattle, WA 98195, USA
* Corresponding author. UW Department of Otolaryngology-HNS, University of Washington Medical Center, 1959 Northeast Pacific Street, UW Box 356515, Seattle, WA 98195.
E-mail address: jruthb@uw.edu

Oral Maxillofacial Surg Clin N Am 36 (2024) 355–368
https://doi.org/10.1016/j.coms.2024.03.002
1042-3699/24/© 2024 Elsevier Inc. All rights reserved.

CURRENT CLASSIFICATION

In 2018, the International Society for the Study of Vascular Anomalies updated the classification system for vascular anomalies with 2 primary vascular lesions: vascular tumors (which are then characterized by biologic behavior: benign, locally-aggressive, or malignant) and vascular malformations (which are classified by originating vessel) (**Table 1**).[4]

VASCULAR TUMORS
Benign Vascular Tumors

Benign vascular tumors include hemangiomas, tufted angiomas, pyogenic granulomas, and others (**Table 2**).[4] Classification is based upon growth pattern: focal, multifocal, segmental, or indeterminate and tissue layers involved: superficial, deep, mixed. Hemangiomas are also frequently reported as part of syndromes such as PHACE (posterior fossa malformation, hemangioma, arterial anomalies, cardiovascular anomalies, eye anomalies). Patients with PHACE syndrome may present with central nervous system impairments such as developmental delay or seizures. Such patients should undergo further imaging of the head, ophthalmologic examination, and cardiac evaluation. Finding a hemangioma should alert the clinician about the potential for other concordant findings.

   Infantile hemangiomas (IHs) are the most common vascular tumors, occurring in as many as 10% of children, with a female preponderance ranging from 2:1 to 3:1.[3,5–7] They also occur more commonly in Caucasian children and premature infants.[8] These lesions present in the following stages: proliferation, plateau, and involution. They are absent at birth, appearing by about 2 weeks of age as a pale macula with telangiectasias. They then grow rapidly and involute, regressing slowly and predictably over the next few years. The lesion's bright red color fades and dulls over time, becoming softer to palpation (**Fig. 1**).

   Involution can occur gradually and may last until the child is approximately 3 years of age. After complete regression, the child's normal skin is restored in about half of cases, while in the other half, increased skin laxity, discoloration, scarring, telangiectasis, or a residual mass may persist.[3,9,10]

   IHs can manifest either superficially or deeply, penetrating through all skin skills and occasionally extending into muscle. About 20% are multifocal and, in these instances, tumors can grow in the brain, liver, lung, spleen, or gastrointestinal tract, a phenomenon called **disseminated hemangiomatosis**.[11] The presence of extensive cutaneous hemangiomas or multiple intrahepatic hemangiomas can result in severe, life-threatening conditions such as congestive heart failure and symptomatic anemia.[10–12] Additionally, when a hemangioma undergoes skin or mucosal breakdown, ulceration and secondary infection may occur.

   The proliferating phase of IHs is characterized by elevated endothelial cell turnover.[13] Capillary endothelial cells exhibit robust growth in tissue culture, forming tubules.[13,14] During this phase, hemangiomas express endothelial markers such as CD31, CD133, and factor VIII–related antigen (von Willebrand factor).[9,14–18] Additionally, angiogenic peptides are upregulated during proliferation, including vascular endothelial growth factor (VEGF), basic fibroblast growth factor, proliferating cell nuclear antigen, and type IV collagenase.[13,16,17]

   As IHs enter involution, certain cell types such as mast cells, other monocytes, and fibroblasts propagate and deposit fibrous tissue around vessels and interstices.[19] Apoptosis starts and peaks by about 2 years. Tissue inhibitor of metalloproteinase 1, which suppresses nascent blood vessel formation, is produced and regulated by an autocrine induction loop.[13] After complete regression, only a few vessels remain in the hemangioma, and a lining of mature endothelial cells surrounded by fibrofatty tissue pad remains.[3,9,15,19]

   IH diagnoses can be confirmed with molecular staining for glucose transporter 1 (GLUT-1), a protein found in erythrocytes, which facilitates differentiation from other vascular anomalies.[20,21]

Table 1
Classification of vascular anomalies

Vascular tumors	Benign Locally aggressive/ borderline Malignant
Vascular malformations	*Simple:* Single distinct vascular malformation *Combined:* 2 or more distinct vascular malformations found in the same lesion *Of major name vessels:* anomalies involving origin, course, number, length, diameter, valve, and communication *Associated with other anomalies:* Vascular malformations in the context of associated syndromes

Table 2
A list of the most common vascular tumors and subcategories

	Behavior	Examples
Vascular tumors	Benign	Congenital hemangioma
		Tufted angioma
		Spindle-cell hemangioma
		Epithelioid hemangioma
		Pyogenic granuloma
		Others
	Locally aggressive/borderline	Kaposiform hemangioendothelioma
		Retiform hemangioendothelioma
		Papillary intralymphatic angioendothelioma
		Composite hemangioendothelioma
		Others
	Malignant	Kaposi sarcoma
		Angiosarcoma
		Epithelioid hemangioendothelioma
		Others

Local tissue hypoxia leads to upregulation of GLUT-1, VEGF, and insulinlike growth factor 2 directly, and indirectly through the renin-angiotensin system. Elevation of these proteins, coupled with the embolization of placental mesenchymal cells, is believed to play a role in promoting endothelial cell proliferation and the progression of IHs. Maternal or infant hypoxic exposure, with preeclampsia and preterm birth, has been theorized to lead to IHs.[22]

Although the term **intraosseous hemangioma** has been used in the literature to describe what can be slow-flow capillary, venous, or mixed capillary-venous-lymphatic vascular malformations, IHs typically do not involve the bone.[9,15,23,24] Skeletal abnormalities, including outer cortex depression, nasal deviation, orbital enlargement, and hypertrophy of the maxilla or mandible, are sporadically observed in association with or following the involution of a sizable cutaneous facial hemangioma. The mechanism underlying this skeletal overgrowth is not well understood but could potentially be linked to heightened blood flow during the tumor's proliferative phase.[9,24]

Congenital hemangiomas may be detected in utero and manifest as fully developed, soft, discolored masses at birth. Often the mass has overlying telangiectasias. These lesions fall into distinct

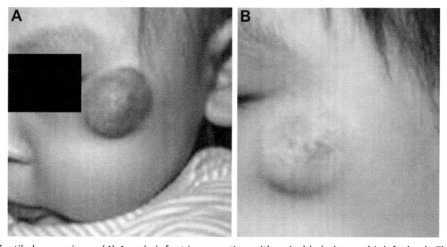

Fig. 1. Infantile hemangioma. (*A*) A male infant is presenting with a sizable lesion on his left cheek. The parents noticed the lesion shortly after birth, concerned over the rapid growth over the subsequent few months. (*B*) This patient was treated with propranolol, which lead to significant reduction in size and redness of the mass. By year 3, a residual fibrofatty mass remained. (Susarla, S., Bly, R., Mulliken, J., & Kaban, L. (2023). Maxillofacial Vascular Anomalies. In L. Kaban (Ed.), Oral and Maxillofacial Surgery in Children (1st ed.). Quintessence Publishing Company, Ltd.).

categories: noninvoluting congenital hemangiomas (NICHs), rapidly involuting congenital hemangiomas (RICHs), and partially involuting congenital hemangiomas (PICHs).[25,26] NICH lesions exhibit gradual, proportionate growth over time without spontaneous regression. In contrast, RICH lesions do not undergo proliferation postnatally and do undergo rapid involution, typically resolving completely by 2 years of age (**Fig. 2**).

PICH lesions are generally singular occurrences located in the head or extremities near joints. Surgical excision is frequently necessary during the preschool years for NICHs, while the management of RICH lesions is usually nonsurgical unless complications such as ulceration or bleeding arise. After involution of RICHs, residual atrophic skin may be present, but not residual fibrofatty tissue. In terms of molecular staining, congenital hemangiomas do not express GLUT-1, while IHs do.

Locally Aggressive/Borderline Vascular Tumors

Locally aggressive vascular tumors and those with borderline behavior primarily include hemangioendotheliomas, the most well-known of which is a kaposiform hemangioendothelioma (KHE). Clinically, KHE appear as cutaneous, violaceous lesions that often present in the head and neck. In 1940, the phrase Kasabach-Merritt syndrome was coined to describe a patient presenting with thrombocytopenia, petechiae, and bleeding with a giant hemangioma.[27] This, however, is not a syndrome, but instead a constellation of coagulopathic phenomena. It may be associated with KHEs and less frequently with tufted angiomas, but not IHs.[17,28,29] Kasabach-Merritt phenomenon includes

profound thrombocytopenia (<10,000 mm^3), low fibrinogen levels, and increased fibrin split products. The prothrombin time and activated partial thromboplastin time can be slightly elevated. Notably, this coagulopathy should **not** be treated with heparin, which may accelerate the growth of the lesion.[30] KHE may also be associated with bone resorption, and can lead to localized osteopenia, or disappearing bone disease.[31]

Kaposi sarcoma (KS) is a low-grade, locally aggressive vascular tumor associated with immunosuppressed states, most commonly as an acquired immunodeficiency syndrome–defining malignancy. KS starts as a macule and grows into plaques, and later into nodules.[32] It typically involves the skin, mucosa, and viscera. There is currently no cure for KS and surgical excision is restricted for severe issues of cosmesis or to alleviate significant discomfort.

Malignant Vascular Tumors

Malignant vascular tumors include angiosarcomas and epithelioid hemangioendotheliomas. Angiosarcoma does not commonly occur in pediatric patients. In adults, these tumors can be appreciated in sun-damaged areas of the head and neck, breast, or the liver.[33] Cutaneous angiosarcoma has been putatively linked to ultraviolet light exposure or prior radiation exposure.[34] Epithelioid hemangioendothelioma has a higher metastatic rate and more aggressive behavior than other hemangioendotheliomas. They typically appear as nonspecific cutaneous nodules, and a vascular tumor may not be suspected at the time of the diagnosis.[35]

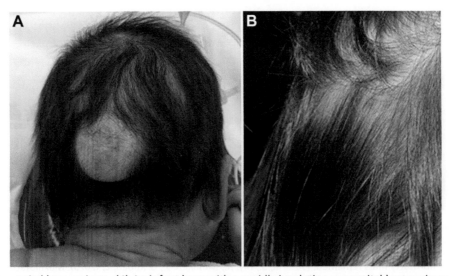

Fig. 2. Congenital hemangioma. (*A*) An infant born with a rapidly involuting congenital hemangioma (RICH) in the posterior scalp. (*B*) Involution was nearly complete by 12 months.

VASCULAR MALFORMATIONS

Vascular malformations arise from dysfunctional morphogenesis of blood and lymphatic vessels (**Table 3**).[36] Although present at birth, many may not manifest clinically until late infancy or childhood.[2,9,15] Malformations typically exhibit proportional growth with the individual, persist throughout life, and may fluctuate due to various inciting factors such as trauma, infection, or endocrine changes (eg, pregnancy and puberty).[9,23] While most vascular malformations were historically characterized as sporadic, some follow an autosomal dominant pattern. Over the past 2 decades, there has been significant progress in understanding the molecular basis of inherited vascular anomalies.[37,38]

Approximately one-third of patients with vascular malformations have corresponding skeletal changes.[24] This may involve primary intraosseous vascular malformations or associated changes in size, shape, or density of bone adjacent to the malformation.[22,24] For example, the most common abnormality occurs when the bone beneath a slow-flow cutaneous vascular malformation grows and expands. On a cellular level, these anomalies exhibit a normal endothelial cell cycle, unless affected by thrombosis, trauma, and endovascular or surgical intervention.

Anatomically, vascular malformations are classified based on the vessels involved and their association with other anomalies. They are also categorized by flow characteristics, with differentiation between slow-flow and fast-flow lesions. Simple lesions involve a single malformation and include capillary, venous, lymphatic, arteriovenous (AV) malformations (AVMs), and AV fistulae. Capillary, venous, and lymphatic malformations are characterized as slow-flow lesions, while AVMs are fast-flow lesions.

Although most vascular malformations are simple, combined malformations involving 2 or more malformations within the same lesion can occur. Vascular malformations are described based on the predominant type(s) of vessel(s) involved. For instance, the port-wine stain, once mistakenly referred to as a capillary hemangioma, should be termed a capillary malformation. Similarly, the terms lymphangioma and cystic hygroma are more accurately described as lymphatic malformations. The old term cavernous hemangioma corresponds to a venous malformation, and hemangiolymphangioma indicates a combined lymphaticovenous malformation. Arterial malformations include aneurysms, ectasias, or stenoses, and AV fistulas and malformations are also observed in the maxillofacial region. Most combined malformations demonstrate slow-flow dynamics.

For pediatric patients, lymphatic malformations are the most common vascular malformation found in the head and neck.[39] They may appear as ballotable masses that range from blue to dark red depending on whether intralesional bleeding is present.[39]

Vascular malformations associated with major named vessels comprise a further subdivision. These lesions, also known as "channel type" or "truncal" malformations, can affect veins, arteries, or lymphatics. Anomalies of major named vessels can have a wide variety of presentations, including alterations in vessel origin or course, number of vessels, or persistence of embryonic vessels. Vascular malformations associated with syndromes are categorized separately.

DIAGNOSIS OF VASCULAR ANOMALIES AND MALFORMATIONS
Clinical Examination

IHs. The diagnosis of IHs is primarily clinical. They may be clinically confounded with capillary

---

Table 3
Vascular malformations

Simple (Single vascular malformation within lesion)	Capillary malformations (low-flow) Lymphatic malformations (low-flow) Venous malformations (low-flow) Arteriovenous malformations (high-flow) Arteriovenous fistula (high-flow)
Combined (2 or more vascular malformations within lesion)	Capillary-venous malformation (CVM) Capillary-lymphatic malformation (CLM) Capillary-arteriovenous malformation (CAVM) Lymphatic-venous malformation (LVM) Capillary-lymphatic-venous malformation (CLVM) Capillary-lymphatic-arteriovenous malformation (CLAVM) Capillary-venous-arteriovenous malformation (CVAVM) Capillary-lymphatic-arteriovenous malformation (CLAVM)

malformations such as port-wine stains, AVMs, dermoid cysts, and pyogenic granulomas.[22] In early stages, superficial IHs appear bright red, while deep lesions may have an absence of cutaneous or mucosal discoloration. There is typically firmness to palpation, and although pulsations are absent, a notable Doppler signal is often observed. These lesions exhibit fast-flow characteristics during the proliferation phase and transition to slow-flow during regression. Frequently, dilated cutaneous veins are visible adjacent to the tumor. As IHs involute, the bright red colorization of superficial lesions deepens, small central areas on the surface turn gray, and the mass softens to palpation. Deep hemangiomas, with intact overlying skin, soften and gradually involute, similarly to bright red superficial lesions.[6] The skin color typically fades to a normal hue, but often there is minor telangiectasia and lost elasticity. After involution, a fibrofatty residual pad may remain in the submucosa.

Vascular malformations. The appearance and structure of vascular malformations vary according to involved vessels. Capillary malformations exhibit a pink hue in infancy, darken during childhood, and take on a deep purple color in older patients. In children, they have a smooth texture resembling normal skin, while in adults, the surface often develops a "pebbly" appearance and becomes slightly raised. Venous malformations appear bluish and are soft, easily compressible, with palpable phleboliths. Venous abnormalities can expand during the Valsalva maneuver or when in a dependent position. Enlargement may occur after injury, partial resection, or be associated with puberty, pregnancy, or the use of medications to suppress ovulation. Lymphatic lesions typically lack color (**Fig. 3**), while combined lymphatic-venous malformations (previously hemolymphangiomas) have a deep purple-blue hue. They may fluctuate in association with upper respiratory tract infections.

Macrocystic lesions of the head and neck (referred to previously as cystic hygromas) can be transilluminated in the clinic and are often identified prenatally due to increased nuchal translucency.[40] Within the oral cavity, pure lymphatic malformations or combined capillary-lymphatic malformations frequently display highly irregular surfaces, featuring clear or dark hemorrhagic bullae and vesicles, with resemblance to salmon eggs. AV lesions (AVMs) are warm, sometimes tender, and may exhibit pulsations and a bruit if macroshunting occurs. Schobinger introduced a clinical staging system for AVMs that is helpful in predicting the natural history.[10,41] Stage I lesions are quiescent; stage II are expansile and exhibit enlargement, pulsations, and a bruit; stage III are destructive; and stage IV lesions are associated with decompensatory cardiac failure (**Table 4**).

Intraorally, the mucosa is stained with concurrent gingival hypertrophy. Bleeding may occur around the necks of teeth adjacent to the malformation, and the teeth may be loose and depressible into the alveolus (**Fig. 4**).

Imaging Studies

Ultrasonography is a useful adjunct for the evaluation of flow characteristics of vascular malformations. It is typically employed as a screening tool, especially for pediatric patients as to avoid utilizing ionizing radiation or sedation.

The standard imaging technique for studying vascular anomalies is MRI with gadolinium enhancement.[42] On T1-weighted images, IHs appear as a soft tissue mass with intermediate intensity, while on T2-weighted images, they exhibit hyperintensity. Flow voids appear around and within the tumor mass indicating high flow and shunting between arteries and veins.[9] Involuting hemangiomas demonstrate less flow and increased lobularity and fatty tissue. MRI is useful in differentiating a deep hemangioma from a lymphatic or venous malformation.[10] Short tau inversion recovery sequencing, which is based on T2 but nullifies fat signaling, is particularly useful in evaluating vascular anomalies (**Fig. 5**). Angiography is not indicated for the diagnosis of hemangiomas, but may be performed prior to endovascular treatment of a vascular malformation.

Plain radiography and computed tomography (CT) detect skeletal changes adjacent to vascular lesions. For example, a large IH may create bony changes due to mass effect or hypertrophy secondary to increased perfusion during the proliferating phase. In contrast, one-third of vascular malformations of the head and neck area show skeletal aberrations.[24,43] Skeletal changes may include underlying bony hypertrophy (or cartilage when lesions involve the external ear), distortion in shape (seen with venous, lymphatic, or combined lesions), or osteopenia and bony destruction (seen with AV lesions).[24,43]

Molecular Studies

Comprehensive management of the patient with a vascular anomaly should include genetic testing as a key component. Identification of genetic variants, when present, can not only establish a conclusive diagnosis but also provide valuable guidance for clinical management. Furthermore, it aids in the screening for additional anomalies

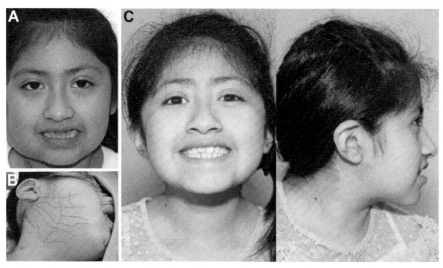

Fig. 3. A female patient with a history of right-sided parotid microcystic lymphatic malformation. (*A*) At 8 years of age with 2 to 3 months of progressive right facial swelling. (*B*) Intraoperative facial nerve monitoring during surgical resection. (*C*) She returned to clinic at 9 years of age after undergoing a right total parotidectomy with lymphatic malformation removal, including a right suprahyoid neck dissection, left upper lip lesion excision, and nasal alar rim lesion excision.

and informs treatment strategy. Notable syndromes with vascular anomalies are listed in **Table 5**.

The predominance of mutations detected in individuals with vascular anomalies affect 2 key intracellular signaling pathways: phosphoinositide 3 kinase/AKT/mammalian (or mechanistic) target of rapamycin (PI3K/AKT/mTOR) and RAS/mitogen activated protein kinase (RAS/MAPK).[38] Each pathway is integral to cell cycle regulation and activating mutations are associated with vascular anomalies and syndromes.

Recent advancements have enabled targeted therapeutic approaches. Patients with overgrowth secondary to vascular anomalies often exhibit somatic activating mutations in PI3K/AKT/mTOR. In such cases, the use of sirolimus, an mTOR inhibitor, has proven effective in curtailing uncontrolled proliferation.[44] Similarly, recent clinical studies highlight the efficacy of MEK1/2 inhibitors, such as selumetinib, in managing AVMs by targeting the RAS/MAPK signaling pathway.[45]

Table 4 Schobinger clinical staging system for arteriovenous malformations	
Stage	**Description**
I (Quiescence)	Pink-bluish stain, warmth, and arteriovascular shunting by continuous Doppler scanning or 20-MHz color Doppler scanning
II (Expansion)	Stage I + enlargement, pulsations, thrill, bruit, and tortuous, tense veins
III (Destruction)	Stage II + either dystrophic skin changes, ulceration, bleeding, persistent pain, or necrosis
IV (Decompensation)	Stage III + cardiovascular collapse

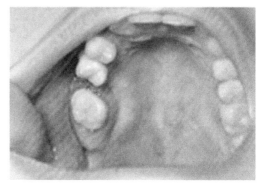

Fig. 4. A patient with a maxillary arteriovenous malformation with localized changes consisting of mucosal staining and gingival hypertrophy.

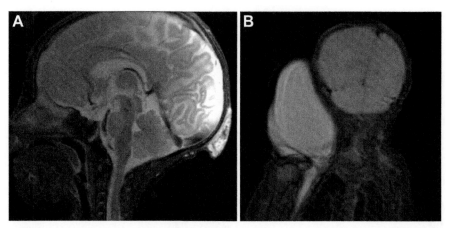

Fig. 5. Use of MRI in various vascular anomalies. (*A*) MRI with short tau inversion recovery (STIR) sequencing of a patient with a rapidly involuting congenital hemangioma (RICH) along the occipital scalp. The lesion is hyperintense, well circumscribed, with no underlying bony changes or intracranial extension. There is early arterial enhancement with multiple prominent occipital vascular flow voids adjacent to the mass in surrounding soft tissue. (*B*) MRI with STIR sequencing demonstrating a hyperintense lesion with a major cystic component (10 x 7 × 9.2 cm) indicative of a large lymphatic malformation.

MANAGEMENT AND TREATMENT OF VASCULAR MALFORMATIONS

IHs are typically managed conservatively being allowed to involute and regress spontaneously. While many lesions in the palate, gum, and lips should be observed, some larger head and neck lesions may require more aggressive management due to concerns of disfigurement or functional compromise. Large lesions may lead to adjacent bony or soft tissue hypertrophy. Management requires a multidisciplinary approach, with a combination of medical, laser, and surgical therapy available.

Systemic corticosteroids were previously employed; however, due to their side effect profile, there is a growing shift toward the use of alternative agents, with propranolol emerging as first-line therapy.[46] Propranolol is a non-selective B1 and B2 adrenergic receptor antagonist and is effective for treating IHs. Potential mechanisms of action include vasoconstriction, inhibition of angiogenesis, or induction of apoptosis. Propranolol dosing is set at 2 to 3 mg/kg/d and divided over 2 to 3 doses. Patient should be monitored continuously for adverse effects such as bronchial hyperactivity, symptomatic bradycardia, hypotension, and hypoglycemia.

Table 5
Notable syndromes associated with vascular anomalies

Syndrome	Clinical Features	Gene
Klippel-Trenaunay	CM + VM ± LM + limb overgrowth	PIK3CA
Parkes Weber	CM + AVF + limb overgrowth	RASA1
Sturge-Weber	Facial + leptomeningeal CM + eye anomalies ± bone and/or soft tissue overgrowth	GNAQ
Maffucci	VM ± spindle-cell hemangioma + enchondroma	IDH1/IDH2
CLOVES	LM + VM + CM ± AVM + lipomatous overgrowth	PIK3CA
Proteus	CM, VM, and/or LM + asymmetrical somatic overgrowth	AKT1
Bannayan-Riley-Ruvalcaba	AVM + VM + macrocephaly, lipomatous overgrowth	PTEN
CLAPO	Lower lip CM + face and neck LM + asymmetry and partial/generalized overgrowth	PIK3CA

Abbreviations: AVF, arteriovenous fistula; AVM, arteriovenous malformation; CLAPO, capillary malformation of the lower lip, lymphatic malformation of the face and neck, asymmetry and partial/generalized overgrowtH; CLOVES, congenital lipomatous overgrowth, vascular malformations, epidermal nevis, spinal/skeletal anomalies/scoliosis; CM, capillary malformation; LM, lymphatic malformation; VM, venous malformation.

For IHs that exhibit ulceration, frequent cleansing and topical antibiotics are recommended. When IHs do not respond to propranolol and when there is associated bleeding, significant functional compromise, airway obstruction, or vision loss, surgical management is recommended, and ideally before a child starts school.

Congenital hemangiomas are ineffectively managed by medical therapy. RICHs are typically observed while NICHs may be managed with laser therapy or surgical intervention.

Venous malformations vary in size, from small, well-localized lesions to diffuse lesions that may involve adjacent bone. Adjacent bone can become distorted in shape and size. In rare cases, the venous malformation may exist within craniofacial bones; the mandible is most frequently involved while the maxilla is less commonly affected.

When venous or combined lymphatic-venous malformations cause secondary bony distortion, without direct intraosseous involvement, orthodontic treatment and orthognathic procedures are recommended and can be performed safely, without fear of excessive bleeding. Patients with intraosseous venous malformations that display microshunting may exhibit major hemorrhage spontaneously or intraoperatively. Any hemorrhage must be differentiated between bleeding from the intraosseous vascular lesion or from coagulopathies.

Venous malformations may induce localized coagulation and, at times, disseminated intravascular coagulopathy due to stagnation and turbulence in blood flow. Hematologic studies demonstrate a normal prothrombin time and partial thromboplastin time while fibrin split products and fibrinopeptide may be elevated, with decreased fibrinogen and platelet levels. Heparin treatment should be considered if indicated. Only after correction of the coagulopathy are surgical procedures feasible. Another approach is to begin giving heparin, followed by antifibrinolytic therapy with ε-aminocaproic acid. Failure to address the chronic consumptive coagulopathy may lead to issues with hemostasis intraoperatively.

In the past, the mainstay of treatment was surgery. However, resection of venous malformations, particularly large lesions, may be associated with significant morbidity or even disfiguration, especially if lesions are diffuse.[47] In this context, resection is recommended for the smaller, well-localized lesions, persistently symptomatic lesions despite sclerotherapy, or those in proximity to critical anatomic structures (ie, sensory or motor nerves) where scarring from sclerosing treatment may complicate surgical excision in the future (**Fig. 6**).

Sclerosing therapy is now recommended for large superficial venous malformations, which requires general anesthesia with concurrent fluoroscopic guidance. Whichever sclerosing agent is utilized (eg, sodium tetradecyl sulfate, ethanol, ethanolamine oleate, bleomycin, or polidocanol) is then injected into the malformation, resulting in an inflammatory reaction and subsequent fibrosis. Usually, several sessions (6–8 weeks apart) are required to reduce large venous malformations. Recanalization is a known phenomenon in venous malformations.[48] Sclerotherapy can be dangerous and should be performed only by experienced interventional radiologists. Complications include local blistering, prolonged pain or swelling at injection site, full-thickness skin necrosis, and nerve damage.[49] Systemic complications include hemolysis, transient hemoglobinuria, and potential for renal toxicity and cardiac arrest.[49,50] Small oral mucosal venous malformations may be treated by injection of 1% sodium tetradecyl sulfate. Notably, malformations are not removed from sclerosing therapy and patients should be counseled that deformities may persist following sclerosing treatment; further treatment may require resection. As more knowledge is gained about genetic etiology, targeted medical therapy is beginning to be an option for these patients.

Commonly, venous and combined lymphatic-venous lesions are associated with intermittent swelling, pain, and fever. For patients with these symptoms, it may be difficult to differentiate between cellulitis, intralesional abscesses, thrombophlebitis, and phlebothrombosis. Upon examination, a local source may be identified (eg, dental caries or a periapical abscess). Management will require appropriate antibiosis (typically penicillin or clindamycin) and subsequent surgical drainage if an abscess is present. Aspirin may be considered in reducing pain if thrombosis is present.[51] In patients who respond to aspirin, the administration of this antiplatelet drug is typically continued indefinitely (325 mg per day).

Lymphatic malformations commonly involve the tongue, floor of mouth, mandible, submandibular, and neck soft tissues. Lymphatic malformations are benign and treatment may be observational unless functional compromise or severe esthetic concerns are present.[52] Common sequelae such as intralesional bleeding are typically managed nonoperatively. However, lymphatic malformations engender a higher risk of developing superinfections. More than 3 infections annually merit consideration for prophylactic antibiotic therapy. For larger lymphatic malformations, macrocystic lesions, or those that are symptomatic, sclerotherapy should be considered.

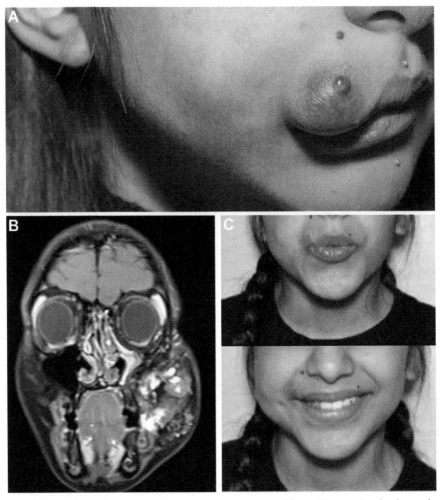

Fig. 6. Venous malformation. (*A*) A patient with right malar venous malformation previously glue embolized by an interventional radiologist. The lesion was subsequently resected transorally through a buccal incision. (*B*) MRI demonstrated hyperintense T2 lesion and hypointense T1 in right subcutaneous tissue and masticator space deeply investing temporalis and masseter. No intraosseous component. Lesionwas measured at 11.4x9.2 × 4.5 cm. (*C*) Postop photographs at 2 months.

Sclerosing treatment involves evacuation of the malformation cavity by aspiration, followed by injection of chemical agents (eg, sodium tetradecyl sulfate, doxycycline, ethanol, bleomycin, and picibanil—OK432) that induce scarring between the walls of the lesion. Sclerotherapy is minimally invasive and has a lower morbidity when compared to surgical resection. Serial treatments, 6 to 8 weeks apart, may be required. Ulceration of the overlying soft tissue is the most common adverse event and most observed when ethanol is used as a sclerosing agent or when lesions are superficial. Due to size, sclerosing agents are less effective with microcystic malformations. Recent advances in targeted molecular therapies have facilitated the introduction of oral medications (eg, sirolimus) for

managing severe microcystic lymphatic malformations. Based upon similar pathophysiologic characteristics, sirolimus has also emerged as a potential treatment for Gorham-Stout disease ("vanishing bone disease").[52]

In some cases, large lymphatic malformations can lead to highly morbid, functional impairments such as airway obstruction and feeding difficulties (**Fig. 7**).

In older children, bony hypertrophy and malocclusion develop adjacent to the lesion.[53] Patients with macroglossia may be prone to developing mandibular prognathism and open bite secondary to the progressive mandibular distortion. Patients with these complications usually undergo multiple surgical procedures, which may consist of cervical

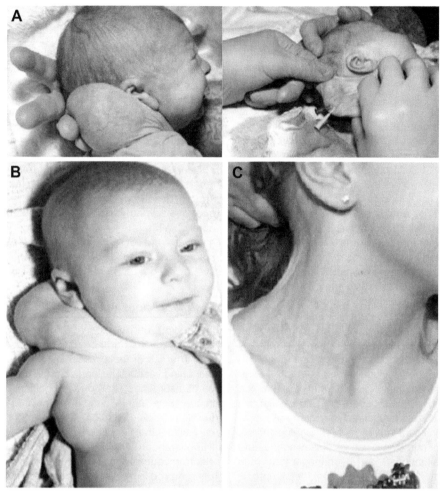

Fig. 7. A female patient with history of a complex cystic lymphatic malformation in the right supraclavicular neck that extended between the sternocleidomastoid and trapezius and inferiorly below her clavicle into her right axilla. She underwent multiple aspirations prior to definitive resection at 18 months. (*A*) At 2 weeks, initial aspiration. (*B*) At 3 months of age, seen in clinic to discuss surgical interventions. (*C*) Age 6 years, presenting for interval follow-up, demonstrating full recovery. She reported no functional deficits, without any breathing or swallowing concerns.

excision, lingual reduction, and various orthognathic surgical procedures. Orthognathic correction is typically performed after the completion of growth, and only if the lingual size and position allow for it, such as in the case of mandibular setback.

Capillary malformations also occur in isolation or in association with lymphatic, venous, or arterial malformations. In such combined vascular anomalies, management is based on the characteristics of the predominant, deeper malformation. Cutaneous capillary malformations may be seen in the mid and upper face and can be associated with Sturge-Weber syndrome (SWS), which can involve capillary malformations in eyes and leptomeninges.[54] High suspicion for SWS warrants a

brain MRI and ophthalmology consultation. Laser therapy has proved to be highly effective for the management of superficial component of capillary malformations. Typically, the use of pulsed dye laser (λ=595 nm) treatment is employed to brighten the lesion. This is performed serially, with treatments spaced 6 weeks apart, until there is a treatment response plateau. As lesions progress to thicker and darker states, pulsed-dye laser treatment becomes less effective. Notable advantages of early treatment (infancy or early childhood) include superior lightning, reduced risk of hyperpigmentation, and the potential for decreased psychological impact.

A rare, hereditary form of vascular malformation occurring intraorally is hereditary hemorrhagic telangiectasia (HHT). It follows an autosomal dominant inheritance pattern.[15] Patients with HHT typically present with difficult-to-control epistaxis, but other organs can be involved in leading to gastrointestinal bleeding, stroke, cardiac failure, among others, with management options varying depending on organs involved.[55] Intraoral manifestations also occur exhibiting characteristic ectasia from extremely thin endothelial walls.

AVMs represent high-flow lesions where shunting occurs between arterial and venous circulations. In the maxillofacial region, they predominately involve the dentoalveolar segment. Sequelae may include loose teeth, gingival bleeding, and potential massive hemorrhage, either spontaneously or intraoperatively. AVMs are slightly more prevalent in females (male to female ratio of 1:1.5), occurring in the head and neck more frequently than in the extremities or trunk. While often noticed at birth, AVMs may be overlooked due to their seemingly innocuous nature, with symptoms becoming evident later in childhood. Patients typically seek evaluation and treatment when AVMs expand and cause symptoms, commonly triggered by trauma, puberty, or pregnancy.

Diagnostic tools include ultrasonography, color Doppler examination, MRI, magnetic resonance angiography, and CT scans.[56] Super-selective arterial embolization reserved for treatment represents a significant advance in managing inflow. Although not curative, it can be lifesaving in acute bleeding situations. AVM management has evolved, emphasizing intervention for symptomatic relief, bleeding control, preservation of function, and improving associated deformities. Cure is rarely achieved due to the extensive involvement of multiple tissue planes.

Asymptomatic AVMs may be observed longitudinally or excised, particularly in anatomically safe regions. Caution must be exercised during surgery to prevent enlargement or collateral flow development. Interventions for higher Schobinger stage lesions (III and IV) aim at palliating pain, bleeding, or congestive heart failure. Ligation or proximal embolization is contraindicated due to rapid collateral flow development.

The current management strategy involves arterial embolization followed by surgical excision 24 to 72 hours after embolization. The timing is crucial to prevent recanalization. Surgical goals include complete resection of the AVM nidus and involved tissue, with soft tissue defects managed through adjacent tissue transfers. In tooth-bearing areas, long-term bleeding control may be challenging. A strategy involving tooth removal, socket packing, and oversewing has been successful. Unfortunately, AVMs often recur, with a reported overall success rate of 60%, varying by Schobinger stage. For stage III lesions, embolization is palliative, and reoperation may not be feasible.

Vascular Lesions Adjacent to the Facial Nerve

Depending on the location, some craniofacial vascular lesions put the facial nerve at significant risk. The risk of facial nerve injury is higher when managing vascular lesions compared to traditional parotid surgeries, likely due to significant alteration in the facial nerve course.[57] The course of the facial nerve is conventionally evaluated during surgery with intraoperative nerve integrity monitoring (NIM) (standard NIM), which performs continuous electromyography at 2 to 4 locations.[58] In 2018, Bly and colleagues performed a retrospective cohort analysis comparing surgical patients receiving NIM or preoperative facial nerve mapping (FNM) and reported significantly less facial nerve injuries in the group with preoperative mapping.[59,60] FNM may also provide the surgeon with a more targeted approach, reducing intraoperative times, and decreasing the need for anterograde approach with main trunk identification (**Fig. 8**).

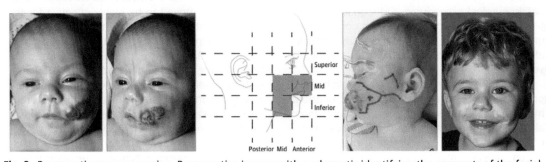

Fig. 8. Preoperative nerve mapping. Preoperative images with a schematic identifying the segments of the facial nerve that is impacted. This infant had an infantile hemangioma that did not respond to propranolol therapy. The lesion was excised directly with peripheral nerve identification and preservation. (*From:* Bly RA, Holdefer RN, Slimp J, et al. Preoperative Facial Nerve Mapping to Plan and Guide Pediatric Facial Vascular Anomaly Resection. *JAMA Otolaryngol Head Neck Surg.* 2018;144(5):418-426. https://doi.org/10.1001/jamaoto.2018.0054)

CLINICS CARE POINTS

- Propranolol has emerged as first-line therapy for managing IHs.

- A combination of sclerotherapy and surgical excision may be necessary in managing large vascular lesions with significant functional impairment.

- Vascular lesions adjacent to the facial nerve may benefit from preoperative FNM.

DISCLOSURE

The authors have nothing to disclose.

REFERENCES

1. Huoh KC, Rosbe KW. Infantile hemangiomas of the head and neck. Pediatr Clin North Am 2013;60(4): 937–49.

2. Mulliken JB, Glowacki J. Hemangiomas and vascular malformations in infants and children: a classification based on endothelial characteristics. Plast Reconstr Surg 1982;69(3):412–22.

3. Mulliken J, Young A. Vascular Birthmarks : hemangiomas and malformations. Philadelphia, PA: Saunders; 1988.

4. 2018 International Society for the Study of Vascular Anomalies. ISSVA Classification of Vascular Anomalies. Available at: issva.org/classification. [Accessed 30 April 2024].

5. Jacobs AH, Walton RG. The incidence of birthmarks in the neonate. Pediatrics 1976;58(2):218–22.

6. Hand JL, Frieden IJ. Vascular birthmarks of infancy: resolving nosologic confusion. Am J Med Genet 2002;108(4):257–64.

7. Enjolras O, Mulliken JB. Vascular tumors and vascular malformations (new issues). Adv Dermatol 1997;13:375–423.

8. Amir J, Metzker A, Krikler R, et al. Strawberry hemangioma in preterm infants. Pediatr Dermatol 1986; 3(4):331–2.

9. Mulliken JB, Fishman SJ, Burrows PE. Vascular anomalies. Curr Probl Surg 2000;37(8):517–84.

10. Finn MC, Glowacki J, Mulliken JB. Congenital vascular lesions: clinical application of a new classification. J Pediatr Surg 1983;18(6):894–900.

11. Burke EC, Winkelmann RK, Strickland MK. Disseminated hemangiomatosis. the newborn with central nervous system involvement. Am J Dis Child 1964; 108:418–24.

12. Cooper AG, Bolande RP. Multiple hemangiomas in an infant with cardiac hypertrophy. postmortem angiographic demonstration of the arteriovenous fistulae. Pediatrics 1965;35:27–35.

13. Takahashi K, Mulliken JB, Kozakewich HP, et al. Cellular markers that distinguish the phases of hemangioma during infancy and childhood. J Clin Invest 1994;93(6):2357–64.

14. Mulliken JB, Zetter BR, Folkman J. In vitro characteristics of endothelium from hemangiomas and vascular malformations. Surgery 1982;92(2):348–53.

15. Cohen MM. Vasculogenesis, angiogenesis, hemangiomas, and vascular malformations. Am J Med Genet 2002;108(4):265–74.

16. Vikkula M, Boon LM, Mulliken JB. Molecular genetics of vascular malformations. Matrix Biol 2001;20(5–6): 327–35.

17. Vikkula M, Boon LM, Mulliken JB, et al. Molecular basis of vascular anomalies. Trends Cardiovasc Med 1998;8(7):281–92.

18. Yu Y, Flint AF, Mulliken JB, et al. Endothelial progenitor cells in infantile hemangioma. Blood 2004; 103(4):1373–5.

19. Glowacki J, Mulliken JB. Mast cells in hemangiomas and vascular malformations. Pediatrics 1982;70(1): 48–51.

20. North PE, Waner M, Mizeracki A, et al. A unique microvascular phenotype shared by juvenile hemangiomas and human placenta. Arch Dermatol 2001; 137(5):559–70.

21. North PE, Waner M, Mizeracki A, et al. GLUT1: a newly discovered immunohistochemical marker for juvenile hemangiomas. Hum Pathol 2000;31(1):11–22.

22. Smith CJF, Friedlander SF, Guma M, et al. Infantile Hemangiomas: An Updated Review on Risk Factors, Pathogenesis, and Treatment. Birth Defects Res 2017;109(11):809–15.

23. Kaban LB, Mulliken JB. Vascular anomalies of the maxillofacial region. J Oral Maxillofac Surg 1986; 44(3):203–13.

24. Boyd JB, Mulliken JB, Kaban LB, et al. Skeletal changes associated with vascular malformations. Plast Reconstr Surg 1984;74(6):789–97.

25. Enjolras O, Mulliken JB, Boon LM, et al. Noninvoluting congenital hemangioma: a rare cutaneous vascular anomaly. Plast Reconstr Surg 2001;107(7):1647–54.

26. Boon LM, Enjolras O, Mulliken JB. Congenital hemangioma: evidence of accelerated involution. J Pediatr 1996;128(3):329–35.

27. Kasabach HH, Merritt KK. CAPILLARY HEMANGIOMA WITH EXTENSIVE PURPURA: REPORT OF A CASE. JAMA Pediatr 1940;59:1063–70. Available at: https://api.semanticscholar.org/CorpusID:71603949.

28. Enjolras O, Wassef M, Mazoyer E, et al. Infants with Kasabach-Merritt syndrome do not have "true" hemangiomas. J Pediatr 1997;130(4):631–40.

29. Enjolras O, Mulliken JB, Wassef M, et al. Residual lesions after Kasabach-Merritt phenomenon in 41 patients. J Am Acad Dermatol 2000;42(2 Pt 1):225–35.

30. Sarkar M, Mulliken JB, Kozakewich HP, et al. Thrombocytopenic coagulopathy (Kasabach-Merritt phenomenon) is associated with Kaposiform hemangioendothelioma and not with common infantile hemangioma. Plast Reconstr Surg 1997;100(6):1377–86.

31. Lee S, Finn L, Sze RW, et al. Gorham Stout syndrome (disappearing bone disease): two additional case reports and a review of the literature. Arch Otolaryngol Head Neck Surg 2003;129(12):1340–3.

32. Radu O, Pantanowitz L. Kaposi sarcoma. Arch Pathol Lab Med 2013;137(2):289–94.

33. Painter CA, Jain E, Tomson BN, et al. The Angiosarcoma Project: enabling genomic and clinical discoveries in a rare cancer through patient-partnered research. Nat Med 2020;26(2):181–7.

34. Shon W, Billings SD. Cutaneous Malignant Vascular Neoplasms. Clin Lab Med 2017;37(3):633–46.

35. Ko JS, Billings SD. Diagnostically Challenging Epithelioid Vascular Tumors. Surg Pathol Clin 2015;8(3):331–51.

36. Kunimoto K, Yamamoto Y, Jinnin M. ISSVA Classification of Vascular Anomalies and Molecular Biology. Int J Mol Sci 2022;23(4). https://doi.org/10.3390/ijms23042358.

37. Greene AK, Goss JA. Vascular Anomalies: From a Clinicohistologic to a Genetic Framework. Plast Reconstr Surg 2018;141(5):709e–17e.

38. Borst AJ, Nakano TA, Blei F, et al. A Primer on a Comprehensive Genetic Approach to Vascular Anomalies. Front Pediatr 2020;8:579591.

39. Fevurly RD, Fishman SJ. Vascular anomalies in pediatrics. Surg Clin North Am 2012;92(3):769–800, x.

40. Defnet AM, Bagrodia N, Hernandez SL, et al. Pediatric lymphatic malformations: evolving understanding and therapeutic options. Pediatr Surg Int 2016;32(5):425–33.

41. Gilbert P, Dubois J, Giroux MF, et al. New Treatment Approaches to Arteriovenous Malformations. Semin Intervent Radiol 2017;34(3):258–71.

42. Samadi K, Salazar GM. Role of imaging in the diagnosis of vascular malformations vascular malformations. Cardiovasc Diagn Ther 2019;9(Suppl 1):S143–51.

43. Williams HB. Facial bone changes with vascular tumors in children. Plast Reconstr Surg 1979;63(3):309–16.

44. Adams DM. Practical Genetic and Biologic Therapeutic Considerations in Vascular Anomalies. Tech Vasc Interv Radiol 2019;22(4):100629.

45. Nikolaev SI, Fish JE, Radovanovic I. Somatic Activating KRAS Mutations in Arteriovenous Malformations of the Brain. N Engl J Med 2018;378(16):1561–2.

46. Drolet BA, Frommelt PC, Chamlin SL, et al. Initiation and use of propranolol for infantile hemangioma: report of a consensus conference. Pediatrics 2013;131(1):128–40.

47. Gurgacz S, Zamora L, Scott NA. Percutaneous Sclerotherapy for Vascular Malformations: A Systematic Review. Ann Vasc Surg 2014;28(5):1335–49.

48. Ali S, Mitchell S. Outcomes of Venous Malformation Sclerotherapy: A Review of Study Methodology and Long-Term Results. Semin Intervent Radiol 2017;34(03):288–93.

49. Aronniemi J, Castrén E, Lappalainen K, et al. Sclerotherapy complications of peripheral venous malformations. Phlebology 2016;31(10):712–22.

50. Cavezzi A, Parsi K. Complications of foam sclerotherapy. Phlebology 2012;27(Suppl 1):46–51.

51. Nguyen JT, Koerper MA, Hess CP, et al. Aspirin therapy in venous malformation: a retrospective cohort study of benefits, side effects, and patient experiences. Pediatr Dermatol 2014;31(5):556–60.

52. Perkins JA, Manning SC, Tempero RM, et al. Lymphatic malformations: review of current treatment. Otolaryngol Head Neck Surg 2010;142(6):795–803, 803.e1.

53. Padwa BL, Hayward PG, Ferraro NF, et al. Cervicofacial lymphatic malformation: clinical course, surgical intervention, and pathogenesis of skeletal hypertrophy. Plast Reconstr Surg 1995;95(6):951–60.

54. Comi AM. Update on Sturge-Weber syndrome: diagnosis, treatment, quantitative measures, and controversies. Lymphat Res Biol 2007;5(4):257–64.

55. Kühnel T, Wirsching K, Wohlgemuth W, et al. Hereditary Hemorrhagic Telangiectasia. Otolaryngol Clin North Am 2018;51(1):237–54.

56. Tanoue S, Tanaka N, Koganemaru M, et al. Head and Neck Arteriovenous Malformations: Clinical Manifestations and Endovascular Treatments. Interventional radiology (Higashimatsuyama-shi (Japan) 2023;8(2):23–35.

57. Lee GS, Perkins JA, Oliaei S, et al. Facial nerve anatomy, dissection and preservation in lymphatic malformation management. Int J Pediatr Otorhinolaryngol 2008;72(6):759–66.

58. Lowry TR, Gal TJ, Brennan JA. Patterns of use of facial nerve monitoring during parotid gland surgery. Otolaryngol Head Neck Surg 2005;133(3):313–8.

59. Bly RA, Holdefer RN, Slimp J, et al. Preoperative Facial Nerve Mapping to Plan and Guide Pediatric Facial Vascular Anomaly Resection. JAMA Otolaryngol Head Neck Surg 2018;144(5):418–26.

60. Susarla S, Bly R, Mulliken J, Kaban L. Chapter 14: Maxillofacial Vascular Anomalies. In: Kaban L, editor. Oral and Maxillofacial Surgery in Children. 1st edition. Batavia, IL: Quintessence Publishing Co; 2023. p. 246–52.

Head and Neck Malignancies in Children

Joseph Lopez, MD, MBA[a,b,*], Anthony P. Tufaro, DDS, MD[c]

KEYWORDS

- Oncology • Pediatric cancer • Head & neck cancer • Children cancer • Thyroid cancer

KEY POINTS

- One in 5 children present with a cancer in the head and neck region and this frequency rate of cancer continues to increase.
- The most common site of cancer in the head and neck region in children is the thyroid.
- Early detection of head and neck cancer in children is difficult. Most presenting symptoms are nonspecific.
- Surgical resection remains the mainstay of treatment for the majority of head and neck cancers in children.

INTRODUCTION

Cancer is of the top causes of death in children in the United States.[1] And unfortunately, the incidence of pediatric cancer continues to increase. A recent report by Steliarova-Foucher et al states that the incidence of cancer in children aged 0 to 14 years was 140.6 per million person-years, a significant increase from the 1980s (124.0 per million person-years).[2] Head and neck (HN) cancer in children has also been reported to be on the rise.[2–4]

EPIDEMIOLOGY OF HEAD AND NECK CANCER

At this time, HN cancers make ~12% of all pediatric cancer.[2] This commonly cited number comes from a 2002 study by Albright and colleagues examining HN cancers in 0 to 19-year-old children from 1973 to 1996.[2] While this study has several limitations including likely underreporting of the true incidence of HN cancer in children in the United States since it examines only patients under 18 years of age and looked at a limited portion of the US population,[5] a more recent national Danish study found the proportion likely to be 15%.[6] A recent National Cancer Institute's Surveillance Epidemiology and End Results (SEER) analysis performed by the authors has found similar results (**Table 1**). The authors' analysis has found that 16.7% of pediatric cancer originates in the head and neck region. Similar to prior studies, their analysis also found that HN cancer in children presents in a bimodal distribution.[2,6] The youngest patients present on average at 1 year of age while another cohort of pediatric HN cancer patients present in their teenage years. Like prior studies, their analysis revealed that the thyroid was the most common primary site accounting for 38.4% of all tumors (Lopez et al. 2024, unpublished). This was a large increase from Albright's findings of 22.1%.[2] When only including ages 0 to 19, the authors' study finds that the proportion of children with thyroid cancer continues to still be much higher at

[a] Department of Children's Surgery, Division of Pediatric Head & Neck Surgery, AdventHealth for Children, Orlando, FL, USA; [b] Department of Children's Surgery, Pediatric Head, Neck, & Thyroid Oncology Center, Florida State University, AdventHealth for Children's Hospital, Orlando, FL, USA; [c] Institute of Plastic Surgey and Dermatology. Cleveland Clinic Foundation, Cleveland, OH, USA
* Corresponding author. Department of Children's Surgery, Pediatric Head, Neck, & Thyroid Oncology Center, Florida State University, AdventHealth for Children's Hospital, Orlando, FL.
E-mail address: josephlopezmdmba@gmail.com
Twitter: @drjosephlopez (J.L.)

Oral Maxillofacial Surg Clin N Am 36 (2024) 369–377
https://doi.org/10.1016/j.coms.2024.04.001
1042-3699/24/© 2024 Elsevier Inc. All rights reserved, including those for text and data mining, AI training, and similar technologies.

Table 1
Pediatric head and neck tumors stratified by primary site

Primary Site	Male	Female	Total
Eye/orbit	1749	1632	3381
Middle Ear	28	19	47
Nasal cavity	146	95	241
Paranasal sinuses	152	140	292
Nasopharynx	540	288	828
Oral cavity	358	334	692
Oropharynx	222	136	358
Hypopharynx	7	5	12
Pharynx other	23	14	37
Larynx	33	33	66
Trachea	4	5	9
Cervical esophagus	0	1	1
Head and neck	6176	4745	10,921
Lymphatics	2646	1650	4296
Soft tissue	772	610	1382
Skeleton	813	577	1390
Skin	838	696	1534
Neural	1084	1204	2288
Other	23	8	31
Salivary glands	468	612	1080
Parotid	402	533	935
Submandibular	45	62	107
Other	21	17	38
Thyroid	2050	9169	11,219
Parathyroid	2	7	9
Total	*11,958*	*17,235*	*29,193*

32.0% (Lopez et al. 2024, unpublished). This increase has also been well documented in other countries including Brazil and Denmark.[7,8]

TYPES OF HEAD AND NECK CANCER

The most common site for pediatric HN cancer is the thyroid (**Fig. 1**). This was confirmed by the authors' SEERs analysis (Lopez et al. 2024, unpublished data). This is followed by lymphatics and the eye/orbit. **Table 2** demonstrates tumor stratification by histology based on the authors' SEERs analysis. The largest category is thyroid carcinoma with 11,118 tumors (38.1%), followed by lymphoma with 6287 tumors (21.5%) and neural malignancies with 5121 tumors (17.5%). As described earlier, the tumors with the lowest average age at diagnosis are retinoblastoma (1.3 year old), neuroblastoma (1.7 years), and germ cell neoplasms (2.1 years). Thyroid carcinoma shows the strongest sex preference with 81.8% of diagnoses in females, while acinar cell carcinoma also has a female preference with 69.8% of tumors diagnoses in females. Tumor types showing a male preference are lymphoma at 62.5% of diagnoses in males and squamous cell carcinoma with 62.2% diagnoses in males. Other tumor types do not show a strong sex preference.

PREOPERATIVE CONSIDERATIONS
Examination

Early detection of head and neck cancer is critical. Unlike other anatomic regions of the upper aerodigestive tract, routine detection of early cancer is feasible. Attention to vague symptoms such as facial/neck swelling, fatigue, fevers, dysphagia, pain, epistaxis, nasal obstruction, nasal discharge otalgia, trismus, dysarthria, and facial numbness can provide clinical information when evaluating for an HN cancer. In fact, a recent study out of Denmark found that the aforementioned symptoms are the most commonly presenting symptoms in children with HN cancer.[6]

Biopsies

The standard of care for establishing a diagnosis is biopsy. This can be performed via a fine-needle aspiration/core-biopsy or incisional biopsy. Depending on the age of the child, a biopsy may be obtained under local anesthesia, monitored-anesthesia, or general anesthesia. The authors strongly believe that a tissue diagnosis needs to be established before surgical intervention in order to provide the optimal treatment plan for children with HN cancer. Frozen section biopsy is not recommended due to the numerous limitations with frozen section analyses including the inability to perform immunostaining.

Imaging

Computed tomography (CT) scan of the head and neck with contrast is the gold standard for staging HN cancer. It has several benefits including its widespread accessibility, short processing times, and ease of interpretation by clinicians. Given the

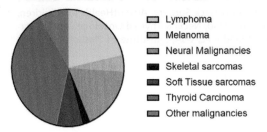

Legend:
- Lymphoma
- Melanoma
- Neural Malignancies
- Skeletal sarcomas
- Soft Tissue sarcomas
- Thyroid Carcinoma
- Other malignancies

Fig. 1. Most common head and neck tumor types.

Table 2
Pediatric head and neck tumors by tumor type

Characteristic	Male	Female	Total	Mean Age
Acinar Cell Carcinoma	105	243	348	17.7
Adenocarcinoma	64	59	123	16.2
Adenoid Cystic Carcinoma	31	44	75	17.3
Germ Cell neoplasms	62	70	132	2.1
Lymphoma	3927	2360	6287	13.1
Hodgkin Lymphoma	1755	1252	3007	15.6
Non-Hodgkin Lymphoma	1157	638	1795	12.8
Other Lymphoma	1015	470	1485	8.6
Melanoma	696	609	1305	16.2
Mucoepidermoid carcinoma	283	387	670	15.4
Neural Malignancies	2537	2584	5121	3.3
Neuroblastoma	101	92	193	1.7
Retinoblastoma	1358	1329	2687	1.3
Other	1078	1163	2241	5.8
Skeletal sarcomas	342	303	645	13.0
Osteosarcoma	113	81	194	14.5
Chondrosarcoma	35	33	68	14.9
Ewing sarcoma	79	67	146	10.8
Other	115	122	237	12.6
Soft Tissue sarcomas	1231	1009	2240	9.4
Rhabdomyosarcoma (RMS)	737	589	1326	7.8
Parameningeal RMS	184	153	337	9.4
Nonparameningeal RMS	553	436	989	7.2
Non-RMS Soft Tissue Sarcomas	494	420	914	11.9
Squamous cell carcinoma	352	214	566	17.1
Thyroid Carcinoma	2020	9098	11,118	17.5
Follicular	119	636	755	17.2
Papillary	1688	8025	9713	17.7
Medullary	122	189	311	13.0
Other Thyroid carcinoma	91	248	339	16.5
Other malignancies	308	255	563	15.0
Total	*11,958*	*17,235*	*29,193*	*13.1*

risk of radiation exposure to children, MRI can also be used for specific anatomic locations such as the paranasal sinus, salivary glands, and oral/oropharynx. An MRI allows for better soft tissue characterization including the evaluation of perineural tumor spread but has several limitations including possible need for sedation/general anesthesia in children due to claustrophobia and duration of scan time. The use of dual-modality imaging such as both CT and MRI may be beneficial in certain situations involving osseous structures, such as the skull base. A CT scan allows for evaluation of cortical erosion and osseous destruction while MRI can detail marrow involvement.[9]

In adults HN patients, detection of cervical lymphadenopathy through CT has been shown to improve the sensitivity (75% for physical examination vs 91% for CT and physical examination).[9] However, imaging for lymph nodes in children can commonly be evaluated with a lymph node ultrasound neck survey. An experienced ultrasonographer can detect cervical lymphadenopathy and provide the information needed for detection of malignancy. Ultrasound lymph node characteristics are critically important to determine lymph node cancer invasion and some of these characteristics include presence of micro calcifications, irregular borders, size, and the lack of fatty hilum.

There are several indications for the use of PET in the setting of initial presentation: assessment of potential distant metastatic disease and evaluation of potential primary sites in the setting of unknown primary cancer.[10] In addition, PET may be helpful in post-treatment surveillance, allowing one to assess local and distant recurrences. However, discerning from post-surgical or post-radiation changes may lead to increased uptake due to inflammation that may be interpreted as tumor recurrence. As such, delaying PET after 12 weeks post treatment is recommended. In addition, certain cancers with low metabolic activity or necrotic tumors are non-fludeoxyglucose (FDG)-avid tumors that may lead to a false-negative result. Therefore, one should be aware that PET imaging has difficulty discerning between inflammation and infectious processes such as radionecrosis.

Staging

The American Joint Committee on Cancer (AJCC) implements a combination the tumor (T = maximum size of tumor), node (N = cervical nodes with metastatic tumor), metastasis (M = evidence of distant metastasis) commonly known as TNM staging classification to classify, prognosticate, and determine treatment of head and neck cancer.[4] For simplicity, small tumors without nodal metastases are considered Stage I and II, whereas large extensive tumors are considered Stage III and IV.

Invasion into surrounding tissue whether into soft tissue, lymphatics, nodes, vascular or neural structures factors into worse prognosis and more extensive treatment. At this time, head and neck cancer in children is staged with the eighth edition of the AJCC guidelines which was introduced in 2017.[11]

TREATMENT/MANAGEMENT
Surgical Resection

With the notable exception of nasopharyngeal carcinoma, surgical resection remains the gold standard for most pediatric head and neck cancer. General surgical principle is to provide clear margins of greater than 5 mm while minimizing morbidity by preserving form and function. Margins greater than 5 mm are deemed adequate in most sites by National Comprehensive Cancer Network guidelines.[12] Literature does support clear pathologic margins as small as 5 mm provide better functional and aesthetic outcomes and quality of life. Choice of treatment such as lip split or neck incision varies based on anatomic accessibility.

Rationale of Neck Dissection

The goal of neck dissection is to remove lympho-fibro-fatty contents of the neck for treatment of cervical lymphatic metastases and to allow for complete staging.

Classification of lymph nodes in the neck is primarily based on the original Memorial Sloan Kettering Cancer Center classification.[13] It has been adopted by the American Head and Neck Society and Committee for Head and Neck Surgery and Oncology of the American Academy of Otolaryngology-Head and Neck Surgery. Neck dissection can be considered therapeutic when there is evidence of local regional disease. It results in aid in staging and management. On the other hand, elective neck dissection is indicated for the removal of possibly undetected regional metastatic disease or confirm N0 status. Elective neck dissection is recommended when perineural or perivascular invasion is found in Stage I and II cases. Prophylactic treatment for N0 neck is to treat any patient whose risk of occult lymph node metastasis is greater than 15% to 20%. Such risk of regional lymph node metastases varies according to the type of cancer, location of the primary site, and stage.

Types of Neck Dissection

One should be familiar with the different types of neck dissections and as to how they have evolved over time:

Radical neck dissection is indicated for advanced neck disease with multiple-level positive lymph nodes, gross extracapsular spread, or infiltration of sternocleidomastoid muscle, cranial nerve XI, or internal jugular vein. It consists of removal of all ipsilateral cervical nodes extending from the inferior border of the mandible to the clavicle. This involves neck levels I through V. The internal jugular vein, sternocleidomastoid muscle, and the spinal accessory nerve are also resected.

A *modified radical neck dissection* is similar to that of the radical neck dissection since it involves removal of all nodes within level I to V. However, it preserves at least 1 or more of the following non-lymphatic structures: sternocleidomastoid (SCM), internal jugular vein, and cranial nerve XI.

A *selective neck dissection* involves preservation of 1 or more node groups which are routinely removed in a radical neck dissection.

A *supraomohyoid neck dissection* involves removal of levels I-III, especially in cases of oral cavity squamous cell carcinoma.

A *central compartment neck dissection* involves selective removal of the level VI nodes. This is usually performed for cancers of the thyroid, hypopharynx, cervical trachea, cervical esophagus, and subglottic larynx.

Radiation therapy

Radiotherapy is a mainstay treatment of HN cancer. Radiation treats cancer cells by its ionization effect within the DNA molecules or by interacting with intracellular water molecules to create free radicals, and thereby indirectly damaging DNA.[14] There are 4 basic principles of radiation biology, the 4 R's: repair, reassortment, repopulation, and reoxygenation. This premise falls on the notion that cancer cells have impaired repair mechanisms. As such, dividing radiotherapy into multiple lower dose treatments otherwise known as "fractionation" exploits the differences in repair capacities between normal tissues and tumors. Therefore, it is hypothesized that hyperfractionation, using 2 or more small doses of radiation per day, would lead to redistribution or reassortment of dividing cells into more radiation-sensitive stages of the cell cycle.[15] Finally, it is also believed that oxygen plays an important role in damaging the double-strands in DNA. Such studies have confirmed that twice the increase in radiation dose is needed to achieve the same cell death in hypoxic tumors compared to well-oxygenated tumors.[16]

Radiation therapy can be used as the primary or adjuvant therapy. Primary therapy may be indicated for patients with unresectable tumors.

Systemic therapy

The use chemotherapy is often employed in children with unresectable HN cancer. The type of chemotherapy that is utilized is highly dependent on the type of cancer. Additionally, children with positive surgical margins or distant metastasis may require adjuvant chemotherapy. It is important to note that all children with HN cancer should be enrolled in clinical trials, if possible, to contribute to ongoing research studying the utility of chemotherapy in HN cancer.

Adjuvant therapy

More recently, the discovery of immune modulation in HN cancer has dramatically improved our understanding and treatment of cancer.[17] In adult HN cancer patients, the development of programmed death 1 (PD-1) immune-checkpoint inhibitors has gained popularity in management of head and neck cancer. The promising results seen with immunotherapy have revolutionized the treatment of HN cancer leading to remission and improved survival leading to recent Food & Drug Administration (FDA) approvals of anti-PD1 antibodies, pembrolizumab, and nivolumab. Although few studies have studied the utility of immunotherapy in pediatric patients, off-label use of these

agents is ongoing and further research is necessary to better delineate their utility in the treatment of HN cancer.

CASE STUDIES
Salivary Cancer: Case 1

A 13-year-old child presented to his pediatrician after his mother noticed facial asymmetry (right fullness > left). The pediatrician ordered an ultrasound which revealed a 3 × 1 × 1 cystic mass with 2 adjacent enlarged lymph nodes. An infection work-up was performed including an evaluation of Epstein Barr virus , cytomegalovirus, and toxoplasmosis and all were negative. The patient was then referred to pediatric head/neck surgery. On examination, a 2 cm palpable, pre-auricular mass was found overlying the inferior border of the zygomatic bone. The inner right-sided buccal mucosa was intact with no evidence of mucosal changes but 2 palpable lymph nodes measuring approximately 1 cm in size were found on level 2. The patient was ordered an MRI which confirmed the presence of a mixed solid-cystic mass that was well circumscribed but heterogeneous and within the superficial lobe of the parotid (**Fig. 2**). Enlargement of the level 2 lymph node was also found on imaging. The patient then underwent a fine-needle aspiration of parotid mass which confirmed malignant cells, specifically mucoepidermoid carcinoma. The patient was then discussed at pediatric tumor board and surgical resection of the tumor with concurrent right selective neck dissection (I–III) was recommended (**Fig. 3**).

Thyroid Cancer: Case 2

A 15-year-old young girl presented to a pulmonologist for multiple sub centimeters nodules throughout

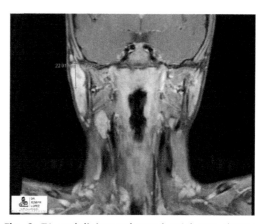

Fig. 2. T1 gadolinium-enhanced axial MRI demonstrating a 3 ×1 cm enhancing mass lesion on the superior portion of the superficial parotid gland.

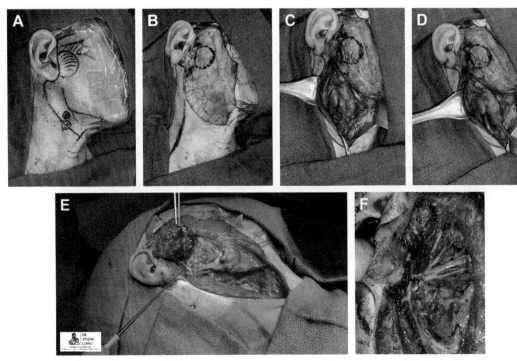

Fig. 3. (*A*) Intra-operative skin margins showing a modified-blair incision (*B*) supra-plastysmal flap elevation with markings of the underlying tumor (*C*) selective neck dissection level I-III (*D*) Removal of lymphatic packet (*E*) Removal of superficial parotidectomy (*E*) Removal of tumor with sacrifice of frontal branch of the facial nerve for perineural invasion (*F*) Frontal branch of the facial nerve with perineural invasion with nerve exhibiting epi-neural vascular changes.

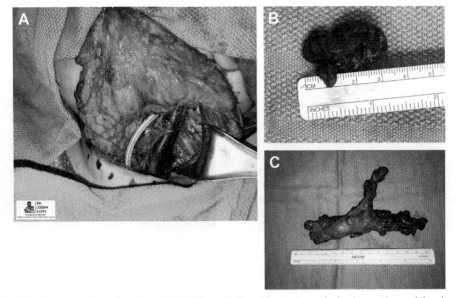

Fig. 4. (*A*) Selective neck dissection Level II-IV (*B*) total thyroidectomy pathologic specimen (*C*) selective neck dissection specimen with multiple pathologic lymph nodes.

the bilateral lungs and multiple left central/lateral neck enlarged lymph nodes. This all occurred after a recent coronavirus disease infection that required hospitalization for respiratory distress. The patient was ordered a thyroid ultrasound as part of the work-up for the cervical lymphadenopathy which revealed a 3-cm hypoechoic nodule with microcalcifications. Further work-up of the lung nodules was not possible to their size. The patient was referred to pediatric head and neck who performed a thyroid nodule biopsy that revealed papillary thyroid carcinoma. Due to history of anxiety and difficulty performing a concurrent left neck lymph node biopsy at the time of the thyroid biopsy, the patient deferred the recommended left-sided neck lymph node biopsy. The patient was presented at pediatric tumor board who recommended a total thyroidectomy, central neck dissection, and excisional biopsy of an enlarged left level 4 lymph node (~3 cm). The patient tolerated the procedure and pathology confirmed multifocal papillary thyroid carcinoma with negative margins and evidence of 8 positive lymph nodes in the central neck. The left-sided level 4 lymph node excisional biopsy also revealed papillary thyroid carcinoma without evidence of extranodal extension. Given these pathologic findings, the patient was represented at pediatric tumor board and a left selective neck dissection (level II-IV) was recommended due to local regional metastasis. The patient underwent a left selective neck dissection 6 weeks post-total thyroidectomy and central neck dissection. Left selective neck dissection pathology revealed a total of 8/40 lymph nodes positive for papillary carcinoma in level II, III, and IV. The patient was then treated with adjuvant radioactive iodine with 154 mCi 3 weeks after the left-sided selective neck dissection. The patient was followed with 3 month ultrasounds and labs which revealed at 1 year follow-up no changes in her pulmonary nodules but a single level 4 lymph node on the right with microcalcifications. This lymph node underwent a fine needle aspiration which revealed a papillary thyroid carcinoma. The patient thereafter underwent a right selective neck dissection (Level II-IV) which revealed 5/42 positive lymph nodes. She is now 6 months post-right selective neck dissection with no evidence of disease (**Fig. 4**).

Rhabdomyosarcoma: Case 3

An 8-year-old male with embryonal rhabdomyosarcoma in the left infratemporal fossa was referred to the authors' institution after developing recurrence 11 months post initial treatment. Cross-sectional imaging demonstrated recurrent disease medial to the left mandibular condyle/

ramus, anterior to the left carotid canal and left internal jugular vein, measuring 2 × 1.5 cm.

The surgical resection was deemed quite challenging due to the tumors proximity to the internal and external carotid arteries (**Fig. 5**). Therefore, a balloon occlusion test was performed to determine if embolization of the left common carotid was feasible and thereby facilitating a safer resection. Since sufficient collateral flow existed through the Circle of Willis, embolization of the internal carotid artery proximal and distal to the tumor was performed in addition to embolization of the external carotid artery (**Fig. 6**A, B).

Surgical resection via an infratemporal fossa approach via lip-split and lower cheek flap was performed. A composite resection involving a segmental mandibulectomy was also performed (**Fig. 6**C, D). The tumor was safely dissected off the internal carotid artery, foramen lacerum, and internal jugular vein and negative pathologic margins were obtained. The infratemporal fossa was reconstructed with a free anterolateral (ALT) flap. The patient tolerated surgery well without any neurologic deficits with no evidence of recurrent disease at 15 months post-operatively.

Osteosarcoma: Case 4

A 13-year-old female presented to her dentist with a swelling in the left mandibular area. The

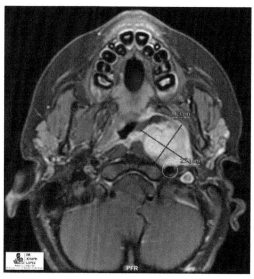

Fig. 5. T1 gadolinium-enhanced axial MRI demonstrating a 3.6 × 2.7 cm enhancing mass lesion centered in the left parapharyngeal/retropharyngeal space. The prevertebral musculature on the left side is displaced medially and the medial lateral pterygoid muscle is displaced laterally. The lesion is directly adjacent to the descending and horizontal portion of the left internal carotid artery (*circled*).

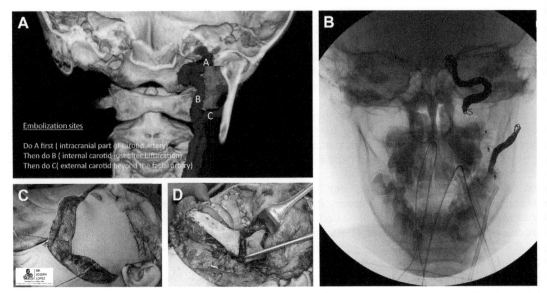

Fig. 6. (*A*) Embolization sites (*B*) Skull X-ray after embolization (*C*) Infratemporal Fossa Lip-Split, Cheek Flap Approach; (*D*) Mandibulectomy via CAD/CAM guide.

associated teeth were stable. A cone beam CT revealed the classic features of an osteogenic sarcoma, a sunburst appearance, periosteal lifting, and formation of new bone in the soft tissues. She was presented to multidisciplinary tumor board and the consensus was to proceed with surgical resection of the tumor. Neo-adjuvant therapy was not considered based on the fact that this was a low-grade tumor. The patient had standard staging work up and the mandible was found to be the only site of disease. She underwent a composite resection of the left mandible and immediate reconstruction with a fibula free tissue transfer. Pre-operative surgical planning included cutting guides for the fibula and the mandible. Custom hardware was used to fix the fibula in place. The patient had an R0 resection and was reviewed in tumor board again and no adjuvant therapy was advised. The patient did very well post-operatively. The authors utilized

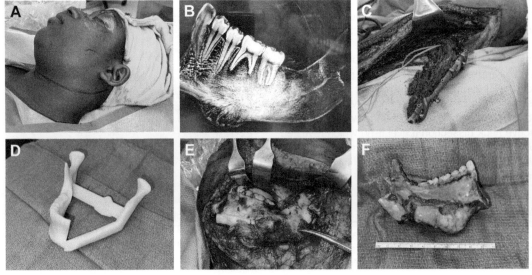

Fig. 7. (*A*) Pre-operative markings (*B*) "sun-burst" appearance of tumor on X-ray (*C*) Fibula-Free Tissue Transfer (*D*) 3D anatomic model of resection and fibula reconstruction (*E*) mandibular tumor in-situ (*F*) composite resection specimen.

guiding elastics in the early post-operative period to maintain perfect occlusion (**Fig. 7**).

SUMMARY

Pediatric HN cancer appears in a bimodal distribution by age and its incidence has continued to increase since 2000. Furthermore, its incidence is increasing at a faster rate than overall pediatric cancer. Future studies are needed to further evaluate underlying factors that cause HN cancer in children.

CLINICS CARE POINTS

- Head & Neck cancer is increasing incidence over the past two decades.
- Management of head and neck cancer in children is supported by lower level evidence studies and requires further investigation to improve best-practices.

DISCLOSURE

Both authors have no conflicts to disclose.

REFERENCES

1. Goldstick JE, Cunningham RM, Carter PM. Current causes of death in children and adolescents in the united states. N Engl J Med 2022;386(20):1955–6.
2. Albright JT, Topham AK, Reilly JS. Pediatric head and neck malignancies: Us incidence and trends over 2 decades. Arch Otolaryngol Head Neck Surg 2002;128(6):655–9.
3. Bernier MO, Withrow DR, Berrington de Gonzalez A, et al. Trends in pediatric thyroid cancer incidence in the united states, 1998-2013. Cancer 2019;125(14):2497–505.
4. Vergamini LB, Frazier AL, Abrantes FL, et al. Increase in the incidence of differentiated thyroid carcinoma in children, adolescents, and young adults: A population-based study. J Pediatr 2014;164(6):1481–5.
5. Hardin AP, Hackell JM, Committee On P, et al. Age limit of pediatrics. Pediatrics 2017;140(3). https://doi.org/10.1542/peds.2017-2151.
6. Lilja-Fischer JK, Schroder H, Nielsen VE. Pediatric malignancies presenting in the head and neck. Int J Pediatr Otorhinolaryngol 2019;118:36–41.
7. de Souza Reis R, Gatta G, de Camargo B. Thyroid carcinoma in children, adolescents, and young adults in brazil: A report from 11 population-based cancer registries. PLoS One 2020;15(5):e0232416.
8. Schmidt Jensen J, Gronhoj C, Mirian C, et al. Incidence and survival of thyroid cancer in children, adolescents, and young adults in denmark: A nationwide study from 1980 to 2014. Thyroid 2018;28(9):1128–33.
9. Hamilton B. Diagnostic imaging. In: Bell RB, Andersen PA, Fernandes RP, editors. Oral, head and neck oncology and reconstructive surgery. 1st edition. St. Louis, MO: Elsevier; 2018. p. 107–18.
10. Evangelista L, Cervino AR, Chondrogiannis S, et al. Comparison between anatomical cross-section imaging and 18FDG-PET in the staging, restaging, treatment response, and long-term surveillance of squamous cell head and neck cancer: a systematic literature overview. Nucl Med Commun 2014;35:123–34.
11. Lydiatt WM, Patel SG, O'Sullivan B, et al. Head and neck cancers—major changes in the American Joint Committee on Cancer eighth edition cancer staging manual. CA Cancer J Clin 2017;67(2):122–37.
12. Miller MC, Goldenberg D. AHNS series: do you know your guidelines? Principles of surgery for head and neck cancer a review of the National Comprehensive Cancer Network guidelines. Head Neck 2017;39:791–6.
13. Amin MB, Greene FL, Edge SB, et al. The eighth edition AJCC cancer staging manual: continuing to build a bridge from a population-based to a more "personalized" approach to cancer staging. CA Cancer J Clin 2017;67:93–9.
14. Elliot DA, Nabavizadeh N, Seung SK, et al. Radiation therapy. In: Bell RB, Andersen PA, Fernandes RP, editors. Oral, head and neck oncology and reconstructive surgery. 1st edition. St. Louis, MO: Elsevier; 2018. p. 268–90.
15. Withers HR. Cell cycle redistribution as a factor in multifraction irradiation. Radiology 1975;114:199–202.
16. Barilla J, Lokajicek M. The role of oxygen in DNA damage by ionizing particles. J Theor Biol 2000;207:405–14.
17. Vermorken JB, Herbst RS, Leon X, et al. Overview of the efficacy of cetuximab in recurrent and/or metastatic squamous cell carcinoma of the head and neck in patients who previously failed platinum-based therapies. Cancer 2008;112:2710–9.

Craniomaxillofacial Fibro-osseous Lesions in Children

Andrea B. Burke, DMD, MD

KEYWORDS

- Fibro-osseous disease • Fibrous dysplasia • McCune–Albright syndrome • Ossifying fibroma
- Cemento-osseous dysplasia

KEY POINTS

- Significant histologic overlap complicates the diagnosis of benign, nonodontogenic, craniofacial fibro-osseous diseases.
- Clinical behavior (quiescent/stable, slow growing, and aggressive) is the most important consideration when managing craniofacial fibro-osseous lesions.
- Treatment objectives are patient-specific, ranging from active surveillance to recontouring of bone or complete resection.

INTRODUCTION

Fibro-osseous lesions (FOLs) encompass a varied range of pathologic conditions in which fibrous tissue replaces normal bone, leading to the development of irregular, woven bone. These lesions involve developmental, reactive, dysplastic, and neoplastic processes.[1] Owing to the diverse etiology and pathogenesis, accurately categorizing these lesions remains a challenging task.[2]

The craniofacial complex is anatomically the most sophisticated structure in the vertebrate skeleton, with most bones forming via intramembranous ossification. FOLs occur commonly in the craniofacial bones, and their clinical behavior is unique compared to that of the axial and appendicular skeleton. Lesions are typically discovered in childhood and, in some cases, can be quite aggressive.

When evaluating a patient with suspected craniofacial FOL, history is important: *Is this lesion something that was noticed recently, has been bothering the patient for some time, or was this an incidental finding?* On presentation, it is important to ask about associated symptoms,

including changes to the surrounding tissues. Be aware of underlying comorbid conditions and genetic factors that can be part of a larger systemic constellation of findings. For instance, fibrous dysplasia (FD) can be part of the McCune–Albright syndrome (MAS), presenting with café-au-lait macules and hyperfunctioning endocrinopathies (**Fig. 1**).

Previous reports state that the average age of diagnosis for pediatric craniofacial FOL is 8 to 12 years.[3–5] Most lesions begin to grow as slow, painless masses, gradually expanding the bone. Depending on their clinical behavior, lesions may be characterized as slow growing, quiescent, or aggressive. The later may be accompanied by pain and paresthesia and more rapid growth/expansion.[3] Furthermore, depending on the location of the lesion, other findings may include trismus, malocclusion, or orbital symptoms (including visual acuity changes and proptosis)

The radiographic examination will be of utmost importance in discovering and diagnosing FOL. Maxillofacial computed tomography (CT), typically without contrast, is the gold standard imaging, but lesions can be discovered on dedicated dental

Department of Oral and Maxillofacial Surgery, University of Washington School of Dentistry, 1959 Northeast Pacific Street, Box 357134, Seattle, WA 98195-7134, USA
E-mail address: abburke@uw.edu

Oral Maxillofacial Surg Clin N Am 36 (2024) 379–390
https://doi.org/10.1016/j.coms.2024.03.004
1042-3699/24/© 2024 Elsevier Inc. All rights reserved.

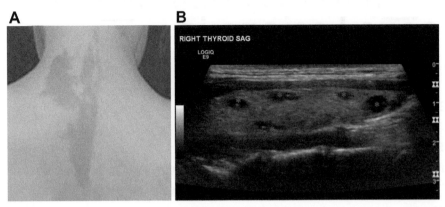

Fig. 1. Extraskeletal findings in fibrous dysplasia. (*A*) Café-au-lait macule with characteristic coast-of-Maine borders and not crossing the midline. (*B*) Thyroid ultrasound depicting multiple cystic nodules (*asterisk*).

films and other studies. In pediatric patients, the development of "black bone" MRI sequencing has proved helpful in minimizing ionizing radiation exposure.[6] Determining the location of the craniofacial FOL can help narrow down the differential diagnosis. As abnormal conditions are more likely to be unilateral, determine whether the bone is affected on one or both sides. Size is extremely important when assessing the clinical behavior of fibro-osseous bony lesions. Take note of whether there is a single lesion or multifocal appearance, as the differential for multifocal lesions is shorter than compared to a solitary lesion. Multifocal bony lesions also tend to be those with systemic implications. Lesions may exist as a radiolucent structure or have various amounts of calcified structures—appearing radiopaque or of mixed radiographic density.[7] Dystrophic calcification can occur ectopically in surrounding soft tissues or within the lesion (such as in cemento-ossifying fibroma [COF]). The effects of FOL on surrounding structures can be subtle or dramatic, with mass effects causing widening of the inferior alveolar nerve (IAN) or cortical destruction. Tooth displacement may occur, or resorption may be noted. Inflammation may cause periosteal reaction or cortical spiculation.[7]

All craniofacial FOL histology is composed of a variation of the following: (1) woven bone admixed with fibrous tissue; (2) bland spindle cells; (3) immature, woven bone (osteoid) in a collagenized fibroblastic stroma; and (4) occasionally, globules of immature bone/cementum (**Fig. 2**). In the jaws, the convention has been to call "bone" anything with trabecular morphology and osteoblasts or osteocytes, and anything with acellular mineralized material, "cementum." However, cementum and osteoid are histologically identical. Therefore, the clinical context (the biopsy location) is important when making a diagnosis.[8]

CLASSIFICATION OF FIBRO-OSSEOUS LESIONS

Classification of benign, nonodontogenic fibro-osseous diseases remains a challenge due to the significant histologic overlap and frequent misdiagnosis of these complex diseases. They have been categorized as benign mesenchymal tumors, including giant cell lesions and associated syndromes (cherubism, Noonan multiple giant cell syndrome), FD (MAS), ossifying fibroma (OF; COF), and cemento-osseous dysplasia (COD; florid, focal).[1,9]

As they are considered a spectrum of benign mesenchymal disease, where bone is replaced by fibrous tissue, other pathologies have been grouped with FOL, including osteoblastoma and myxoma.[9] All FOLs have the characteristic bony changes and various proliferation of hematopoietic giant cells and angiogenesis.[10]

Previous attempts at categorization have placed craniofacial FOLs into "Odontogenic" category, "Tumors of Undefined Neoplastic Nature," "Bone-related lesions," and more recently "Fibro-osseous tumors and dysplasias."[2,11] This most recent WHO classification (2022)[12] includes segmental odontomaxillary dysplasia (SOD), both juvenile trabecular and psammomatoid OF, and familial gigantiform cementoma (not discussed here). Other classifications have included FOLs and giant cell lesions in a "Benign Mesenchymal Tumor" category.[3,13]

Much of the confusion stems from archaic terminology, applied to the diagnosis and descriptions of lesions, but not considering their biologic behavior. For example, some FOLs can be aggressive, but some are not. Chuong and colleagues[3] developed a classification specific to GCT but this can be loosely translated to all the FOLs. Yet, the issue is that treatment decisions, including

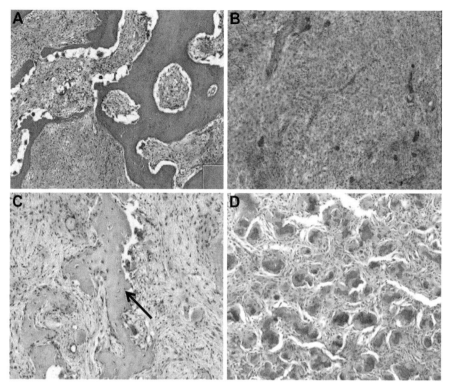

Fig. 2. Fibro-osseous lesion histology. (*A*) General characteristics include a background stroma of fibrous tissue admixed with woven bone. (*B*) Areas of bland spindle cells in sheets may be present. (*C*) Immature, woven bone or osteoid (*arrow*), and (*D*) globules of cementum (cementicles) may be seen.

surgical management, are based on this confusing nomenclature while not taking into account the overall *clinical behavior* of the FOL. Plus, the added complexity of tooth-bearing bone makes for a broader differential. The author has identified some examples of FOL and FO-related lesions based on recent classification.

Simple Bone Cyst

Simple bone cysts (traumatic bone, unicameral bone, or idiopathic bone cysts) are not true cysts, as they do not have an epithelial lining. They are empty, commonly fluid-filled cavities within the bone that occur in childhood (**Fig. 3**). While not an FOL per se, they share similar features, including occasional multinucleated giant cells along the bony surface (Howship's lacunae), indicating bone resorption. Their etiology remains unknown, but trauma or a low-flow vascular malformation was previously suspected as the cause.[1] Thought to be on the same pathophysiologic spectrum as FOL, they can occur within an FOL or may be associated with the misdiagnosis of FOL.

More common in young female individuals, these lesions are most common in the posterior mandible. Radiographically, a multilocular radiolucency is present, with lesions showing cortical thinning and sometimes displacement of teeth.[7] Surgical exploration and curettage yields a blood-filled cavity with no discernible lining. Bone will fill in these lesions, and recurrence, especially in children, is rare.[9]

Aneurysmal Bone Cyst

Existing along this spectrum of bony diseases, aneurysmal bone cysts (ABCs) are also pseudo-cysts which can occur within FOL. They have been observed either as solitary lesions or in conjunction with existing FOLs. These lesions are most commonly found in young people (>30 years of age), with a female prevalence.[1] Occurrence has been noted in the spine, femur, and tibia, with rare occurrences in the craniofacial skeleton. ABCs are expansive vascular bony lesions characterized by blood-filled channels, enveloped by cellular fibrous connective tissues and reactive woven bone. Their etiology is unknown, with some similar speculation around trauma or low-flow venous malformations.

ABCs may be aggressive, exhibiting rapid growth and swelling, leading to pain and destruction of

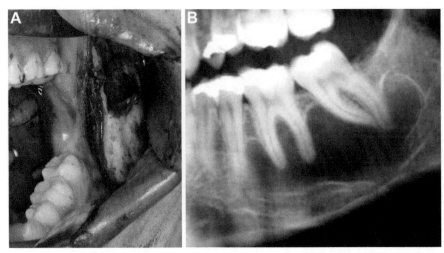

Fig. 3. Simple bone cyst. (*A*) Blood-filled cavity noted on surgical exploration of the left posterior mandible. (*B*) Well-defined radiolucency of the left mandible, scalloping around the roots of the teeth, and displacing the inferior alveolar canal.

surrounding structures. Consequently, pain, paresthesia, and cortical expansion are common presentations. Dental examination may reveal tooth resorption and malocclusion due to the expansive nature of ABCs. Radiographically, these lesions appear as unilocular or multilocular radiolucencies with cortical expansion and "eggshell" thinning. CT or MRI often reveals the characteristic "fluid-fluid" level, indicative of layered old and new blood, which is considered pathognomonic (**Fig. 4**).[7]

Histologically, ABCs exhibit cortical bone thinning, occasional perforation, and lack a true endothelial or cystic lining. The lesion typically contains unclotted blood, sometimes actively bleeding, with minimal fibroblastic tissue that may include multinucleated giant cells. Trabeculae of osteoid (immature bone) form a lacy pattern of calcification. Treatment involves curettage and enucleation of contents, often coupled with peripheral osteotomy

or cryogenic treatment to prevent recurrence.[1] Recurrence rates vary but can be as high as 50%, particularly in the presence of coexisting lesions. In rare cases, surgical resection may be necessary for complete ABC removal. Follow-up typically reveals bony defect filling within 6 to 12 months.[9]

Cytogenetic abnormalities, such as the gene fusion between osteoblast cadherin (CDH11) on chromosome 16q22 and ubiquitin-specific protease 6 (transferrin receptor-like protein-2 [Tre2] or ubiquitin carboxyl-terminal hydrolase 6 [USP6]), have been identified in ABCs. Some reports note giant cell lesions in the jaw with the USP6 rearrangement.[14]

Giant Cell Lesion/Central Giant Cell Granuloma

Typically, true giant cell tumors (GCT) predominantly manifest in the epiphyses of long trabecular

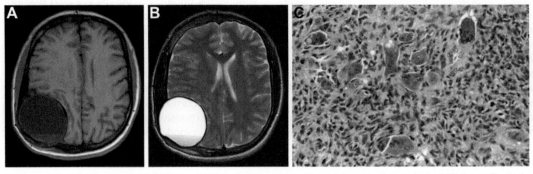

Fig. 4. Aneurysmal bone cyst. (*A*) T1- and (*B*) T2-weighted MR images of a large aneurysmal bone cyst within fibrous dysplasia bone of the calvarium. Note the characteristic layering of old and new blood within the lesion and the significant expansion. (*C*) High-power hematoxylin and eosin stain shows fibrous background with multinucleated giant cells.

bones. Conversely, giant cell lesions (central giant cell granuloma [CGCG]) that are observed in the jaws are considered non-neoplastic; however, they can exhibit aggressive behavior akin to neoplastic conditions. In addition to CGCG and GCT, they can be classified as brown tumor of hyperparathyroidism. Most cases stem from secondary hyperparathyroidism in conjunction with renal failure, which elevates parathyroid hormone (PTH), thereby causing osteoclastic bony resorption.[1,9] Laboratory values may also show elevated serum alkaline phosphatase and calcium levels, with low phosphorus (**Fig. 5**).

CGCGs predominantly affect female individuals before the age of 30 years, and the majority of cases are found in the anterior mandible, often crossing the midline. Clinically, these lesions are categorized as either nonaggressive or aggressive.[3] Aggressive lesions, characterized by pain, rapid growth, significant swelling, paresthesia, root resorption, cortical perforation, and recurrence, are more prevalent in a younger age group. They are typically larger at the time of diagnosis (size exceeding 4 cm at presentation) and have a higher recurrence rate. On the other hand, nonaggressive lesions exhibit slow growth, lack of pain, variable expansion on presentation, and no evidence of resorption.[3] Radiographically, these lesions present as expansile unilocular or multilocular radiolucencies with a noncorticated but well-defined appearance. Nonaggressive lesions are commonly found incidentally on dental radiographs or as a nonpainful jaw swelling.

Histologically, these lesions display a dense population of multinucleated giant cells set against a backdrop of actively proliferating mesenchymal cells that are ovoid to spindle-shaped, accompanied by bony destruction and heightened vascularity. There is some indication that these giant cells may indeed represent osteoclasts (**Fig. 5**).[10]

The standard treatment involves surgical enucleation and curettage. For nonaggressive lesions, this should be sufficient. However, locally aggressive and destructive lesions are similar to the GCT of long bones and have a high rate of recurrence, with no inclination to metastasize. Aggressive lesions necessitate additional therapies such as interferon-alpha2a, RANKL inhibition (denosumab), calcitonin, steroids, or other antiangiogenic drugs. Brown tumors respond to the correction of the underlying endocrinopathy, usually with parathyroidectomy or treatment of renal disease.[9]

When observed in multiple quadrants, potential differential diagnoses should encompass conditions such as cherubism and Noonan syndrome. Cherubism is an uncommon disorder resulting from autosomal dominant or spontaneous gain-of-function mutations in the SH3 Domain Binding Protein 2 (SH3BP2) gene, promoting osteoclastogenesis.[15] This condition manifests as painless bilateral swelling in the upper and lower jaws, leading to cheek fullness and, in some cases, an upturned appearance of the eyes resembling a cherub or angel—hence the name "Cherubism." In severe instances, significant expansion may involve most of the mandible and/or maxilla. Intraorally, the lesions exhibit clinical features consistent with giant cell lesions, causing tooth displacement or occasionally resulting in missing teeth. Additional clinical features may include submandibular lymphadenopathy and elevated serum

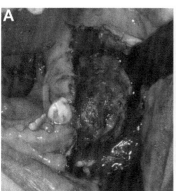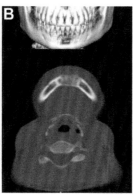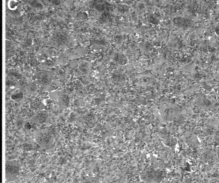

ig. 5. Giant cell lesion. (*A*) Intraoperative enucleation in a child showing a specimen with the characteristic purplish hue. (*B*) Maxillofacial CT imaging of a giant cell lesion in the anterior mandible, as seen in the 3D reformat (*above*) and the axial slice (*below*). Note the poorly-defined, destructive nature which erodes the cortex. (*C*) Low-power hematoxylin and eosin stain showing the presence of large multinucleated giant cells, with multiple nuclei dispersed throughout the cytoplasm. These giant cells are surrounded by a stroma of mononuclear spindle-shaped cells and areas of hemorrhage.

alkaline phosphatase levels.[9] Typically, the giant cell lesions associated with cherubism regress after skeletal maturity or puberty, as the condition is usually self-limiting. In cases of aggressive disease, interventions such as tooth extraction, surgical contouring, or curettage of lesions may be deemed necessary.

Noonan syndrome with multiple giant cell lesions represents a phenotypic variation of the autosomal dominant condition characterized by craniofacial anomalies (including ptosis, hypertelorism, downslanting palpebral fissures, and low-set, posteriorly rotated ears), pulmonary valve stenosis and/or hypertrophic cardiomyopathy, short stature, pectus carinatum/excavatum, short webbed neck, mild developmental delay, cryptorchidism, lymphatic dysplasia, and coagulation factor deficiency. The mutation identified in Noonan syndrome with multiple giant cell lesions is in the PTPN11 gene.[16] Additionally, giant cells are also observed in other syndromes associated with the rat-sarcoma virus (Ras)/mitogen-activated protein kinases (MAPK) pathway.

Fibrous Dysplasia

The most extensively studied FOL is FD, an uncommon mosaic disease affecting bone marrow stromal cells due to a postzygotic somatic activating mutation in the GNAS gene. Fibro-osseous tissue replaces normal bone and marrow, leading to potential complications such as fractures, deformities, functional limitations, and bone pain.[17] Clinically, FD can manifest in the craniofacial, axial, and/or appendicular skeleton, with onset typically in childhood. Even though painless swellings are typically noted on clinical examination, patients can experience bone pain, which may be related to their disease burden or extent of bony involvement. There is no discernible gender preference, and most clinically evident bone lesions emerge by age 10 years.[4] Importantly, FD is not heritable, and lesions will not spread to other uninvolved bones as the child grows.

When the mutation affects a single bone, it is termed monostotic; if it involves multiple bones, it is polyostotic. In the craniofacial skeleton, the most commonly affected bones are the midface and skull base. Isolated cases may not be discovered until later in life due to their asymptomatic nature.[18]

During embryogenesis, GNAS mutations can involve tissues derived from the ectoderm, mesoderm, or endoderm. In isolated FD, only specific mesodermal tissues are affected. However, MAS describes the cases of FD associated with extraskeletal features such as café-au-lait macules (ectoderm) and endocrinopathies (endoderm). These endocrinopathies may include testicular or ovarian lesions (linked to gonadotropin-independent precocious puberty), thyroid lesions (with or without hyperthyroidism), excess growth hormone, neonatal hypercortisolism, and fibroblast growth factor-23 (FGF23)-mediated phosphate wasting (with or without hypophosphatemia).[19] The GNAS mutation has been identified in intraductal papillary mucinous neoplasms of the pancreas in individuals with MAS, an area of active research.[20,21]

In radiographic terms, these lesions characteristically exhibit a "ground-glass" appearance; however, their appearance can span from radiolucent at a young age, evolving to sclerotic and heterogeneous at older ages.[18,22] Many cases are incidentally discovered, and the distinctive radiographic features may render biopsy unnecessary. Craniofacial lesions often extend across sutures, and noteworthy features include cortical expansion without perforation. Technetium-99m bone scans prove highly valuable in diagnosis, with CT imaging regarded as the gold standard for detailed lesion clarification (**Fig. 6**).

Diagnosis of FD is established through histologic analysis; however, sampling errors can occur depending on where the biopsy specimen is taken from. Like many other FOL, there is a background of loosely arranged fibrous tissue, alongside irregularly shaped bony structures known as trabeculae, historically (and erroneously) described as "Chinese characters." These trabeculae often lack connections and may or may not exhibit osteoblastic rimming. Occasionally, there are noticeable osteoid globules interspersed with fibrous stroma and highly vascularized tissue. Collagen fibers, called Sharpey's fibers, typically grow perpendicular to the sites of bone formation. Unlike OF, there is no clear demarcation where the affected bone meets normal bone. While some studies suggest variations in maturity and ossification between skull/jaw bones and axial/appendicular skeleton lesions, these findings lack consistent replication due to small sample sizes.

While GNAS mutation testing is considered the gold standard for diagnosis of FD, its value is limited. First, given the mosaic nature of the disease, only affected tissue can be tested. Second, standard polymerase chain reaction techniques are inadequate in testing mutations in the serum and skin.[23] Last, it has been seen that mutation levels within affected tissue also can change over time, with older individuals carrying less mutation-bearing cells.

The definitive approach to treating FD is surgical, but for many craniofacial lesions, the current

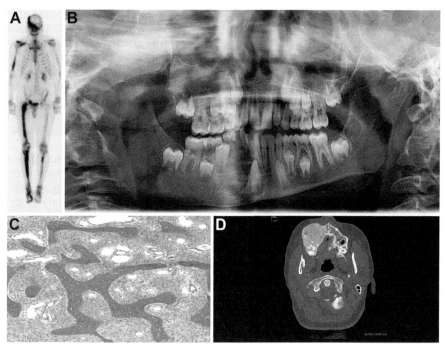

Fig. 6. Fibrous dysplasia. (*A*) Technetium-99 bone scan of a subject with McCune–Albright syndrome. All the affected bones (dark black) are on the right side. (*B*) Panoramic radiograph of a child with polyostotic fibrous dysplasia affecting both the right maxilla and mandible. Obvious expansion of the bones is noted, with opacification of the right maxillary sinus. (*C*) H&E stain showing the characteristic woven bone pattern with dense fibroblastic stroma. (*D*) Axial cut maxillofacial CT scan showing ground-glass appearance of the right maxilla with cortical expansion, involving the alveolar bone.

management trend relies on close observation until skeletal maturity for many patients. Frequently, conservative debulking and recontouring surgeries are performed, although they can be complicated by recurrence of the lesion after surgery.[19,24] Previous research indicates that around 68% of operations experienced regrowth, particularly in patients with untreated growth hormone excess. Therefore, it is strongly recommended that any underlying endocrine issues be identified and addressed before surgery. The reasons behind the postoperative regrowth of some FD lesions remain unclear, and predicting recurrence is still challenging. Studies on craniofacial FD surgery have shown that biopsies are not linked to regrowth and recurrence, unlike more extensive surgical procedures. To reduce the likelihood of recurrence, many elective procedures are delayed until skeletal maturity when FD lesions tend to become less active.[19] Additionally, although resection and reconstruction surgeries carry higher risks, they seem to have lower recurrence rates compared to reshaping procedures, with rates of 45% and 82%, respectively.[24]

Special attention is paid to optic neuropathy in the context of FD, which is one of the most feared

complications of the condition, although it is rare.[25] Prophylactic optic nerve decompression is no longer recommended for treating FD of the optic canal as it has been found to increase the risk of vision loss.[18] The preferred approach for patients with FD affecting the optic canal involves close monitoring, including regular ophthalmologic assessments with optical coherence tomography and evoked potentials, along with medical management for growth hormone excess if present. According to a meta-analysis of the National Institutes of Health (NIH) patient cohort, surgery in asymptomatic patients is associated with a worse prognosis compared to those managed conservatively. Visual impairment was observed in patients with growth hormone excess who delayed treatment until adulthood; however, none of the subjects with growth hormone excess treated during childhood experienced visual disturbances.[26] Routine hearing tests are also advised, along with periodic maxillofacial CT scans to monitor changes.[27]

Because of the complicated nature of FD/MAS, dental needs may sometimes be overlooked, leading practitioners to delay or sometimes avoid dental procedures. Dental procedures are safe in patients with FD and do not adversely impact the progression of the disease. Individuals with craniofacial FD often show a tendency toward malocclusion, and there are no absolute contraindications to orthodontic treatment in FD. Successful cases of orthognathic surgery and dental implants have been reported in patients with FD.[19]

Nonsteroidal anti-inflammatory drugs and supportive care are recommended for diffuse and/or chronic bone pain, or in severe cases, bisphosphonates or RANKL inhibition may be employed.[28] In MAS, medically addressing FGF23-mediated hypophosphatemia and other endocrine abnormalities is essential.[27] While malignant transformation to osteosarcoma has been documented, it is exceedingly rare.[17,29]

Ossifying Fibroma/Cemento-ossifying Fibroma

OF and COF are considered true neoplasms, and the Juvenile ossifying fibroma variant is recognized for its notable aggressiveness. Clinically, these lesions are more commonly identified in the mandible, affecting all age ranges, but predominantly in female individuals in their third to fourth decades.[1] Small lesions may be discovered incidentally. While typically painless, these lesions may lead to expansion, causing the obliteration of surrounding structures and displacement of teeth.[13]

Radiographically, they exhibit a distinct margin of lucency surrounding a radiopaque, heterogeneous lesion. Histologically, both ossifying and cemento-ossifying forms share similarities, featuring variable trabeculation, osteoid material in the former, and cementicles in the latter (**Fig. 7**).[2,8] They are often misidentified for COD or FD, though FD tends to be more uniform in histologic appearance. Remarkably, these lesions may be easily separated from the bone during surgical excision and may be encapsulated. Aggressive lesions may be treated with en bloc resection. Recurrence is infrequent, except for the juvenile variant, which shows a higher propensity for recurrence.[30]

The juvenile variant of juvenile ossifying fibroma (JOF) (or COF) may be either trabecular or psammomatoid in nature, presenting as well-circumscribed radiolucencies. The trabecular form has been reported more frequently in younger children and has a predilection for the jaw bones. The COF form tends to occur in the mandible, causing radiographically well-defined expansion (**Fig. 8**).[7,13] The psammomatoid type occurs in slightly older children and adolescents and is found in other craniofacial bones in the naso-orbito-ethmoidal complex. In general, the younger the patient, the more aggressive is the OF lesion. However, not every young patient with OF has the juvenile variant.[31]

Juvenile OF is not encapsulated and often exhibits histology with abundant and dense fibrous connective tissue. Since the behavior is more like a true neoplasm, these lesions will outwardly expand and impinge upon neighboring structures. Trabecular forms have strands of osteoid with irregular osteocytes; psammomatoid variants often have spherical ossicles. ABC formation has been reported within JOF, in a largely hemorrhagic stroma rich in osteoclasts. These ABCs tend to occur in younger children with aggressive maxillary lesions. JOF lesions are best treated with enucleation and peripheral ostectomy. Malignant transformation has not been noted, but JOF may exhibit recurrence, largely due to inability to completely resect the lesion. There is no correlation between age and recurrence.[31]

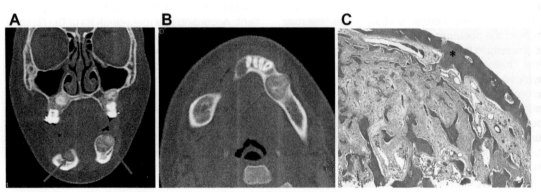

Fig. 7. Ossifying fibroma. Maxillofacial CT showing coronal (*A*) and axial (*B*) slices of a pediatric patient with bilateral mandibular ossifying fibromas. The lesion is causing expansion of the cortical bone. (*C*) Low-power hematoxylin and eosin slide showing the typical findings of a fibro-osseous lesion, with notable encapsulation (*asterisk*) of the specimen.

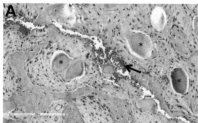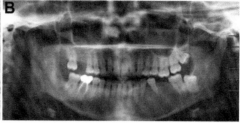

Fig. 8. Cemento-ossifying fibroma. (*A*) 20X view of a hematoxylin and eosin statin, showing prominent globules of cementum—"cementicles" (*asterisk*), admixed with trabecular bone and a fibrous stroma. Hemorrhage is also noted (*arrow*). (*B*) A large cemento-ossifying fibroma in the left body of the mandible. The teeth and surrounding structures are being displaced by this lesion that underwent rapid expansion during childhood.

Osseous Dysplasia/Cemento-osseous Dysplasia

Osseous dysplasia, also known as COD, remains the most prevalent fibro-osseous ailment affecting the jaws and alveolar bone.[13] Among its 3 forms, the periapical and florid types are relatively straightforward to diagnose based on clinical and radiographic characteristics. Conversely, the focal type often requires a biopsy for a conclusive diagnosis due to its broad range of potential differential diagnoses. The origin of these lesions remains unclear, with a suggested association with the periodontal ligament due to its close proximity. They are typically not seen in the pediatric population.

The focal form typically involves a solitary site, usually in the posterior mandible. In contrast to the periapical and florid variants, the focal form is more frequently observed in Caucasian female individuals. Radiographically, the lesion is well defined, often displaying a mixed radiolucent and radiopaque pattern, frequently accompanied by a radiolucent rim (**Fig. 9**).[7] Biopsy may be warranted because these solitary lesions share a broad range of potential diagnoses, including periapical diseases. This form may also be considered a predecessor to the more advanced florid COD.

Periapical COD primarily affects the anterior mandible and is linked to vital teeth. It is most commonly observed in women of African descent. Typically asymptomatic, it is usually discovered incidentally in middle-aged adults.[1] Radiographically, it begins as a well-circumscribed radiolucent lesion, gradually increasing in density to become more radiopaque. Treatment is generally unnecessary, apart from periodic surveillance, as most of these lesions do not cause cortical expansion and do not exhibit growth.

Florid COD resembles the periapical variant but may involve multiple quadrants, presenting bilaterally. It may be discovered incidentally, though secondary infections may occur, leading to pain or evidence of an alveolar sinus tract.

Radiographically, these lesions resemble the periapical form but with a more widespread appearance, affecting both dentate and edentulous regions.[7]

Histologically, these lesions exhibit cellular mesenchymal tissue comprising spindle-shaped fibroblasts and collagen fibers, along with a mixture of woven bone. The lesions also contain a concentration of small blood vessels. As the lesion becomes more sclerotic, there is less fibrous tissue present, and increased mineralization is noted. In some lesions, inflammation and multinucleated giant cells can also be observed.[2,13] Treatment typically involves observation unless there is concern for another underlying process. Biopsy may be indicated because these solitary lesions have a broad differential diagnosis that includes periapical diseases.

Segmental Odontomaxillary Dysplasia

As its name suggests, SOD is a developmental disturbance, causing asymptomatic, unilateral expansion of the maxilla. In addition to the bone, teeth are affected, with eruption disorders, congenitally missing premolars and spacing. It is most commonly diagnosed within the first decade of life, with a slight male gender predilection.[32] SOD was initially reported in 1987 by Miles and colleagues as hemimaxillofacial dysplasia, but the name was subsequently changed. It has also been associated with HATS (hemimaxillary enlargement, asymmetry of the face, hypodontia, teeth abnormalities, and skin findings) when hyperpigmentation is present. Many cases also involve lip clefting on the affected side and ipsilateral facial hypertrichosis.[33] Mild facial asymmetry may also accompany the maxillary expansion. SOD is often misdiagnosed or undiagnosed and is frequently confused for monostotic FD.

Radiographically, it appears as a mixed radiopaque lesion and can cause diminution of the maxillary sinus. Premolars are often absent in the

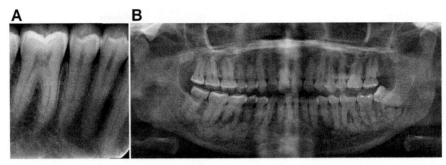

Fig. 9. Cemento-osseous dysplasia: focal (*A*) and florid (*B*) types. In a younger patient, the focal lesions often appear radiolucent and ill-defined (*A*), later progressing to radiopaque later in age (*B*).

affected area, and the roots of other teeth may be affected (**Fig. 10**). Thick trabecular and immature woven bones, with the absence of lamellar bone and osteoblastic rimming, are noted. Dental alteration is also seen, with fibrous enlargement of the pulp in primary teeth and irregular dentinal tubules. It is speculated that the alterations in bony development lead to the changes seen in the dentition. Mucosal changes are not specific and show collagenous fibrous connective tissue with myxoid changes. Owing to its rarity, it is unclear whether SOD is a self-limiting disease, as report of follow-up is limited. Recontouring may be performed but is rarely indicated, and treatment is often limited to orthodontia and/or restorative procedures.[32]

GENERAL TREATMENT CONSIDERATIONS

Finally, treatment of craniofacial FOLs is extremely variable, spanning from active surveillance to recontouring and complete resection in some cases. Surgeons should consider underlying medical conditions that may be contributing to the appearance of bone, including workup for endocrinopathies (ie, hyperparathyroidism, growth hormone excess).[19] Workup may include technetium or PET scans to identify polyostotic disease. Laboratory data may be informative, such as alkaline

phosphatase, bone turnover markers, vitamin D, PTH, calcium, and phosphorus. Referral to a multidisciplinary center with bone specialists should be considered, particularly if other examination findings are present. Many pathologists do not have expertise in bone histology, and it is crucial that a trusted pathologist review both the FOL histology and the radiographic findings.[2] Further, sampling bias and processing of bone may only give a snapshot of the histology or cause errors in processing a specimen. For instance, there may be giant cell-rich area of the specimen or other spots indicative of inflammation—how can you be sure that you got the best sampling?

Treatment goals are often patient-specific, closely related to the age of the patient and the clinical behavior of the FOL. If an FOL is behaving aggressively, nomenclature is not going to guide the treatment. Clinical behavior can be divided into categories—quiescent/stable, slow growing, and aggressive—as adapted from the Chuong–Kaban classification of GCT in 1986.[3] The highlighted features of aggressive lesions include 1 primary criterion or 3 secondary criteria, based on size and recurrence. This is extremely important to take into consideration, because if the behavior is slow, close observation in a reliable patient may be the best treatment.

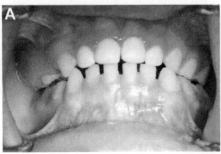
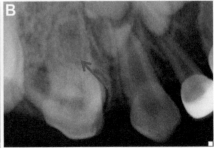

Fig. 10. Segmental odontomaxillary dysplasia. (*A*) Intraoral photo showing obvious expansion of the right posterior maxillary alveolar ridge. (*B*) Periapical radiograph showing the absence of a developing tooth bud (*arrow*).

The most widely studied craniofacial fibro-osseous lesion (CF-FOL) often FD will be discovered incidentally; based on its characteristic radiographic appearance, a biopsy is not necessary in most cases. An example of overtreatment is optic nerve decompression for FD involving the bony orbit, a treatment that had been advocated for decades without clinical evidence.[25] Studies have since looked at the case for optic nerve decompression and noted that despite significant disease, the vast majority of patients were not going blind and could be managed with active surveillance.[26] Those patients who were being followed closely and had significant changes were then referred to surgery as needed. This drastically changed how a rare disease was treated, and improved quality of life, for what is usually a surgery with high morbidity.

Generally, resection and reconstruction, with complete removal of the affected bone and mutant cells, will lead to reduced recurrence. As mentioned in CF-FD, regrowth has been significantly associated with growth hormone excess in the MAS subgroup, following surgery.[24] This is likely because the surgeons did not consider endocrinopathy to play a role in their outcomes.

Finally, based on the clinical behavior of lesions, we can consider targeted therapies. Previous work has shown that greater skeletal disease burden in FD is associated with higher levels of RANKL expression.[23] Thus, in aggressive lesions, DMAB has been trialed off-label as an adjuvant therapy with positive effect, causing the bone to involute and become more sclerotic.[28]

SUMMARY

The term "fibro-osseous lesion" should be considered a working diagnosis. All clinical, radiologic, and histopathologic data are needed to establish a diagnosis. Despite notable patterns, many FOL will not present "by the book," and should be treated based on their clinical behavior. Much remains unknown about CF-FOL and their unique properties. Further research into molecular mechanisms will help identify common pathways underlying the pathophysiology of craniofacial bone diseases, including FOLs.

DISCLOSURE

The author has nothing to disclose.

REFERENCES

1. Neville BW DDACCAC: Oral and maxillofacial pathology. Fourth edition. St. Louis, MO: Elsevier; 2016.

2. Eversole RS, Su L, ElMofty S. Benign fibro-osseous lesions of the craniofacial complex. A review. Head Neck Patho 2008;2:177.

3. Chuong R, Kaban LB, Kozakewich H, et al. Central giant cell lesions of the jaws: a clinicopathologic study. J Oral Maxillofacial Surg 1986;44:708.

4. Hart ES, Kelly MH, Brillante B, et al. Onset, progression, and plateau of skeletal lesions in fibrous dysplasia and the relationship to functional outcome. J Bone Miner Res 2007;22:1468.

5. Zhang J, Troulis MJ, August M. Diagnosis and treatment of pediatric primary jaw lesions at Massachusetts General Hospital. J Oral Maxillofac Surg 2021;79:585.

6. Zhen Low X, Chin Lim M, Nga V, et al. Clinical application of "black bone" imaging in paediatric craniofacial disorders. Br J Radiol 2021;94(1124):20200061.

7. White SC. Oral radiology: principles and interpretation. Edition 7. St. Louis: Elsevier; 2014.

8. El-Mofty S. Regarding the use of the term "Cementum" in Fibro-Osseous lesions of the craniofacial skeleton. Head Neck Pathol 2018;12:631.

9. Kaban L. Pediatric Oral and Maxillofacial Surgery. Philadephi, PA: W.B. Saunders; 2004.

10. Brooks PJ, Glogauer M, McCulloch CA. An overview of the derivation and function of multinucleated giant cells and their role in pathologic processes. Am J Pathol 2019;189:1145.

11. Wright JM, Vered M. Update from the 4th Edition of the World Health Organization Classification of Head and Neck Tumours: Odontogenic and Maxillofacial Bone Tumors. Head Neck Pathol 2017;11(68).

12. Vered M, Wright JM. Update from the 5th Edition of the World Health Organization Classification of Head and Neck Tumors: Odontogenic and Maxillofacial Bone Tumours. Head Neck Pathol 2022;16(63).

13. Nelson BL, Phillips BJ. Benign fibro-osseous lesions of the head and neck. Head Neck Pathol 2019;13:466.

14. Brooks PJ, Chadwick JW, Caminiti M, et al. Primary aneurysmal bone cyst of the mandibular condyle with USP6-CDH11 fusion. Pathol Res Pract 2019;215:607.

15. Reichenberger EJL, Levine MA, Olsen BR, et al. The role of SH3BP2 in the pathophysiology of cherubism. Orphanet J Rare Dis 2012;7(Suppl 1).

16. Karbach J, Coerdt W, Wagner W, et al. Case report: Noonan syndrome with multiple giant cell lesions and review of the literature. Am J Med Genet 2012;158A:2283.

17. Boyce AM, et al. In: Adam MPAH, Pagon RA, et al, editors. Fibrous dysplasia/McCune-Albright syndrome. Seattle (WA): University of Washington, Seattle; 2015. p. 1993–2019. GeneReviews® [Internet].

18. Lee JS, FitzGibbon EJ, Chen YR, et al. Clinical guidelines for the management of craniofacial fibrous dysplasia. Orphanet J Rare Dis 2012;7(1).

19. Burke AB, Collins MT, Boyce AM. Fibrous dysplasia of bone: craniofacial and dental implications. Oral Dis 2017;23:697.

20. Wood LD, Noë M, Hackeng W, et al. Patients with McCune-Albright syndrome have a broad spectrum of abnormalities in the gastrointestinal tract and pancreas. Virchows Arch 2017;470:391.

21. Collins MT. Spectrum and natural history of fibrous dysplasia of bone. J Bone Miner Res 2007;22.

22. Kushchayeva YS, Kushchayev SV, Glushko TY, et al. Fibrous dysplasia for radiologists: beyond ground glass bone matrix. Insights Imaging 2018;9:1035.

23. Castro LF de, Burke AB, Wang HD, et al. Activation of RANK/RANKL/OPG pathway is involved in the pathophysiology of fibrous dysplasia and associated with disease burden. J Bone Miner Res 2019; 34:290.

24. Boyce AM, Burke A, Cutler Peck C, et al. Surgical Management of polyostotic craniofacial fibrous dysplasia: long-term outcomes and predictors for postoperative regrowth. Plast Reconstr Surg 2016; 137:1833.

25. Lee J, FitzGibbon E, Butman JA, et al. Normal vision despite narrowing of the optic canal in fibrous dysplasia. N Engl J Med 2002.

26. Amit M, Collins MT, FitzGibbon EJ, et al. Surgery versus watchful waiting in patients with craniofacial fibrous dysplasia - a meta-analysis. PLoS One 2011;6.

27. Javaid MK, Boyce A, Appelman-Dijkstra N, et al. Best practice management guidelines for fibrous dysplasia/McCune-Albright syndrome: A consensus statement from the FD/MAS international consortium. Orphanet J Rare Dis 2019;14.

28. Raborn LN, Burke AB, Ebb DH, et al. Denosumab for craniofacial fibrous dysplasia: duration of efficacy and post-treatment effects. Osteoporos Int 2021;32(9):1889–93.

29. Wagner VP, Carlos R, Romañach MJ, et al. Malignant transformation of craniomaxillofacial fibroosseous lesions: A systematic review. J Oral Pathol Med 2019;48:441.

30. Baumhoer D, Haefliger S, Ameline B, et al. Ossifying fibroma of non-odontogenic origin: a fibro-osseous lesion in the craniofacial skeleton to be (Re-)considered. Head Neck Pathol 2022;16:257.

31. Chrcanovic BR, Gomez RS. Juvenile ossifying fibroma of the jaws and paranasal sinuses: a systematic review of the cases reported in the literature. Int J Oral Maxillofac Surg 2020;49:28.

32. González-Arriagada WA, Vargas PA, Fuentes-Cortés R, et al. Segmental odontomaxillary dysplasia: report of 3 cases and literature review. Head Neck Pathol 2012;6:171.

33. Whitt JC, Rokos JW, Dunlap CL, et al. Segmental odontomaxillary dysplasia: Report of a series of 5 cases with long-term follow-up. Oral Surg Oral Med Oral Pathol Oral Radiol Endod 2011;112.

Pediatric Odontogenic Infections

Lindsey Teal, MD, MPH[a,1], Barbara Sheller, DDS, MSD[b], Harlyn K. Susarla, DMD, MPH[b,*]

KEYWORDS

• Odontogenic infection • Dental caries • Oral surgery • Health disparities

KEY POINTS

• Odontogenic infections arise from the teeth and/or periapical and periodontal tissue and often result from untreated dental caries, periodontal conditions, or other pathology.
• If left untreated, odontogenic infections can spread to surrounding deep spaces in the face and neck and can lead to fatal complications.
• Definitive treatment of odontogenic infections includes extraction of the affected tooth and surgical debridement.
• Odontogenic infections are polymicrobial and are treated with antibiotics that target facultative anaerobic, obligate anaerobic, and aerobic bacteria.
• Odontogenic infections contribute to a large health care burden and are associated with oral health disparities.

INTRODUCTION

Odontogenic infections are infections that originate from the teeth or their supportive structures. Infections frequently arise from periapical and periodontal tissue, with common causes including dental caries, periodontal disease (gingivitis), and trauma. Dental caries and periodontal diseases have a large global burden and are the most common noncommunicable disease worldwide.[1] Data collected in the United States from 2017 to 2020 found that over 1 in 5 adults have untreated dental caries.[2] Dental caries in pediatric populations (age 2–11 years) in the United States from 2011 to 2020 were found to be less prevalent at 12%.[3] However, despite the decreased prevalence in pediatric populations, dental caries in both pediatric and adult populations disproportionately affect low socioeconomic groups and racial/ethnic minority groups.[2,3]

When these preventable diseases are left untreated, the infection has the potential to invade the alveolar bone and ultimately spread to surrounding anatomic regions, including the oral cavity, neck, lower face, and periocular region. This can lead to devastating complications, including sinusitis, cellulitis, soft-tissue abscesses, multi-compartment involvement of sublingual, submental, and submandibular spaces (Ludwig angina), periorbital infections, airway obstruction, cavernous sinus thrombosis, mediastinitis, sepsis, and necrotizing soft-tissue infections (NSTIs). Therefore, it is imperative that clinicians evaluating these patients understand the relevant anatomy, pathway of spread, microbiome, presentation, workup, and treatment of odontogenic infections to provide optimal care for these patients.

MICROBIOLOGY

Odontogenic infections are often polymicrobial and arise from endogenous oral flora. Infections are comprised of facultative anaerobic, obligate

a Division of Plastic Surgery, Department of Surgery, University of Washington Medical Center, 325 9th Avenue, Seattle, WA 98013, USA; b Department of Dentistry, Seattle Children's Hospital, 4800 Sand Point Way NE, Seattle, WA 98105, USA
1 Present address: 1600 2nd Avenue Apartment 2511, Seattle, WA 98101.
* Corresponding author. Department of Dentistry, Seattle Children's Hospital, 4800 Sand Point Way NE, Seattle, WA 98105.
E-mail address: harlyn.susarla@seattlechildrens.org

Oral Maxillofacial Surg Clin N Am 36 (2024) 391–399
https://doi.org/10.1016/j.coms.2024.03.005
1042-3699/24/© 2024 Elsevier Inc. All rights reserved, including those for text and data mining, AI training, and similar technologies.

anaerobic, and aerobic bacteria. Approximately 70% to 96% of odontogenic infections involve mixed flora.[4,5] Common facultative anaerobic strains include *Streptococcus viridans*, *Streptococcus anginosus*, and *Staphylococcus aureus*. Prevalent obligate anaerobic bacteria include *Fusobacterium*, *Prevotella*, and anaerobic cocci.[6] Aerobic bacteria are found to a lesser extent, with the most common bacteria being *Neisseria*.[7] Improvements in molecular diagnostic techniques, including 16s ribosomal RNA sequencing, have enabled detection of new bacteria not previously cultured, including *Dialister pneumosintes* and *Eubacterium brachy*.[8] The polymicrobial nature of these infections should be considered when selecting antibiotics for treatment.

PATHWAY OF SPREAD

Infections often arise from the periapical or periodontal tissue. Periapical diseases are caused by inflammation and subsequent infection of the pulp at the root tip. Common causes of periapical disease include dental caries, dental trauma, or unsuccessful pulpal treatment. Periodontal diseases are caused by inflammation of the surrounding gingiva and bone that support the teeth. In early stages, this presents as gingivitis, or inflammation of the gingiva, and later progresses to periodontitis, which leads to bone and tissue resorption and can house infection. If these local infections are left untreated, they spread to invade the surrounding alveolus cancellous bone. Once the infection penetrates the cortical plate, it can then spread to surrounding potential spaces. The stages of infection usually start with inoculation (edema, inflammation), then progress to cellulitis (pain, induration), and later to an abscess (fluctuance, fever).

Primary potential spaces are those directly affected by spread from odontogenic infections. Infections from maxillary teeth can spread lingually to the palatal space, buccally to the vestibular and buccal space, or superiorly to the infraorbital (canine) space. Mandibular teeth infections can spread buccally to the vestibular and buccal space or lingually to the sublingual, submandibular, and submental spaces. Persistence of infection in these primary spaces can progress to spread into secondary spaces. These include masticator (submasseteric, pterygomandibular, superficial, and deep temporal), lateral pharyngeal, and retropharyngeal spaces.

Uncontrolled infections within the sublingual, submental, submandibular, retropharyngeal, or lateral pharyngeal spaces can lead to airway compromise due to their proximity to the airway.

The retropharyngeal space is the most inferior of the secondary spaces and uncontrolled infections in this area can lead to mediastinitis. The infraorbital space houses the infraorbital vein and if infection seeds the vein in this space, it can spread to the cavernous sinus. Similarly, the infratemporal space, the most inferior aspect of the deep temporal space, houses the pterygoid plexus. Infections in this space can also spread to the cavernous sinus, leading to cavernous sinus thrombosis. It is important that clinicians understand the anatomy and clinical significance of infections present in these potential spaces (**Table 1**).

CLINICAL ASSESSMENT

Obtaining a detailed history and physical history assists in determining the origin of the infection and severity of symptoms. Important questions regarding the history of the present illness include timeline of dental pain, dental caries, dental trauma, dental hygiene, recent dental procedures, and any previous antibiotic treatment for this condition. This may provide a better understanding of the origin of the infection and duration. A shorter duration of symptoms with a high degree of pain or rapid spread is concerning for a more aggressive infection and requires immediate attention. Symptoms that should heighten concern include rapid progression of pain, rapid swelling to face or neck, fever, dyspnea, dysphagia, odynophagia, trismus, ocular pain, vision changes, or severe headache.

Upon clinical evaluation, the airway should first be assessed. Stridor, or respiratory distress, necessitates urgent treatment and stabilization of the airway. Vital signs should be obtained and tachycardia, hypotension, or fever should prompt immediate treatment due to concern for sepsis. A full craniofacial examination should then be performed. Examine the head and neck for areas of swelling or erythema. Erythema with induration, swelling, and tenderness is consistent with cellulitis. Clinical representation of buccal and infraorbital cellulitis is depicted in **Fig. 1**. However, if the area of swelling is associated with fluctuance, this may indicate an underlying abscess. Evaluate the neck for signs of tracheal deviation and assess the contours of the mandible and cheek to evaluate for blunting of the inferior mandible or the nasolabial fold. Lymph nodes of the head and neck should be palpated to evaluate for lymphadenopathy. Intraorally, assess the maximal incisal opening, which should be greater than 25 mm without trismus in healthy patients. Examine the soft tissues for areas of swelling or discharge, including palatal edema, raised floor of mouth/tongue (**Fig. 2**),

Table 1
The anatomic location, clinical symptoms, and clinical relevance of primary and secondary potential spaces in the head and neck

	Potential Spaces	Anatomic location	Clinical symptoms	Clinical relevance
P R I M A R Y	**Maxillary and Mandibular**			
	Vestibular	Between buccal mucosa and gingiva	Tenderness, vestibular fluctuance	
	Buccal	Between buccal mucosa and skin	Cheek edema, obliteration of nasolabial fold	
	Maxillary			
	Palatal	Hard palate	Palatal edema	
	Infraorbital	Between levator labii superioris and oral mucosa	Periorbital edema, obliteration of nasolabial fold	Infection can spread from the infraorbital vein to the cavernous sinus
	Mandibular			
	Sublingual	Between the floor of the mouth and mylohyoid	Floor of mouth/tongue elevation, dysphagia, drooling	
	Submandibular	Between the inferior surface of the mandible and digastric muscles	Blunting of inferior mandibular border, floor of mouth edema, dysphagia, drooling	Involved in Ludwig angina, risk of compromised airway
	Submental	Between mylohoid and the deep cervical fascia	Submental edema and erythema	
S E C O N D A R Y	Submasseteric	Between the zygomatic arch, inferior border of the mandible, masseter, and ramus	Mandibular angle edema/blunting, trismus	
	Pterygomandibular	Between the lateral and medial pterygoid, the pterygomasseteric sling, and ramus	Trismus	
	Superficial temporal	Between the temporalis fascia and temporalis muscle, the zygomatic arch	Trismus	
	Deep temporal	Between the temporal bone, temporalis, and the lateral pterygoid	Edema over sigmoid notch, trismus	Communicates with the cavernous sinus via the pterygoid plexus
	Lateral pharyngeal	Between the pharynx, masticator space, parotid, and the retropharyngeal space	Deviation of uvula, dysphagia, drooling	High risk of airway compromise
	Retropharyngeal	Between the base of the skull, the posterior mediastinum, the prevertebral space, and the buccopharyngeal fascia	Dysphagia, dyspnea, drooling	Mediastinitis results from the spread from the retropharyngeal space, high risk of airway compromise

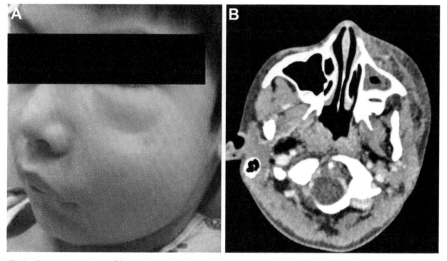

Fig. 1. (*A*) Clinical presentation of buccal and infraorbital space cellulitis. (*B*) Stranding and thickening of subcutaneous fat in buccal and infraorbital space without underlying fluid collection, consistent with cellulitis.

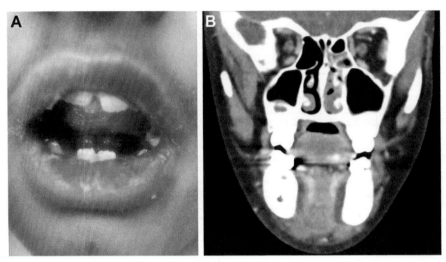

Fig. 2. (*A*) Clinical presentation of sublingual space abscess depicted by elevated floor of mouth and tongue. (*B*) Well-defined fluid collections between the floor of the mouth, lingual aspect of mandible, and mylohyoid, consistent with bilateral sublingual space abscesses.

vestibular swelling (**Fig. 3**) or deviation of the uvula. Examine the teeth for areas of sensitivity to pressure or temperature, caries, or trauma. An ocular examination includes evaluation for proptosis, pupillary response, visual acuity, and extraocular movements.

Odontogenic infections can present with symptoms that overlap those associated with odontogenic cysts or odontogenic tumors. Odontogenic infections typically have a quicker onset, often over several days, and can cause skin erythema, fever, and trismus, which are less frequently seen with odontogenic cysts and tumors. Odontogenic cysts and tumors are distinguished from odontogenic infections in that they have a slower onset, often presenting over several months, and cause cortical expansion and displacement of teeth. Odontogenic infections, cysts, and tumors can cause both intraoral and potential space swelling, and therefore all have the potential for airway compromise (**Table 2**).

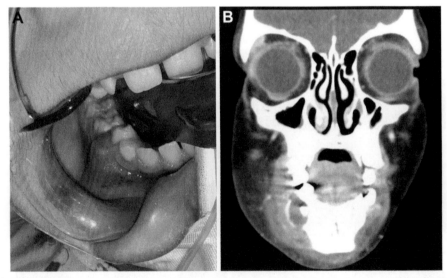

Fig. 3. (*A*) Clinical presentation of an infected odontogenic cyst within the vestibular space. (*B*) Well-defined fluid collection between the buccal mucosa and the alveolus, consistent with vestibular space abscess. The abscess is associated with carious deciduous right mandibular first molar and involved a radiolucent lesion (the final pathology was consistent with dentigerous cyst) associated with the first premolar.

Table 2
Comparison of the symptoms and timeline of presentation of odontogenic infections, cysts, and tumors

	Odontogenic Infections	Odontogenic Cysts/Tumors
Intraoral swelling	+	+
Potential space swelling	+	+
Pain	+	+
Potential for airway compromise	+	+
Trismus	+	-
Fever	+	-
Erythema	+	-
Cortical expansion	-	+
Displacement of teeth	-	+
Timeline	Quick(days)	Slow (months)

IMAGING

Various imaging studies can be useful for further evaluation and the modality is dependent on findings from the clinical examination. Dental panoramic radiographs assist in screening for an odontogenic source (ie, periapical abscess). A radiolucent area at the dental apex on radiographs may indicate a periapical abscess. If there is concern for soft-tissue fluid collection, a point-of-care ultrasound can be obtained.[9] Ultrasound is a quick, low-cost tool that correctly identifies 84% of odontogenic deep space infections.[10] In infections involving the buccal, infraorbital, submandibular, submental, and submasseteric spaces, ultrasound produced the same results as MRI.[10] However, MRI was found to be superior in sublingual, masticator, lateral pharyngeal, and retropharyngeal spaces. If there is concern for deep space involvement that is unable to be evaluated by clinical examination, a computed tomography (CT) scan or MRI of the head and neck should be obtained.[11] On CT scan, the thickening and stranding of subcutaneous tissue is consistent with cellulitis (see **Fig. 2**A), whereas a well-defined fluid collection is consistent with an abscess (see **Figs. 2**B and **3**B). Clinical examination findings that best predict need for an infection indicated for a CT scan include blunting of the inferior border of the mandible, maximum incisal opening of less than 25 mm, trismus, dysphagia, odynophagia, raised floor of mouth, lymphadenopathy, tachycardia, and swelling.[12,13] If there is concern for mediastinal involvement, a chest CT should be obtained. It is important to note that if there is any concern for a compromised airway, the airway should be secured prior to obtaining imaging.

TREATMENT

Patients with the following symptoms concerning for deep space infections warrant immediate evaluation by an oral and maxillofacial surgeon (OMS) with hospital privileges: odynophagia, dysphagia, limited maximal incisal opening with trismus, raised floor of mouth, and deviation of the uvula.[14] If there is concern for airway compromise (stridor), fever, tachycardia, or hypotension, the patient should receive immediate care in a hospital setting.

Definitive treatment of odontogenic infections includes surgical drainage of abscess and removal of the infectious source (**Fig. 4**A).[15] Removing the nidus of the infection is often accomplished by timely extraction or root canal treatment of the affected tooth (**Fig. 4**B).[16] Most odontogenic infections can be accessed intraorally by making an incision at the highest point of swelling. The infected space should be probed with blunt dissection to avoid damage to surrounding structures and should be adequately irrigated. A drain is left to prevent infection from reaccumulating in the affected space.[16] For deep neck abscesses, incision and drainage is recommended in the setting of an unstable airway or poorly defined loculation.[17] However, in patients with a stable airway and well-defined fluid collection, ultrasound-guided aspiration performed by interventional radiology is a safe and effective treatment method.[17]

A systematic review and randomized control trial found resolution of odontogenic infection after surgical treatment with or without antibiotics.[18,19] Antibiotics alone have not been proven to prevent the spread of infection.[20] Therefore, clinicians should ensure these patients receive immediate care from a dentist or oral maxillofacial surgeon as opposed to delaying care by prescribing antibiotics in lieu of surgical care.

While antibiotics are not used as the primary form of treatment in odontogenic infections, they are often used in combination with surgical treatment. They should be administered to patients demonstrating local spread of infection or systemic symptoms of infection. Due to the polymicrobial nature of odontogenic infections, antibiotics that are effective against facultative anaerobes, obligate anaerobes, and aerobes should be used. A systematic review found that no one antibiotic is superior to another.[21] In the outpatient setting, amoxicillin, clindamycin, or azithromycin are often used, with amoxicillin being the most common first-line antibiotic prescribed.[22] However, due to the wide use of beta-lactam antibiotics, there has been increased concern with prescribing beta-lactam antibiotics alone, given the increased resistance to these antibiotics. A prospective study conducted in 2021 found that 13% to 39% of odontogenic infections included bacteria that generate beta-lactamase.[23] Despite this growing resistance, many providers still prescribe first-line beta-lactam antibiotics, which may further emphasize the fact that surgical debridement is the most important aspect of treatment. The American Dental Association published guidelines in 2019 regarding the choice of antibiotics in patients with periapical pain and intraoral swelling and recommend beta-lactam antibiotics (amoxicillin) treatment alone for 3 to 7 days.[24] However, other studies propose that if there are local antimicrobial resistance patterns to amoxicillin, then amoxicillin combined with clavulanic acid or amoxicillin with metronidazole can be considered.[15] In patients with a penicillin allergy, clindamycin, azithromycin, or moxifloxacin therapy are recommended.[21] In hospitalized patients, ampicillin/sulbactam, clindamycin, penicillin with metronidazole, or ceftriaxone are recommended.[21] It is important to emphasize that, in the era of increased antibiotic stewardship, providers should exercise careful judgment in selecting the right antibiotic for the type of infection and keeping the course as short as possible. Surgical treatment remains the mainstay of management for odontogenic infections.

COMPLICATIONS

Early diagnosis and treatment of odontogenic infections is imperative to prevent complications from arising, such as Ludwig angina, mediastinitis, cavernous sinus thrombosis, and sepsis. Ludwig angina is a result of rapid spread of cellulitis to the submandibular, sublingual, or submental spaces. Expansion of these spaces can lead to life-threatening complications such as airway obstruction. Stridor, dyspnea, hoarseness, dysphagia, drooling, and blunting of mandibular angle are often present and should raise concern for Ludwig angina.[25] The mainstay of treatment is to secure the airway, which should not be delayed for imaging. After the airway has been secured, CT of the neck may be obtained followed by antibiotics, steroid treatment, and surgical drainage.

Descending necrotizing mediastinitis is a potentially fatal complication of odontogenic infections and results from spread from the retropharyngeal secondary space. Clinical examination findings include fever, tachycardia, hypotension, retrosternal pain, cough, and Hamman sign (crunching sound in precordium synchronous with pulse).[26] A CT scan of the chest is useful in diagnosis and treatment includes urgent surgical intervention to

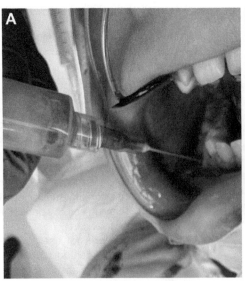
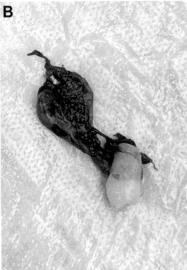

Fig. 4. (*A*) Needle aspiration of vestibular abscess to obtain sample for microbiologic analysis. (*B*) Gross view of associated infected dentigerous cyst and right mandibular first premolar.

drain infected fluid from the chest and repair esophageal perforation, if indicated.[27]

Cavernous sinus thrombosis results from spread of the infection from the facial vein or pterygoid plexus to the cavernous sinus.[28] The structures housed within the cavernous sinus include the oculomotor nerve (cranial nerve [CN] III), trochlear nerve (CN IV), ophthalmic nerve (CN V1), maxillary nerve (CN V2), abducens nerve (CN VI), and the internal carotid artery. Therefore, symptoms associated with cavernous sinus thrombosis include ophthalmoplegia, or weakness with extraocular movements. Other symptoms include headache, periorbital edema, and proptosis. CT or MRI are used as diagnostic imaging studies. Treatment includes surgical drainage and antibiotics. However, there is a high mortality rate of 14% to 30% even with treatment.[29]

Progression to sepsis with odontogenic infections is rare but occurs when the infection spreads to the bloodstream.[30] Clinical findings include tachycardia, hypotension, fever, and malaise. These patients should be referred to a hospital immediately and be treated with intravenous antibiotics, fluids, and surgical debridement and source control.

NSTI is an aggressive bacterial infection that quickly destroys fascia and subcutaneous tissue. Early recognition and management improve mortality. A systematic review of NSTIs found that broad-spectrum antibiotics and surgical debridement within 6 hours resulted in a mortality of 19%, compared to those treated after 6 hours with a mortality rate of 32%.[31] Clinical examination findings include rapidly expanding erythema, tenderness expanding beyond the zone of erythema, bulla formation, crepitus, and skin necrosis. It is estimated that 1% of odontogenic infections progress to NSTIs.[32] Therefore, given the rapid progression of this disease, it is important that providers are aware of these findings to expedite treatment.

PUBLIC HEALTH IMPACT

Odontogenic infections are a public health concern that have a significant impact on hospital resources and are associated with disparities in access to oral health care. The annual cost of hospitalization for pediatric dental infections is $162 million.[33] A cost analysis of 200 patients seen in the emergency room for odontogenic infections found nearly half required inpatient admission, 16% spent at least 1 day in the intensive care unit, and on average their hospital stays cost $15,500.[34] This results in a significant health care burden for the treatment of odontogenic infections, which are largely caused by preventable diseases, such as dental caries. This emphasizes the importance of preventative care and early treatment of caries and periodontal disease.[35] However, not all Americans are able to receive routine access to dental care, as access to dental care is limited in low-income, uninsured, racial/ethnic minority, immigrant, and rural patients.[36] For many of these patients, the emergency department is where they receive their dental care when problems arise. Seven percent of individuals in the United States receive dental care only from physicians.[37] However, emergency medicine providers are not trained to provide comprehensive oral health care. A survey of pediatric emergency physicians found that only 19% felt confident in treating dental trauma.[38] Therefore, members of these populations are likely receiving substandard dental care.

SUMMARY

Odontogenic infections frequently occur from untreated periapical or periodontal diseases, such as dental caries and gingivitis. These largely preventable infections incur a significant cost to the health care system and disproportionately affect members of ethnic/racial minorities and low-income/uninsured groups due to lack of access to dental care. Odontogenic infections can spread to deep spaces and can be life threatening. Patients presenting with signs of early sepsis (fever, tachycardia, hypotension), airway compromise (stridor, dyspnea), rapid spread of infection, ocular symptoms, or limited maximal incisal opening should be urgently evaluated. The gold standard of treatment includes extraction of the affected teeth and surgical drainage of the associated infected fluid. Continued efforts should be made to increase access to dental care to low-income, uninsured, racial/ethnic minority, immigrant, and rural groups.

CLINICS CARE POINTS

- The gold standard of treatment for serious odontogenic infections is timely removal of the source of infection (extraction of the affected tooth) and incision and drainage of any infected fluid collections.

- Patients with the following red flag symptoms should be seen urgently by an OMS with hospital privileges: odynophagia, dysphagia, limited maximal incisal opening with trismus, raised floor of mouth, or deviation of the uvula.

- Patients with the following symptoms should be urgently referred to a hospital: stridor, labored breathing, rapid spread of infection, fever, tachycardia, and hypotension.

DISCLOSURE

The authors have nothing to disclose.

REFERENCES

1. Jepsen S, Blanco J, Buchalla W, et al. Prevention and control of dental caries and periodontal diseases at individual and population level: consensus report of group 3 of joint EFP/ORCA workshop on the boundaries between caries and periodontal diseases. J Clin Periodontol 2017;44(Suppl 18): S85–93.

2. Bashir NZ. Update on the prevalence of untreated caries in the US adult population, 2017-2020. J Am Dent Assoc 2022;153(4):300–8.

3. Bashir NZ. Trends in the prevalence of dental caries in the US pediatric population 2011-2020. J Clin Pediatr Dent 2022;46(5):51–7.

4. Sebastian A, Antony PG, Jose M, et al. Institutional microbial analysis of odontogenic infections and their empirical antibiotic sensitivity. J Oral Biol Craniofac Res 2019;9(2):133–8.

5. Böttger S, Zechel-Gran S, Schmermund D, et al. Microbiome of odontogenic abscesses. Microorganisms 2021;9(6):1307.

6. Robertson D, Smith AJ. The microbiology of the acute dental abscess. J Med Microbiol 2009;58(Pt 2):155–62.

7. Słotwińska-Pawlaczyk A, Orzechowska-Wylęgała B, Latusek K, et al. Analysis of the clinical status and treatment of facial cellulitis of odontogenic origin in pediatric patients. Int J Environ Res Public Health 2023;20(6):4874.

8. Flynn TR, Paster BJ, Stokes LN, et al. Molecular methods for diagnosis of odontogenic infections. J Oral Maxillofac Surg 2012;70(8):1854–9.

9. Mardini S, Gohel A. Imaging of Odontogenic Infections. Radiol Clin North Am 2018;56(1):31–44.

10. Ghali S, Katti G, Shahbaz S, et al. Fascial space odontogenic infections: Ultrasonography as an alternative to magnetic resonance imaging. World J Clin Cases 2021;9(3):573–80.

11. Yonetsu K, Izumi M, Nakamura T. Deep facial infections of odontogenic origin: CT assessment of pathways of space involvement. AJNR Am J Neuroradiol 1998;19(1):123–8.

12. Christensen BJ, Park EP, Suau S, et al. Evidence-Based Clinical Criteria for Computed Tomography Imaging in Odontogenic Infections. J Oral Maxillofac Surg 2019;77(2):299–306.

13. Weyh A, Busby E, Smotherman C, et al. Overutilization of Computed Tomography for Odontogenic Infections. J Oral Maxillofac Surg 2019;77(3):528–35.

14. Gray S, Moore K, Callahan N, et al. The role of the pediatric and general dentist in management of odontogenic infections: an algorithmic approach from triage to management. J Dent Child 2023; 90(1):39–47.

15. Robertson DP, Keys W, Rautemaa-Richardson R, et al. Management of severe acute dental infections. BMJ 2015;350:h1300.

16. Jevon P, Abdelrahman A, Pigadas N. Management of odontogenic infections and sepsis: an update. Br Dent J 2020;229(6):363–70.

17. Biron VL, Kurien G, Dziegielewski P, et al. Surgical vs ultrasound-guided drainage of deep neck space abscesses: a randomized controlled trial: surgical vs ultrasound drainage. J Otolaryngol Head Neck Surg 2013;42(1):18.

18. Matthews DC, Sutherland S, Basrani B. Emergency management of acute apical abscesses in the permanent dentition: a systematic review of the literature. J Can Dent Assoc 2003;69(10):660.

19. Fouad AF, Rivera EM, Walton RE. Penicillin as a supplement in resolving the localized acute apical abscess. Oral Surg Oral Med Oral Pathol Oral Radiol Endod 1996;81(5):590–5.

20. Brennan MT, Runyon MS, Batts JJ, et al. Odontogenic signs and symptoms as predictors of odontogenic infection: a clinical trial. J Am Dent Assoc 2006;137(1):62–6.

21. Flynn TR. What are the antibiotics of choice for odontogenic infections, and how long should the treatment course last? Oral Maxillofac Surg Clin North Am 2011;23(4):519–vi.

22. Ahmadi H, Ebrahimi A, Ahmadi F. Antibiotic Therapy in Dentistry. Int J Dent 2021;2021:6667624.

23. Umeshappa H, Shetty A, Kavatagi K, et al. Microbiological profile of aerobic and anaerobic bacteria and its clinical significance in antibiotic sensitivity of odontogenic space infection: A prospective study of 5 years. Natl J Maxillofac Surg 2021;12(3):372–9.

24. Lockhart PB, Tampi MP, Abt E, et al. Evidence-based clinical practice guideline on antibiotic use for the urgent management of pulpal- and periapical-related dental pain and intraoral swelling: A report from the American Dental Association. J Am Dent Assoc 2019;150(11):906–21.e12.

25. Bridwell R, Gottlieb M, Koyfman A, et al. Diagnosis and management of Ludwig's angina: An evidence-based review. Am J Emerg Med 2021;41:1–5.

26. Elagami MM, Ghrewati M, Sharaan A, et al. Acute descending mediastinitis: an unusual presentation. Cureus 2022;14(7):e27302.

27. Elsahy TG, Alotair HA, Alzeer AH, et al. Descending necrotizing mediastinitis. Saudi Med J 2014;35(9): 1123–6.

28. DiNubile MJ. Septic thrombosis of the cavernous sinuses. Arch Neurol 1988;45(5):567–72.

29. Yeo GS, Kim HY, Kwak EJ, et al. Cavernous sinus thrombosis caused by a dental infection: a case report [published correction appears in J Korean Assoc Oral Maxillofac Surg. 2014 Oct;40(5):258. Kim,

HyunYoung [corrected to Kim, Hyun Young]]. J Korean Assoc Oral Maxillofac Surg 2014;40(4): 195–8.

30. Neal TW, Schlieve T. Complications of Severe Odontogenic Infections: A Review. Biology 2022;11(12): 1784.

31. Nawijn F, Smeeing DPJ, Houwert RM, et al. Time is of the essence when treating necrotizing soft tissue infections: a systematic review and meta-analysis. World J Emerg Surg 2020;15:4.

32. Zemplenyi K, Lopez B, Sardesai M, et al. Can progression of odontogenic infections to cervical necrotizing soft tissue infections be predicted? Int J Oral Maxillofac Surg 2017;46(2):181–8.

33. Allareddy V, Nalliah RP, Haque M, et al. Hospital-based emergency department visits with dental conditions among children in the United States: nationwide epidemiological data. Pediatr Dent 2014;36(5):393–9.

34. Eisler L, Wearda K, Romatoski K, et al. Morbidity and cost of odontogenic infections. Otolaryngol Head Neck Surg 2013;149(1):84–8.

35. Monse B, Heinrich-Weltzien R, Benzian H, et al. PUFA–an index of clinical consequences of untreated dental caries. Community Dent Oral Epidemiol 2010;38(1):77–82.

36. Northridge ME, Kumar A, Kaur R. Disparities in Access to Oral Health Care. Annu Rev Public Health 2020;41:513–35.

37. Lewis C, Lynch H, Johnston B. Dental complaints in emergency departments: a national perspective. Ann Emerg Med 2003;42(1):93–9.

38. Cully M, Cully J, Nietert PJ, et al. Physician Confidence in Dental Trauma Treatment and the Introduction of a Dental Trauma Decision-Making Pathway for the Pediatric Emergency Department. Pediatr Emerg Care 2019;35(11):745–8.

Facial Nerve Pathology in Children

Natalie Derise, MD[a], Craig Birgfeld, MD[b], Patrick Byrne, MD[c], G. Nina Lu, MD[a],*

KEYWORDS

- Facial paralysis • Mobius syndrome • Pediatric facial palsy • Facial nerve pathology

KEY POINTS

- Facial paralysis is rare in the pediatric population and occurs 2 to 4 times less frequently than in adults.
- Congenital causes dominate facial nerve pathology in the pediatric population.
- Dynamic restoration of function is the treatment of choice for pediatric patients.

INTRODUCTION

The facial nerve is a complex cranial nerve responsible for the movement of the muscles of facial expression, salivation, tearing, and taste. Its fundamental role in nonverbal communication profoundly impacts social interactions and the negative psychosocial impact of facial palsy is well-reported.[1,2] Control of facial movements not only allows for emotional expression and nonverbal communication, but also serves a critical role in eye protection, nasal airway stability, oral competence, and speech.

Facial nerve pathology in the pediatric population differs from the adult population in several important ways. Facial paralysis is rare in the pediatric population and occurs 2 to 4 times less frequently than in adults.[3] In comparison to the incidence of approximately 30 per 100,000 in adults, 2.7 in 100,000 children under the age of 10 and 10.1 in 100,000 of children over the age of 10 are affected by acute facial nerve paralysis each year.[4,5] Pediatric facial nerve pathology can be classified into three categories: congenital (ie, present at birth), acquired, and idiopathic. Unlike in adults, congenital facial palsy is more common than acquired facial palsy in the pediatric population. The underlying etiology is critical in helping to determine the prognosis and treatment strategies for pediatric patients. It is important that practitioners can recognize facial paralysis and associated syndromes in children and also understand some of the nuances and differences of facial paralysis in the pediatric patient population.

ANATOMY

The facial nerve, also known as the seventh cranial nerve, is composed of motor, general sensory, special sensory, and autonomic components originating from the facial motor and superior salivatory nuclei within the pons. Functionally, this translates to control of facial expression, taste of the anterior two-thirds of the tongue, sensation of the concha bowl and external auditory canal, dampening of loud sounds, and secretion of the lacrimal, nasal, and salivary glands.[6] After exiting the brainstem at the pontomedullary junction, the nerve enters the internal auditory canal through the internal auditory meatus in the petrous part of the temporal bone. The facial nerve then begins its course within the fallopian canal and is accompanied by the vestibulocochlear nerve (CN VIII) in the first (labyrinthine) segment. This portion is the narrowest segment of the fallopian canal and likely the site of greatest facial nerve injury in the setting

a Department of Otolaryngology – Head and Neck Surgery, University of Washington, Seattle, WA, USA; b Department of Surgery, Division of Plastic Surgery, University of Washington, 325 9th Avenue, Seattle, WA 98105, USA; c Department of Otolaryngology – Head and Neck Surgery, Cleveland Clinic Foundation, 9500 Euclid Avenue, Cleveland, OH 44106, USA
* Corresponding author.
E-mail address: ninalu@uw.edu

Oral Maxillofacial Surg Clin N Am 36 (2024) 401–409
https://doi.org/10.1016/j.coms.2024.02.004
1042-3699/24/© 2024 Elsevier Inc. All rights reserved.

of inflammatory conditions such as Bell's Palsy, Ramsey Hunt syndrome.[7] In adults, the facial nerve occupies up to 83% of the fallopian canal in the labyrinthine segment.[8] Saito and colleagues demonstrated that in children, this ratio was closer to 50% in cadaveric specimens. This larger relative space allows more room for nerve swelling following an insult and offers an explanation to why the incidence of acquired facial nerve palsy is lower in children.[9]

After traveling within the labyrinthine segment of the fallopian canal for 3 to 5 mm, the facial nerve makes its first turn, or genu, at the geniculate ganglion.[8] This ganglion is located just distal to the nerve's exit from the internal auditory canal, at the transition point from the labyrinthine to the tympanic component of the fallopian canal. The ganglion contains cell bodies of sensory neurons that form the greater superficial petrosal nerve (GSPN), which provides parasympathetic innervation to the lacrimal gland. Tethering of the facial nerve at the site of the geniculate by the GSPN contributes to traction injury of the nerve in the setting of a temporal bone fracture (**Fig. 1**).

After the first genu, the nerve traverses the tympanic cavity (tympanic segment) before turning inferiorly at the second genu to become the mastoid or vertical segment. The nerve to the stapedius and chorda tympani branch from this segment. The chorda tympani travels back across the tympanic cavity, lateral to the incus to enter the petrotympanic suture, whereby it eventually joins with the lingual nerve to provide taste to the anterior two-thirds of the tongue.

Upon exiting the skull via the stylomastoid foramen, the facial nerve branches out to innervate the muscles responsible for facial expressions. Before entering the parotid gland, the facial nerve sends branches to the occipitalis, posterior belly of the digastric, and the stylohyoid. The nerve enters into the parotid gland, dividing it into superficial and deep lobes. Within the parotid, the nerve divides into 2 main divisions at the pes anserinus. The traditional teaching is that the nerve ends in 5 main branches (temporal, zygomatic, buccal, marginal mandibular, and cervical).[7] (**Fig. 2**) This is an oversimplification, however, as there are multiple interconnections, redundancy, and overlap between these nerves, as evidenced by patients who develop synkinesis.[10]

EMBRYOLOGY AND ETIOLOGY
Embryology

The facial nerve arises from the second branchial arch as do the muscles that it innervates. The muscles include the mimetic muscles,

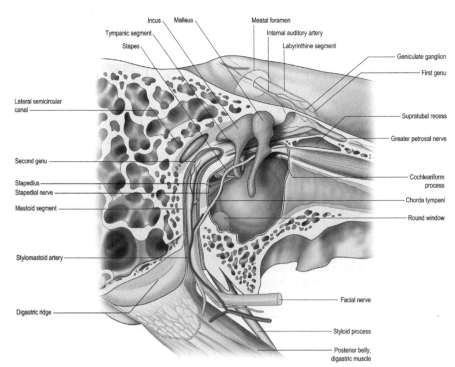

Fig. 1. The facial nerve course through the temporal bone. Note the take off of the Greater Petrosal Nerve from the geniculate ganglion tethering the facial nerve within the fallopian canal. (Reprinted from Gray's Anatomy, 42nd edition, Standring S. et al., Chapter 42 External and Middle Ear. Figure 42.12, 735-751.e1., Copyright 2021 with permission from Elsevier.)

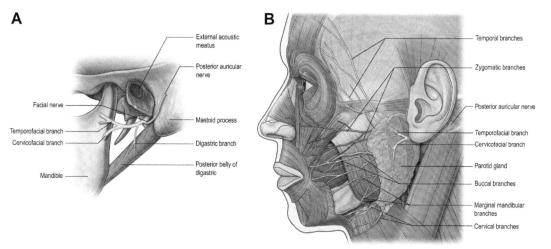

Fig. 2. Extratemporal branching pattern of facial nerve after exit from stylomastoid foramen. (*A*) Facial Nerve main trunk at exit from stylomastoid foramen. (*B*) Branching of facial nerve within and extending from the parotid gland. (With permission from Drake RL, Vogl AW, Mitchell A (eds) Gray's Anatomy for Students, 2nd ed. Elsevier, Churchill Livingstone. Copyright 2010.)

stapedius, the posterior belly of the digastric, and the stylohyoid. The facial nerve and the mimetic muscles begin developing within the first 3 months of gestation and the nerve does not reach full maturation until approximately 4 years of life. By 9 weeks of gestation, the muscles of the 2nd branchial arch are formed and continue to mature. The peripheral facial nerve branches continue to develop over weeks 10 to 15. Although the facial nerve is a contiguous structure at the time of birth, it continues to mature and does not reach its final anatomic location until approximately age 4.[11] During the first 4 years of life, the mastoid has the most rapid rate of growth and pneumatization, doubling in size.[12] Prior to mastoid pneumatization, the extratemporal segment of the facial nerve is much more superficial and at greater risk of injury with birth trauma and with parotid surgery.[13]

The development of the facial nerve has a layer of complexity given its close relation to cranial nerve VIII (auditory nerve) and the formation of the fallopian canal. Before 16 weeks of gestational age, the otic capsule will invaginate around the facial nerve and enclose it within the fallopian canal. The close relationship between the facial nerve and the otic capsule gives insight into why many congenital facial nerve anomalies coincide with inner ear deformities. Concurrent stapes anomalies are also common, as its suprastructure is also derived from the 2nd branchial arch. In many cases whereby the facial nerve is dehiscent, it has occurred during 22 to 25 weeks of gestation when the fallopian canal typically

completely ossifies and fuses around the facial nerve.

There is a wide array of facial nerve anomalies that have been described, with facial nerve dehiscence on the least severe side of the spectrum. Nerve dehiscence can be associated with normal anatomic location, with the anterolateral displacement of the nerve, or with aberrant intratemporal branching, all of which can put the nerve at risk during otologic surgeries.

In congenital facial nerve palsy, the underlying pathophysiology can be due to agenesis of partial or entirety of the nerve, aberrant branching of the nerve, or agenesis of the facial muscles themselves.

Etiology

Broadly, facial nerve pathology can be divided into congenital causes and acquired causes. Congenital facial palsy is defined as the presence of facial palsy at the time of birth and acquired facial paralysis is defined with normal facial function at birth.

Congenital Facial Nerve Paralysis

The incidence of congenital facial nerve palsy has been reported up to 6.9% of all live births, with the most common etiology being birth trauma.[14] Birth trauma occurs from direct physical injury to the facial nerve. The facial nerve in infants is particularly at risk during when forceps are used to aid in delivery.[15] The underlying cause is typically due to a neuropraxis with normal facial nerve and muscle anatomy. Thus, patients generally have favorable outcomes and often have a complete return of function without intervention.[16,17]

Congenital unilateral lower lip palsy, or CULLP is a congenital anomaly in which patients are born with the agenesis of the depressor labii inferioris and/or depressor anguli oris, resulting in weakness of unilateral lower lip depression that presents as an asymmetric smile with crying.[18] The mentalis muscle is typically not involved. This affects 1 per 160 live births and is commonly associated with cardiovascular anomalies.[19]

This differs from Moebius syndrome, which is the agenesis of the facial nerve and/or muscle itself. This often occurs in conjunction with agenesis of the abducens nerve. This can be unilateral or bilateral and is associated with a high incidence of concurrent congenital deformities.[20,21] (Fig. 3)

Other congenital syndromes have well-documented correlations with facial palsy, but the most common are those within the spectrum of craniofacial microsomia.[22,23] Several other syndromes and genetic mutations may be associated with facial palsy. Syndromic causes include Mobius syndrome, Goldenhaar-Gorlin syndrome, CHARGE association, Arnold Chiari malformation, and syringobulbia. Genetic causes include hereditary myopathies, 3q21 to 22 mutation, and 10q21.3 to 22.1 mutation.[17,20,24]

Acquired Facial Nerve Paralysis

As patient age increases, the distribution of facial nerve etiologies begins to mirror those of the adult population, although occurring much less frequently. Idiopathic facial nerve palsy, also known as Bell's palsy, is not as prevalent in the pediatric population as in the adult population: Bell's palsy affects 20 to 30 per 100,000 adults but only

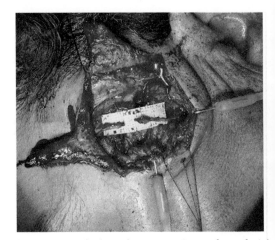

Fig. 4. Frontal branch transection after facial laceration.

6.1 per 100,000 of children aged 1 to 15 are affected.[4,17] Particularly in younger children, facial nerve paralysis can be a propagation of acute otitis media and subsequently mastoiditis. Other common infectious causes include Lyme disease, HSV, Varicella, Mumps, and Coxsackievirus.

Behind idiopathic and infectious causes, trauma is the next most common cause of pediatric facial nerve paralysis. Trauma can range from individual branches to all branches depending on the level of injury (**Fig. 4**). Surgical trauma due to intervention within the head, neck, or brain are potential causes and presents similarly to the adult population. Inflammatory causes include Henoch-Schonlein purpura and Kawasaki disease. Less commonly, the cause of pediatric facial nerve palsy is a neoplastic process, particularly schwannomas, hemangiomas, rhabomyosarcoma, and parotid tumors. **Table 1** provides an abbreviated list of the most common causes of pediatric facial nerve paralysis.

TREATMENT

The etiology of facial nerve paralysis guides the treatment pathway for each case. This is particularly important in children as more recent studies have shown that more than 70% of facial paralysis cases have an identifiable underlying cause.[16] When facial nerve paralysis is caused by a known entity, such as an infection or tumor, the underlying disease process should be treated first. The use of steroids in children presenting with acute idiopathic FNP has historically been poorly studied, but the recovery rate for this patient population has been reported in up to 100% at 3 months regardless of intervention. A recent

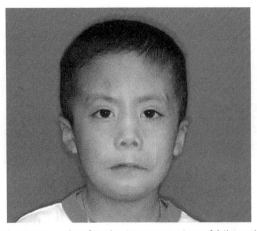

Fig. 3. Example of a classic presentation of bilateral mobius syndrome.

Table 1 Etiologies of facial nerve paralysis	
Congenital	**Acquired**
Syndromic/genetic	Idiopathic
• Moebius	• Bell's palsy
• Craniofacial	Infectious
microsomia	• Otitis media/
○ Goldenhaar	mastoiditis
• DiGeorge	• Meningitis
• CHARGE	• Ramsay-Hunt (Vari-
• VACTERYL	cella-Zoster Virus)
• Arnold-Chiari	• Lyme disease
• Syringobulbia	• Mumps
Asymmetric crying	• Tuberculosis
facies	Neoplastic
• Birth trauma	• Parotid tumors
• CULLP	• Facial nerve
	schwannoma
	• Acoustic neuroma
	• Rhabdomyosarcoma
	Systemic disease
	• Guillain-Barre
	• Vasculitis
	○ Kawasaki disease
	○ Henoch-Schnloein
	purpura
	• Melkersson-Rosen-
	thal syndrome
	• Arterial
	hypertension
	Iatrogenic
	Traumatic

multicenter placebo-controlled randomized trial (n = 187) supported increased recovery rates at 1, 3, and 6 months when pediatric Bell's palsy patients were treated with prednisolone within 72 hours of onset compared with placebo.[25] Other factors to consider when determining the appropriate treatment include the degree of palsy and the duration of palsy.

Treatment Goals

Across all approaches to facial nerve rehabilitation, the main focus is to restore dynamic function when able, but this is particularly salient in the pediatric population. Children with facial nerve palsy typically have normal life expectancy with few medical comorbidities and long-lasting, dynamic treatment options are the treatment of choice when available. Static procedures may be used in conjunction with dynamic procedures to restore eye closure for corneal protection, improve resting symmetry, and correct nasal valve and oral competence. With contemporary advances in functional free muscle transfer, rarely are static

procedures alone selected for the treatment of pediatric facial palsy.

Nonsurgical Treatment Options

In patients with partial palsy, postparalytic facial palsy syndrome, and synkinesis, targeted facial nerve therapy and chemodenervation should be considered. Facial nerve therapy aims to retrain any functioning muscles on the affected side, controlling synkinesis, and relieving excess muscle tension. These therapies require deliberate action and regular practice, so the patient must be mentally willing to participate in the exercises.[5] Chemodenervation with onabotulinum toxin is effective in improving static and dynamic facial symmetry in patients with post paralytic facial palsy synkinesis. However, this requires an injection administered every 3 months and may not be a reasonable treatment option for younger patients.

Surgical Treatment Options

In the setting of acute, traumatic, or iatrogenic facial nerve injury, the aim should be toward immediate (<72 hrs) primary neurorrhaphy or the placement of a cable nerve graft when there is insufficient length for tension free anastomosis.[26] Early primary repair is preferred to optimize outcomes. Nerve transfers may be considered in situations whereby there is viable distal facial nerve and muscle complex but an insufficient proximal nerve source. Donor sources for nerve transfer include trigeminal (masseteric, deep temporal), hypoglossal, and cross-facial nerve grafting. Reinnervation of facial muscle motor end plates is feasible up to 24 months, but after this time frame, results are unreliable.[27] If no viable distal facial nerve and muscle complex is available for reinnervation, both static and dynamic facial reanimation procedures can be considered. Luckily, due to higher peripheral and central nerve plasticity in children, they have higher rates of success with reanimation procedures. Some children who receive masseter to CN VII transfers have developed spontaneous movement related to this neuroplasticity.[22]

Upper face

The primary goals of upper face reanimation are to prevent corneal surface keratopathy and correcting brow asymmetry. Visual field deficits from brow ptosis on the paretic side are less commonly seen in the pediatric population compared with adults, as a child's skin and connective tissues are tenacious enough to combat any gravitational effects until later in life.[7] When a frozen brow is

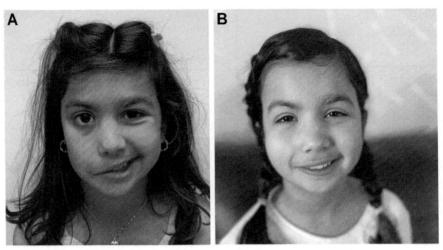

Fig. 5. Demonstrates the restoration of lower eyelid orbicularis oculi contraction during smile. (*A*) Patient with right-sided congenital facial palsy prior to surgery. (*B*) After multivector gracilis free flap for restoration of smile and lower eyelid contraction. (Reprint from: Byrne PJ, Novinger LJ, Genther DJ. Tri-Vector Gracilis Microneurovascular Free Tissue Transfer with Periocular Component to Achieve a Duchenne Smile in Patients with Facial Paralysis. Facial Plast Surg Aesthet Med. 2022 Nov-Dec;24(6):494–496. https://doi.org/10.1089/fpsam.2022.0180. Epub 2022 Oct 19.)

noticeable or aesthetically bothersome to a patient, weakening the contralateral side with botulinum toxin can be considered, although less readily pursued by the pediatric population due to injection discomfort and frequency. Similarly, other static procedures such as brow lift, tarsal strip procedures, and eyelid weights are less commonly required in the pediatric population owing to the preservation of resting symmetry from skin-soft tissue support.

Dynamic procedures have been described to restore the protective blink reflex in children. Terzis and Karypidis introduced the idea of dynamic eye reanimation, describing multiple approaches, from the direct neurotization of the orbicularis muscle, to cross-face nerve grafting from the contralateral zygomaticotemporal branch.[28,29] The addition of a vector of muscle within the lower eyelid during gracilis free muscle transfer as described by Byrne and colleagues can provide the dynamic movement of the lower eyelid during smile (**Fig. 5**).[30]

Mid face

The midface is the main focus of facial reanimation due to its dominant role in smile production, oral competence, and speech. Additionally, a lack of nasalis tone can result in nasal valve insufficiency and nasal position asymmetry. Unlike adults, children tend to have fewer issues with nasal valve obstruction and midface symmetry at rest due to improved skin and soft tissue support. Static midface suspension with autologous fascia lata can help restore the nasolabial fold and nasal valve

position if necessary. Autologous grafting is preferred over allograft which has much higher rates of infection and extrusion. Although fascia slings add can improve facial symmetry at rest, static correction as a single modality will not restore symmetry during facial movement. The failure rate/need for revision for static slings is relatively high in the adult population, and extrapolating this to the pediatric population may mean multiple revision surgeries in a patient's future. The aim is to provide facial reanimation results with longevity.[7] Dynamic reanimation that simultaneously restores resting tone obviates the need for static support.

The standard in pediatric midface reanimation is therefore the reinnervation or restoration of dynamic movement, particularly of the smile. Reinnervation allows for continued midface tone to counteract the eventual facial drooping caused by gravitational effects. Given congenital etiologies involve the absence of a distal facial nerve and muscle complex, situations amenable to nerve transfers are less common compared with the adult population. These situations typically arise in the iatrogenic resection of the proximal facial nerve source or central loss of the ipsilateral facial nucleus. Both regional and free muscle tissue transfers have been used in children. Use of the temporalis muscle has been described with various modifications, such as lengthening temporal myoplasty (LTM) and orthodromic temporalis tendon transfer (T3). Regional temporalis transfer procedures only

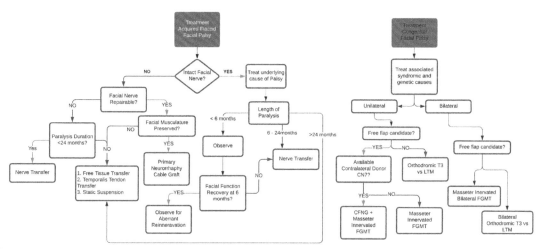

Fig. 6. Treatment algorithm for pediatric patients with acquired and congenital facial palsy. Note the acquired pathway is very similar to the treatment pathway for adults. CFNG, Cross Facial Nerve Graft; LTM, Lengthening Temporal Myoplasty; T3, Temporalis Tendon Transfer.

require a single procedure with immediate visible improvement. Smile excursion can be achieved with the T3 and LTM, but there is little potential for spontaneous smile.[31] Therefore, the shift has been toward free tissue transfer as the gold standard for pediatric facial nerve rehabilitation, given the durable improvement in smile, facial asymmetry and quality of life.[28,32]

The use of the gracilis, pectoralis minor, and latissimus has been described, with the gracilis most widely used in both the pediatric and adult population.[5] This procedure can either be performed in a single stage or 2 stages, depending on the underlying etiology of the facial nerve paralysis. In cases of bilateral facial nerve paralysis (most commonly Moebius syndrome), the free muscle transfer is performed in one stage and the donor innervation is most commonly the ipsilateral masseteric nerve. Spinal accessory nerve, deep temporal nerve, and hypoglossal nerve donor sources have also been described.

When there is a functioning contralateral facial nerve, a cross-face graft will typically be used. A sural nerve graft is most commonly used given its length and relatively benign sensory deficit after harvest. The cross-face graft is coapted to smile-eliciting nerves on the healthy side and used either alone or in conjunction with the masseteric nerve as innervation for the free muscle transfer. The use of dual innervation with masseter and cross-facial grafting significantly improves the success rates of dynamic free muscle transfer. The cross-face graft connection to the contralateral facial nerve is responsible for achieving spontaneous smiles with the free muscle transfer. **Fig. 6** presents the authors' preferred

treatment algorithm in acquired and congenital facial palsy.

Lower face

The asymmetries in the lower face are mostly attributed to the insufficiency of the depressor anguli oris, depressor labii oris, and platysma. These muscles all play a role in depression of the lower lip. Many therapies have been aimed toward weakening the contralateral/normal lip depressors to improve lower lip symmetry. Botulinum toxin to the functioning DAO and DLI have been the mainstays of treatment. Selective myectomy is another popular choice to improve lower lip symmetry. Through an intraoral incision, the DLI on the nonaffected side is resected to create symmetry by reducing asymmetric depression of the lower lip on the normal side.[18,28] Dynamic reanimation via regional muscle transfers of the anterior belly of the digastric and platysma has been described but uncommonly used given variable outcomes. An additional muscle vector to replicate the DLI during gracilis free muscle transfer has been described by Ein and colleagues to restore lower lip depression during smile.[33]

SUMMARY

Facial nerve pathology in children has devastating functional and psychosocial consequences and are most commonly related to congenital agenesis of the facial nerve-muscle complex. Restoration of dynamic movement is a priority in the pediatric population. Fortunately, durable facial reanimation options exist and improve the quality of life for patients long-term.

CLINICS CARE POINTS

- The incidence of acquired acute facial nerve palsy in children is 3 to 10 times lower than in adults.
- The mastoid bone is underdeveloped in the first 4 years of life, leaving the extratemporal facial nerve more susceptible to traumatic injury.
- The close relationship of the facial nerve and otic capsule in embryologic development contributes to why many congenital facial nerve anomalies coincide with inner ear deformities.
- Children with facial paralysis generally have few medical comorbidities and a normal life expectancy. Young children are also less likely to participate in facial retraining. Durable, spontaneous, and dynamic functional restoration is the treatment of choice. Static procedures are considered only after dynamic options are exhausted.

DISCLOSURE

Dr P. Byrne is the co-Founder of Hale, Inc which does not pose a conflict of interest for the subject of this review article. All other authors have no commercial or financial conflicts of interest or funding sources to report.

REFERENCES

1. Japee S, Jordan J, Licht J, et al. Inability to move one's face dampens facial expression perception. Cortex 2023;169:35–49.
2. Hotton M, Huggons E, Hamlet C, et al. The psychosocial impact of facial palsy: A systematic review. Br J Health Psychol 2020;25(3):695–727.
3. El-Hawrani AS, Eng CY, Ahmed SK, et al. General practitioners' referral pattern for children with acute facial paralysis. J Laryngol Otol 2005;119(7):540–2.
4. Cha CI, Hong CK, Park MS, et al. Comparison of Facial Nerve Paralysis in Adults and Children. Yonsei Med J 2008;49(5):725.
5. Malik M, Cubitt JJ. Paediatric facial paralysis: An overview and insights into management. J Paediatr Child Health 2021;57(6):786–90.
6. Dulak D, Naqvi IA. Neuroanatomy, Cranial Nerve 7 (Facial). In: StatPearls. StatPearls Publishing; 2023. Available at: http://www.ncbi.nlm.nih.gov/books/NBK526119/. [Accessed 17 December 2023].
7. Sharma PR, Zuker RM, Borschel GH. Perspectives in the reconstruction of paediatric facial paralysis. Curr Opin Otolaryngol Head Neck Surg 2015;23(6):470–9.
8. Myckatyn TM, Mackinnon SE. A Review of Facial Nerve Anatomy. Semin Plast Surg 2004;18(1):5–11.
9. Saito H, Takeda T, Kishimoto S. Facial nerve to facial canal cross-sectional area ratio in children. Laryngoscope 1992;102(10):1172–6.
10. Rink S, Bendella H, Akkin SM, et al. Experimental Studies on Facial Nerve Regeneration. Anat Rec 2019;302(8):1287–303.
11. Mehta M. Embryology and Development of Facial Nerve. In: Thieme, editor. Atlas of facial nerve surgeries and reanimation procedures. DELHI: THIEME PUBLISHERS; 2023. p. 1–13.
12. Aladeyelu OS, Olaniyi KS, Olojede SO, et al. Temporal bone pneumatization: A scoping review on the growth and size of mastoid air cell system with age. PLoS One 2022;17(6):e0269360.
13. Farrior JB, Santini H. Facial Nerve Identification in Children. Otolaryngol Neck Surg 1985;93(2):173–6.
14. Al Tawil K, Saleem N, Kadri H, et al. Traumatic Facial Nerve Palsy in Newborns: Is It Always Iatrogenic? Am J Perinatol 2010;27(09):711–4.
15. Deramo PJ, Greives MR, Nguyen PD. Pediatric facial reanimation: An algorithmic approach and systematic review. Arch Plast Surg 2020;47(5):382–91.
16. Shargorodsky J, Lin HW, Gopen Q. Facial Nerve Palsy in the Pediatric Population. Clin Pediatr (Phila). 2010;49(5):411–7.
17. Ciorba A. Facial nerve paralysis in children. World J Clin Cases 2015;3(12):973.
18. Krane NA, Markey JD, Loyo M. Neuromodulator for the Treatment of Congenital Unilateral Lower Lip Palsy. Ann Otol Rhinol Laryngol 2019;128(1):62–5.
19. Saylam E, Arya K. Congenital Unilateral Lower Lip Palsy. In: StatPearls. StatPearls Publishing. 2023. Available at: http://www.ncbi.nlm.nih.gov/books/NBK560695/. [Accessed 17 December 2023].
20. Monawwer SA, Ali S, Naeem R, et al. Moebius Syndrome: An Updated Review of Literature. Child Neurol Open 2023;10. 2329048X231205405.
21. Palmer C.A., Mobius Syndrome, Available at: https://emedicine.medscape.com/article/1180822-overview?ecd=ppc_google_rlsa-traf_mscp_emed_md_us&gad_source=1&gclid=CjwKCAiA1fqrBhA1EiwAMU5m_3TDzZn1oxZKr335lr7acbTPpknFeqiSopXMkF48iYEKJAzql_RWNRoCmyIQAvD_BwE, 2023. (Accessed 1 February 2024).
22. Reddy S, Redett R. Facial Paralysis in Children. Facial Plast Surg 2015;31(02):117–22.
23. Brandstetter KA, Patel KG. Craniofacial Microsomia. Facial Plast Surg Clin N Am 2016;24(4):495–515.
24. Hadford SP, Genther DJ, Byrne PJ. Pediatric Facial Reanimation. Facial Plast Surg Clin N Am 2024;32(1):169–80.
25. Babl FE, Herd D, Borland ML, et al. Efficacy of Prednisolone for Bell Palsy in Children: A Randomized, Double-Blind, Placebo-Controlled, Multicenter Trial.

Neurology 2022;99(20). https://doi.org/10.1212/WNL.0000000000201164.

26. Kannan RY, Hills A, Shelley MJ, et al. Immediate compared with late repair of extracranial branches of the facial nerve: a comparative study. Br J Oral Maxillofac Surg 2020;58(2):163–9.

27. Fliss E, Yanko R, Zaretski A, et al. Facial Nerve Repair following Acute Nerve Injury. Arch Plast Surg 2022;49(04):501–9.

28. Banks CA, Hadlock TA. Pediatric Facial Nerve Rehabilitation. Facial Plast Surg Clin N Am 2014;22(4):487–502.

29. Terzis JK, Karypidis D. The Outcomes of Dynamic Procedures for Blink Restoration in Pediatric Facial Paralysis. Plast Reconstr Surg 2010;125(2):629–44.

30. Byrne PJ, Novinger LJ, Genther DJ. Tri-Vector Gracilis Microneurovascular Free Tissue Transfer with Periocular Component to Achieve a Duchenne Smile in Patients with Facial Paralysis. Facial Plast Surg Aesthetic Med 2022;24(6):494–6.

31. Leboulanger N, Maldent JB, Glynn F, et al. Rehabilitation of congenital facial palsy with temporalis flap – Case series and literature review. Int J Pediatr Otorhinolaryngol 2012;76(8):1205–10.

32. Greene JJ, Tavares J, Mohan S, et al. Long-Term Outcomes of Free Gracilis Muscle Transfer for Smile Reanimation in Children. J Pediatr 2018;202:279–84.e2.

33. Ein L, Hadlock TA, Jowett N. Dual-Vector Gracilis Muscle Transfer for Smile Reanimation with Lower Lip Depression. Laryngoscope 2021;131(8):1758–60.

Conceptual Principles in Pediatric Craniomaxillofacial Reconstruction

Andrew D. Linkugel, MD[a,b], Michael R. Markiewicz, DDS, MPH, MD[c],
Sean Edwards, DDS, MD[d], Srinivas M. Susarla, DMD, MD, MPH[a,b,e],*

KEYWORDS

- Pediatric • Reconstruction • Craniomaxillofacial • Cranioplasty • Free tissue transfer • Tissue flaps
- Bone grafts

KEY POINTS

- Pediatric patients require a satisfactory reconstructive outcome during continued development and lifetime durability of their reconstruction.
- Reconstruction with autologous tissue and the use of resorbable fixation both promote growth.
- Achieving symmetry with contralateral structures, in the context of growth, should guide reconstruction.

INTRODUCTION: GENERAL RECONSTRUCTIVE PRINCIPLES AND RECONSTRUCTIVE LADDER AS APPLIED TO CHILDREN

Reconstructive goals of pediatric craniomaxillofacial structures include restoring structure and function in the setting of continued growth. Beginning in embryogenesis, growth of the head and face continues through infancy, childhood, and adolescence, with the face reaching a mature size about 2 years earlier in females than in males.[1] The rate of growth of the skull in infancy and early childhood has been studied extensively.[2–4] The volume of the skull is about 25% of the adult maximum at birth, 55% at 1 year old, and 80% at 5 years old. The midface grows more slowly, and the mandible is the last craniofacial structure to reach adult size. In general, after the eruption of the permanent dentition in a given area, that area of the mandible has reached most of its adult size. The differential growth of the craniomaxillofacial skeleton is summarized in **Fig. 1**. As an example of application of growth principles, permanent (titanium, and so forth) fixation can be used to stabilize reconstruction when an area of the skeleton has finished growing. Likewise, alloplastic implants can be used in this setting. When growth is not complete, resorbable/removable fixation and autologous grafts/flaps are better choices.

Overall, reconstruction of the pediatric craniofacial structures, like many areas of the body, can be organized around the principle of "replace like with

[a] Craniofacial Center, Seattle Children's Hospital, 4800 Sand Point Way NorhtEast, Seattle, WA 98105, USA; [b] Division of Plastic Surgery, Department of Surgery, University of Washington School of Medicine, Seattle, WA, USA; [c] Department of Oral and Maxillofacial Surgery, University at Buffalo School of Dental Medicine, 3435 Main Street, 112 Squire Hall, Buffalo NY 14214, USA; [d] Department of Oral & Maxillofacial Surgery, University of Michigan School of Dentistry, 2200 Vinewood Boulevard, Ann Arbor, MI 48104, USA; [e] Department of Oral and Maxillofacial Surgery, University of Washington School of Dentistry, Seattle, WA, USA
* Corresponding author. Craniofacial Center, Seattle Children's Hospital, 4800 Sand Point Way NE, Seattle, WA 98105.
E-mail address: srinivas.susarla@seattlechildrens.org

Oral Maxillofacial Surg Clin N Am 36 (2024) 411–424
https://doi.org/10.1016/j.coms.2024.03.006

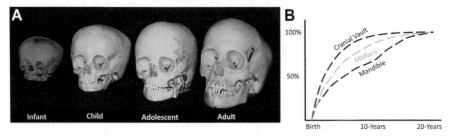

Fig. 1. Craniofacial growth. While the volume of the cranial vault increases from 25% to 80% of the adult maximum over the first 5 years of life, the midface and mandible continue to grow through childhood and adolescence (*A*, *B*). Therefore, at school age, the development of the calvarium is nearly complete while the facial skeleton will, on average, still double in size.

like." The reconstructive ladder, with increasing technical complexity and donor site morbidity at each rung, is a common framework for organizing reconstructive techniques. When applied to children, each level has new considerations. While some wounds may heal satisfactorily in adults with prolonged wound care or negative pressure wound therapy, the extended use of these modalities in young children can be associated with acute stress disorder[5] or excessive exposure to sedating agents.[6] Split-thickness and full-thickness skin grafting are mainstays of soft tissue reconstruction. Because the total body surface area increases as the square of height, the available skin for grafting can be severely limited in young children. Tissue expansion has been used in both the scalp and the face/neck in pediatric patients,[7] but the discomfort associated with repeated expansion can have the same deleterious effects as prolonged wound care. In addition, intentional or accidental manipulation of the device by pediatric patients can lead to mechanical failure. Local 2-stage flaps (ie, forehead, nasolabial) are core procedures for adult facial soft tissue reconstruction and have been successfully performed in children,[8] but also require attention to wound care in the intermediate stage as detailed earlier. Free tissue transfer can be reliably performed even in very young children[9] with attention to special technical considerations and the intense early postoperative period.[10] For all children, minimizing the effect of surgical interventions on critical periods of their social and emotional development as much as possible is paramount. The pediatric reconstructive ladder with special considerations is depicted in **Fig. 2**.

SPECIFIC CONSIDERATIONS BY REGION: CRANIAL VAULT
Cranial Vault Bone Reconstruction

Congenital or acquired defects of the pediatric skull must be reconstructed with consideration

given to the age of the patient and need for lifetime durability of the reconstruction. The dura has reliable osteogenic potential in young (less than 2 years old) children,[11,12] although there are reports of spontaneous calvarial reossification in older individuals.[13,14] For young children with full-thickness defects including dura and older children, cranioplasty with autologous or alloplastic material is required. In general, autologous bone is considered the primary option for pediatric cranioplasty.[15] A sample case of split calvarial reconstruction of the frontal bone and orbit is illustrated in **Fig. 3**. For most types of pediatric cranial vault pathology, bone resected through the primary craniectomy is not suitable for replacement. However, autologous bone from elsewhere on the

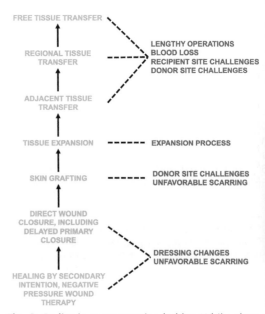

Fig. 2. Pediatric reconstructive ladder. While almost all adult reconstructive techniques are technically possible to perform in children, pediatric patients present unique challenges at each rung of the reconstructive ladder.

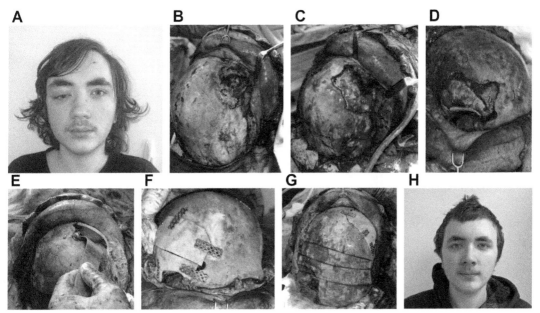

Fig. 3. Erosive lesion of the skull base. This 15-year-old patient presented with the acute onset of vision changes and hypoglobus (*A*) and was found to have a lytic lesion in the right frontal bone (*B*). Resection of the mass resulted in a defect of the right anterior cranial vault, orbital roof, and lateral orbit (*C–D*). Full-thickness contralateral parietal bone graft was harvested, split, and contoured to recreate the orbit, supraorbital rim, and frontal bone (*E–G*). The donor site was reconstructed with the remaining split bone. Final pathology showed intraosseous epidermoid cyst with an associated aneurysmal bone cyst. Post-operatively, the patient had satisfactory improvement in visual symptoms with preserved forehead and brow contour (*H*).

skull, rib, and iliac crest can all be donor sites. Splitting the inner table from the outer table of the calvarial bone can facilitate reconstruction of both the defect and the donor site, and this can be performed in children as young as 1 year old.[16] **Fig. 4** shows split calvarial autograft used in a 2-year-old child. A related technique, exchange (or switch) cranioplasty,[17] involves fixation of a full-thickness calvarial bone graft in the defect. In this case, the donor site is reconstructed with placement of particulate bone graft harvested from the inner table of the craniectomy. Both particulate and cortical bone grafts have the greatest chance for viability when placed over unscarred dura.[18] Furthermore, resorption is reduced when

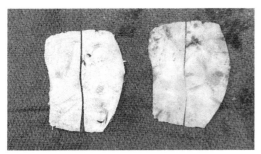

Fig. 4. Calvarial bone split for use as autograft to reconstruct a skull defect in a 2-year-old child.

cortical calvarial bone grafts are placed with rigid fixation.[19] Rigid fixation in children can be accomplished with either titanium or resorbable plating systems. Resorbable plating systems have less potential for growth restriction and are less likely to need to be removed.[20] For children with large defects or defects otherwise not amenable to autologous bone reconstruction, alloplastic materials can be considered. Titanium mesh, while used frequently in adults, is used less often in pediatric patients.[21] It is available "off the shelf" and does not require preoperative customization. Compared to other alloplastic materials, titanium mesh has lower short-term,[22] but a higher long-term[23] complication rate, especially in cases with tenuous soft tissue coverage. Customized synthetic alloplasts include porous polyethylene and polyetheretherketone (PEEK). Porous polyethylene implants used for pediatric cranioplasty do not seem to disturb growth in relatively short-term follow-up.[24] Advantages of porous polyethylene include surrounding tissue ingrowth[25] (although not osteoconduction)[26] and decades of experience in other craniofacial applications.[27,28] PEEK has tensile strength approaching that of autologous bone[29] and was first used in craniofacial surgery in 2007.[30] A PEEK cranioplasty performed for a young patient is shown in **Fig. 5**.

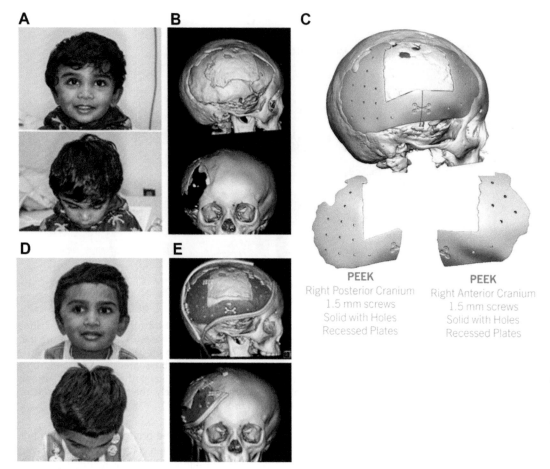

Fig. 5. Polyetheretherketone (PEEK) cranioplasty. This 4-year-old boy had a complicated right-sided calvarial defect after partial resorption of the autologous bone graft after craniotomy for intraventricular hemorrhage (*A–B*). Virtual planning was used to mirror the unaffected side and design a 2-piece PEEK implant (*C*), which provided brain protection and restoration of symmetry (*D–E*).

Cranial Vault Reconstruction: Pericranial Flap

Soft tissue coverage is critical to the durability of any skull reconstruction. While the overlying skin and galea can be spared during resection of many cranial vault pathologies, soft tissue defects may require coverage throughout the reconstructive ladder, from local tissue rearrangement to free tissue transfer. In situations with tenuous soft tissue coverage, the pericranial flap is a local, technically simple source of vascularized tissue for interposition between bony reconstruction and the skin. The pericranium has axial pedicles throughout the skull. It is supplied anteriorly by the supratrochlear and supraorbital vessels, laterally by the superficial temporal artery and deep temporal branches of the maxillary artery, and posteriorly by the occipital and great auricular arteries.[31] This redundant blood supply provides excellent versatility for transposition of the pericranium over a variety of defects. For situations where augmentation is necessary but pericranium is not available, many types of skin substitutes and wound matrices have been used in the scalp.[32]

Scalp Reconstruction

Reconstruction of pediatric scalp can involve each rung of the reconstructive ladder, from wound care to replantation of scalp avulsions.[33] In general, exposure of calvarial bone can be treated most simply by burring to the diploic space followed by application of a skin graft or skin substitute. However, this results in a suboptimal esthetic result (scar alopecia). Defects or areas of scar involving up to 50% of the hair-bearing scalp[34] can be adequately reconstructed with staged tissue expansion. For reconstruction in a single stage, the elasticity of neonatal skin and/or galeal

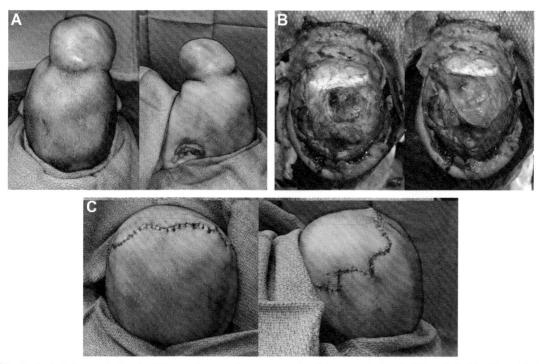

Fig. 6. Occipital encephalocele. This newborn underwent repair of the encephalocele (*A*) early in life. The critical defect was covered with a pericranial flap, and barrel staves were created to address the patient's biparietal narrowing (*B*). The scalp was closed primarily with improvement in the patient's head shape (*C*).

scoring can facilitate closure by primary intention or with local tissue rearrangement. **Fig. 6** depicts the use of a pericranial flap and the creation of barrel staves to improve head shape in a patient with an occipital encephalocele. Similarly, an atretic encephalocele at the vertex was treated with rotational scalp flaps (**Fig. 7**).

SPECIFIC CONSIDERATIONS BY REGION: ORBIT AND MIDFACE
Orbital Reconstruction

In a similar pattern to skull growth, the orbit is about half the adult size at birth and increases to 77% of the adult size by 5 years old.[35] The thin bones that comprise the orbit are generally not amenable to reduction and fixation, so the overall most common presentation for orbital reconstruction is trauma. The typical location of orbital fracture changes with age: at about 7 years of age, the incidence of orbital floor fracture surpasses the incidence of orbital roof fracture.[36] Because of continuing growth, the pediatric orbit is more commonly reconstructed with autologous bone and resorbable material (as compared to permanent implants like titanium and porous polyethylene).[37] In pediatric defects after oncologic resection, reconstructive goals include

separation of the orbit from the intracranial contents, globe support, soft tissue coverage, and the maintenance of orbital size and shape.[38] Orbital roof defects greater than one-third of the roof should be rigidly reconstructed to prevent pulsatile exophthalmos.[38] A case of a newborn patient who underwent reconstruction after resection of a sarcoma with a temporalis muscle and fat pad flap is presented in **Fig. 8**. **Fig. 9** shows immediate reconstruction of the orbital floor and infraorbital nerve[39] after ossifying fibroma extirpation.

Midface Reconstruction

Reconstruction of composite defects in the midface must provide a rigid framework to recreate the facial buttresses, support the maxillary dentition, and provide or support the soft tissue to achieve symmetric facial width and projection. Other midface functions to consider in reconstruction are nasal airway patency, speech, and separation of the pharynx from the skull base. The anatomy of midfacial soft tissue and its evolution over time are complex. Both atrophy and ptosis of soft tissue are thought to drive facial aging,[40] and these both can be accelerated in traumatic or oncologic defects. The importance of resuspension of the midfacial soft tissues is well

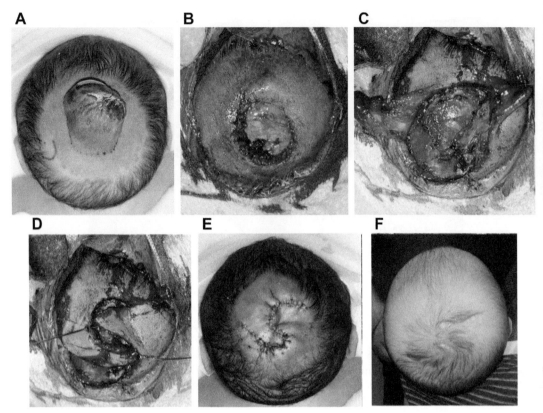

Fig. 7. Vertex atretic encephalocele. This neonate presented with an atretic encephalocele at the vertex (*A*). Resection of the encephalocele resulted in an approximately 5 × 4cm defect with exposed dura after resection of the affected tissue (*B*). Rotational scalp flaps were created (*C*) and advanced (*D*) into the defect to allow closure without tension. Note the significant reactive erythema immediately following closure—this is the typical response of neonatal skin to manipulation (*E*). The wound healed uneventfully (*F*).

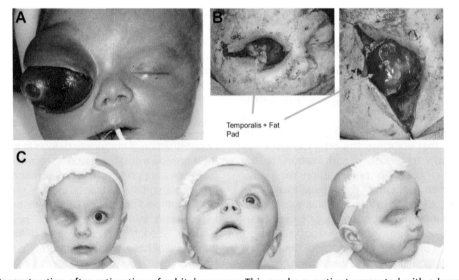

Temporalis + Fat Pad

Fig. 8. Reconstruction after extirpation of orbital sarcoma. This newborn patient presented with a large orbital sarcoma (*A*). Adjuvant radiation therapy was planned after resection. The defect was reconstructed with a temporalis muscle and fat pad flap (*B*) for durable soft tissue coverage in this setting. After radiation, the patient had maintained orbital size and shape to facilitate the placement of an orbital prosthesis (*C*).

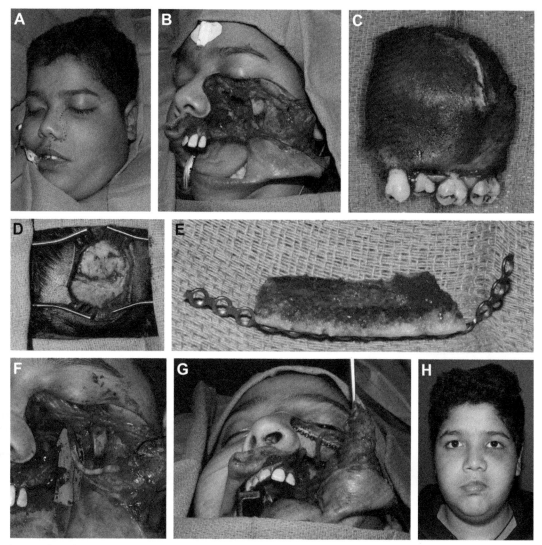

Fig. 9. Orbital floor reconstruction after maxillectomy. This 11-year-old patient presented with a left midface ossifying fibroma and underwent excision through a transfacial approach (*A*). The hemimaxillectomy defect included the infraorbital nerve and orbital floor (*B, C*). A small piece of outer table of the calvarium was harvested (*D, E*) for orbital floor reconstruction. The infraorbital nerve was reconstructed with acellular nerve allograft (*F*), and the calvarial bone graft was fixated to reconstruct the orbital floor (*G*). The patient maintained symmetric globe position postoperatively (*H*).

established in the trauma population.[41] In addition to esthetic deformity, midface ptosis can lead to ectropion and exposure keratopathy. **Fig. 10** shows a case of post-reconstructive midface ptosis treated with secondary resuspension. After extirpation of midface tumors, flap selection is guided by the extent of resection and need for adjuvant radiation therapy. Of malignancies affecting the pediatric midface, sarcoma has the highest incidence and is frequently associated with neoadjuvant or adjuvant radiation therapy.[42] Resection can also be planned virtually, allowing the fabrication of patient-specific cutting guides and implants. **Fig. 11** shows resection with

immediate reconstruction of a midface ameloblastoma with a free fibula flap. A suggested algorithm for the timing of flap reconstruction of the pediatric midface is shown in **Fig. 12**.

SPECIFIC CONSIDERATIONS BY REGION: MANDIBLE, TEMPOROMANDIBULAR JOINT, AND LOWER FACE
Mandible and Temporomandibular Joint Reconstruction

In addition to establishing facial height and lower facial width, the mandible and associated soft

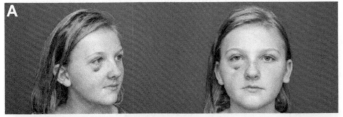

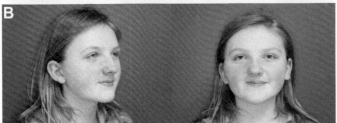

Fig. 10. Repair of midface ptosis. This young patient presented with hardware exposure, soft tissue descent, and mild cicatricial ectropion following outside resection and reconstruction of a maxillary myxoma (*A*). She underwent resuspension of her midfacial soft tissue to her orbital floor implant resulting in improved symmetry (*B*).

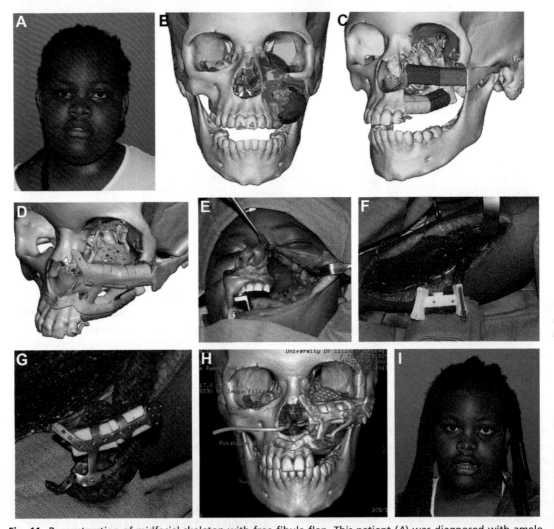

Fig. 11. Reconstruction of midfacial skeleton with free fibula flap. This patient (*A*) was diagnosed with ameloblastoma. Using virtual planning (*B*), the tumor (*red*) and planned resection (*green*) were segmented. Reconstruction was planned virtually with a free fibula flap (*C*), with vascularized fibula used for the alveolar ridge and nonvascularized fibula used for the zygoma. A patient-specific implant, also incorporating reconstruction of the orbital floor, was designed (*D*). The planned resection was completed (*E*), and a custom cutting guide was used to harvest the fibula flap (*F*). The construct was assembled with the flap still perfused on the leg (*G*). The full reconstruction is shown on the postoperative computed tomography (*H*), and the patient demonstrated good facial symmetry postoperatively (*I*).

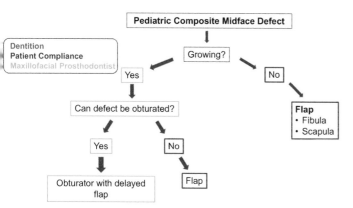

Fig. 12. Reconstructive algorithm for the pediatric midface.

Whenever possible, staged reconstructions should be avoided to lessen burden of care for children

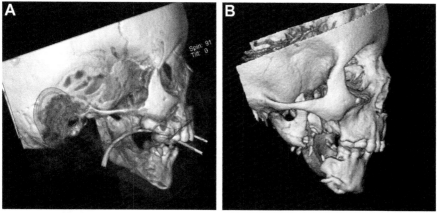

Fig. 13. Spontaneous regeneration after traumatic condylectomy. This patient presented with a traumatic hemi-mandibulectomy from a dog bite injury (*A*). At interval follow-up, regeneration of the condyle, coronoid, and a portion of the body of the mandible was evident on computed tomography (*B*).

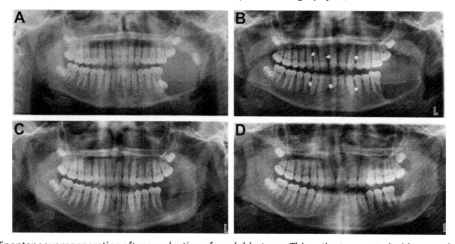

Fig. 14. Spontaneous regeneration after enucleation of ameloblastoma. This patient presented with an ameloblastoma in the left mandibular angle (*A*) and underwent enucleation with sacrifice of the buccal cortex and periosteum. The lingual periosteum and pterygomasseteric sling were maintained. There was a sizable defect 1 week postoperatively (*B*). Progressive spontaneous ossification of the defect was seen at 3 months postoperatively (*C*) with full healing at 1 year postoperatively (*D*).

tissue serve critical functions in airway,[43] speech,[44] and mastication. Restoration of dentition and occlusion in mandible reconstruction are important considerations. Spontaneous regeneration of the mandible, thought to be driven by osteoprogenitor cells in the periosteum,[45] is an additional rung in the reconstructive ladder. Some examples of spontaneous regeneration of the mandible involving the condyle (**Fig. 13**) and tooth-bearing segments (**Fig. 14**) are shown.

Reconstruction is required for persistent or larger defects. The Kaban-Pruzansky classification[46] remains the dominant classification scheme for congenital mandibular hypoplasia and also is a useful framework for considering traumatic and oncologic defects of the ramus-condyle unit in children. There is controversy regarding the need for vascularized versus non-vascularized bone grafting in pediatric mandible reconstruction, with the size of defect, location, associated soft tissue loss, and presence of adjuvant radiation all playing a role.[47] The iliac crest, ribs, and calvarium can provide ample bone graft. For nonvascularized reconstruction of the ramus-condyle unit and temporomandibular joint, costochondral grafts are the most common

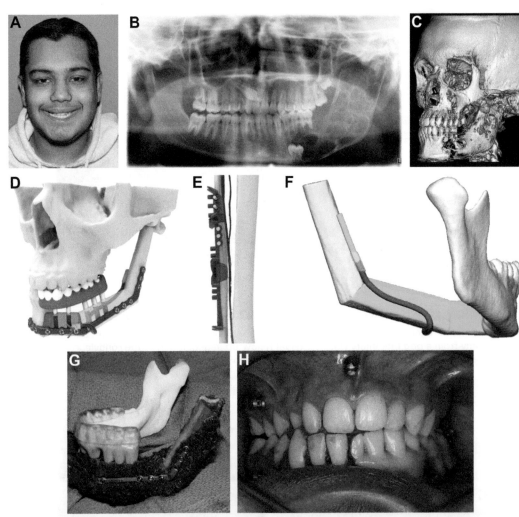

Fig. 15. Mandible reconstruction with free fibula flap. This 14-year-old boy presented with an ameloblastic fibro-odontoma of the left mandible (*A*). Panorex (*B*) and computed tomography (*C*) showed an expansile, multilocular, osteolytic lesion involving the left mandibular body, ramus, coronoid, and condyle. A hemimandibulectomy was recommended, and a free fibula flap, immediate dental implants with prosthesis, and allograft reconstruction of the inferior alveolar nerve (IAN) was planned (*D*). A custom osteotomy and dental implant placement guide was used for the fibula flap harvest (*E*). The planned nerve allograft (*purple*) coaptation to the residual IAN (*green*) is shown (*F*). The 3-piece fibula construct, including dental implants and prosthesis, was assembled using a patient-specific reconstruction plate on the leg with a printed model and splint as reference (*G*). The patient demonstrated premorbid occlusion with the prosthesis postoperatively (*H*).

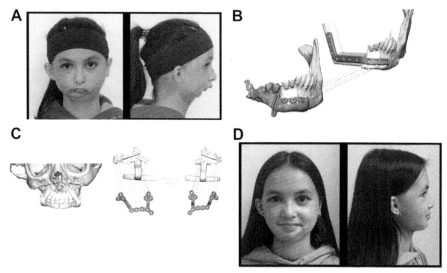

Fig. 16. Mandible reconstruction with free fibula flap and staged orthognathic surgery. This patient underwent multiple resections and adjuvant radiation for a desmoid tumor as a young child. At age 13, she presented with a hemimandibular defect with chin point deviation and maxillary asymmetry related to her prior radiation (*A*). She underwent staged reconstruction, first with free fibula flap reconstruction of the right hemi-mandible with customized cutting guides and plate (*B*). A portion of de-epithelialized skin paddle was interposed between the fibula and temporal fossa to reconstruct the temporomandibular joint. Also at the first stage, she underwent contralateral sagittal split osteotomy for additional improvement of her mandible asymmetry. As a second stage, she underwent LeFort I osteotomy, again with custom cutting guides and plates, to address her maxillary asymmetry (*C*). For soft tissue reconstruction, she has undergone right lower buccal sulcus vestibuloplasty and fat grafting to the lower face (*D*).

technique.[48] For vascularized bone reconstruction of the mandible, the free fibula flap is used most commonly.[49]

Lower Face: Adjunct Procedures

For persistent soft tissue asymmetry after adequate bony reconstruction, fat grafting is a versatile soft

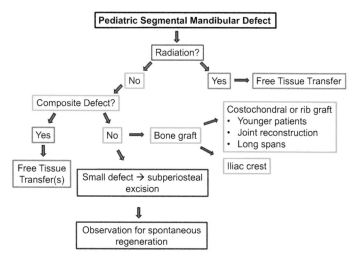

Fig. 17. Reconstructive algorithm for the pediatric mandible.

tissue filler for the lower face and elsewhere in children.[50] For pediatric patients who have finished growing, porous polyethylene or other implants can be added to the bony reconstruction for improved contour and symmetry.[28] The critical sensory function provided by the inferior alveolar nerve (IAN) can significantly affect quality of life if not adequately reconstructed, and full sensory recovery can be achieved with relatively long segments of nerve allograft.[51] A sample case of mandible reconstruction with free fibula flap including IAN reconstruction in presented in **Fig. 15**. **Fig. 16** illustrates several principles in a single patient who underwent staged reconstruction of a complex midface and lower face bone and soft tissue defect in the setting of adjuvant radiation. A suggested algorithm for reconstruction of the pediatric mandible is shown in **Fig. 17**.

SUMMARY

Reconstructive surgery is necessarily guided by application of principles rather than identical procedures, given that each defect and normal appearance is unique. To protect critical structures, maintaining compartmentalization between the cranium, orbit, sinuses, and pharynx is critical. Staging reconstruction throughout growth may be required to achieve the most precise definitive outcome.

CLINICS CARE POINTS

- Of the craniofacial skeleton, the calvarial vault reaches adult size most quickly in children, with the midface growing at an intermediate rate and the mandible growing the most slowly.

- Application of various strategies from the reconstructive ladder to pediatric patients requires extra attention to the burden of care on children and their families.

- Pediatric cranioplasty is best performed with split calvarial bone autograft.

- Orbital roof defects comprising greater than one-third of the orbital roof should be rigidly reconstructed to prevent pulsatile exophthalmos.

- Soft tissue in the midface is vulnerable to ptosis with facial aging and should be supported in the primary reconstruction.

- The restoration of occlusion in children often requires a staged approach with initial reconstruction followed by definitive orthognathic surgery at skeletal maturity.

DISCLOSURE

The authors have nothing to disclose.

REFERENCES

1. Farkas LG, Posnick JC, Hreczko TM. Growth patterns of the face: a morphometric study. Cleft Palate-Craniofacial J 1992;29(4):308–15.
2. Dekaban AS. Tables of cranial and orbital measurements, cranial volume, and derived indexes in males and females from 7 days to 20 years of age. Ann Neurol 1977;2(6):485–91.
3. Libby J, Marghoub A, Johnson D, et al. Modelling human skull growth: a validated computational model. J R Soc Interface 2017;14(130):20170202.
4. Liang C, Profico A, Buzi C, et al. Normal human craniofacial growth and development from 0 to 4 years. Sci Rep 2023;13(1):9641.
5. Woolard A, Hill NTM, McQueen M, et al. The psychological impact of paediatric burn injuries: a systematic review. BMC Publ Health 2021;21:2281.
6. Yabrodi M, Shieh Yu J, Slaven JE, et al. Safety and efficacy of propofol- and ketamine-based procedural sedation regimen in pediatric patients during burn repetitive dressing change: 10 years single center experience. J Burn Care Res 2023;44(4):931–5.
7. Gosain AK, Turin SY, Chim H, et al. Salvaging the unavoidable: a review of complications in pediatric tissue expansion. Plast Reconstr Surg 2018;142(3):759–68.
8. Giugliano C, Andrades PR, Benitez S. Nasal reconstruction with a forehead flap in children younger than 10 years of age. Plast Reconstr Surg 2004; 114(2):316.
9. Upton J, Guo L. Pediatric free tissue transfer: a 29-year experience with 433 transfers. Plast Reconstr Surg 2008;121(5):1725.
10. Burns HR, Skochdopole AJ, Zeledon RA, et al. Pediatric microsurgery and free-tissue transfer. Semin Plast Surg 2023;37(04):231–9.
11. Hobar PC, Schreiber JS, McCarthy JG, et al. The role of the dura in cranial bone regeneration in the immature animal. Plast Reconstr Surg 1993;92(3): 405–10.
12. Gosain AK, Santoro TD, Song LS, et al. Osteogenesis in calvarial defects: contribution of the dura, the pericranium, and the surrounding bone in adult versus infant animals. Plast Reconstr Surg 2003; 112(2):515.
13. Thombre BD, Prabhuraj AR. Spontaneous bone formation in a large craniectomy defect. Childs Nerv Syst 2018;34(8):1449–50.
14. González-Bonet LG. Spontaneous cranial bone regeneration after a craniectomy in an adult. World Neurosurg 2021;147:67–9.
15. Bykowski MR, Goldstein JA, Losee JE. Pediatric cranioplasty. Clin Plast Surg 2019;46(2):173–83.

16. Vercler CJ, Sugg KB, Buchman SR. Split cranial bone grafting in children younger than 3 years old: debunking a surgical myth. Plast Reconstr Surg 2014;133(6):822e–7e.

17. Rogers GF, Greene AK, Mulliken JB, et al. Exchange cranioplasty using autologous calvarial particulate bone graft effectively repairs large cranial defects. Plast Reconstr Surg 2011;127(4):1631.

18. Rogers GF, Greene AK. Autogenous bone graft: basic science and clinical implications. J Craniofac Surg 2012;23(1):323.

19. LaTrenta GS, McCarthy JG, Breitbart AS, et al. The role of rigid skeletal fixation in bone-graft augmentation of the craniofacial skeleton. Plast Reconstr Surg 1989;84(4):578–88.

20. Branch LG, Crantford C, Cunningham T, et al. Long-term outcomes of pediatric cranial reconstruction using resorbable plating systems for the treatment of craniosynostosis. J Craniofac Surg 2017;28(1):26.

21. Ma IT, Symon MR, Bristol RE, et al. Outcomes of titanium mesh cranioplasty in pediatric patients. J Craniofac Surg 2018;29(1):99–104.

22. Abu-Ghname A, Banuelos J, Oliver JD, et al. Outcomes and complications of pediatric cranioplasty: a systematic review. Plast Reconstr Surg 2019;144(3):433e.

23. Kwiecien GJ, Rueda S, Couto RA, et al. Long-term outcomes of cranioplasty: titanium mesh is not a long-term solution in high-risk patients. Ann Plast Surg 2018;81(4):416–22.

24. Lin AY, Kinsella CRJ, Rottgers SA, et al. Custom porous polyethylene implants for large-scale pediatric skull reconstruction: early outcomes. J Craniofac Surg 2012;23(1):67.

25. Oliveira RV, de Souza Nunes LS, Filho HN, et al. Fibrovascularization and osteogenesis in high-density porous polyethylene implants. J Craniofac Surg 2009;20(4):1120.

26. Tark WH, Yoon IS, Rah DK, et al. Osteoconductivity of porous polyethylene in human skull. J Craniofac Surg 2012;23(1):78.

27. Lacey M, Antonyshyn O. Use of porous high-density polyethylene implants in temporal contour reconstruction. J Craniofac Surg 1993;4(2):74–8.

28. Yaremchuk MJ. Facial skeletal reconstruction using porous polyethylene implants. Plast Reconstr Surg 2003;111(6):1818.

29. Zhang J, Tian W, Chen J, et al. The application of polyetheretherketone (PEEK) implants in cranioplasty. Brain Res Bull 2019;153:143–9.

30. Scolozzi P, Martinez A, Jaques B. Complex orbito-fronto-temporal reconstruction using computer-designed PEEK implant. J Craniofac Surg 2007;18(1):224.

31. Argenta LC, Friedman RJ, Dingman RO, et al. The versatility of pericranial flaps. Plast Reconstr Surg 1985;76(5):695.

32. Depani M, Grush AE, Parham MJ, et al. Use of biologic agents in nasal and scalp reconstruction. Semin Plast Surg 2022;36(1):17–25.

33. Gur E, Tiftikcioglu YO, Isık Y. Replantation of pediatric scalp avulsions. J Craniofac Surg 2023;34(1): e22.

34. Manders EK, Schenden MJ, Furrey JA, et al. Soft-tissue expansion: concepts and complications. Plast Reconstr Surg 1984;74(4):493–507.

35. Bentley RP, Sgouros S, Natarajan K, et al. Normal changes in orbital volume during childhood. J Neurosurg 2002;96(4):742–6.

36. Koltai PJ, Amjad I, Meyer D, et al. Orbital fractures in children. Arch Otolaryngol Head Neck Surg 1995; 121(12):1375–9.

37. Azzi J, Azzi AJ, Cugno S. Resorbable material for pediatric orbital floor reconstruction. J Craniofac Surg 2018;29(7):1693.

38. Skochdopole AJ, Layon SA, Hashemi ASA, et al. Cranio-orbital oncoplastic reconstruction in pediatric population: single-institution's experience of 10 cases. FACE 2024;5(1):88–98.

39. Callahan N, Miloro M, Markiewicz MR. Immediate reconstruction of the infraorbital nerve after maxillectomy: is it feasible? J Oral Maxillofac Surg 2020; 78(12):2300–5.

40. Gosain AK, Klein MH, Sudhakar PV, et al. A volumetric analysis of soft-tissue changes in the aging midface using high-resolution MRI: implications for facial rejuvenation. Plast Reconstr Surg 2005;115(4):1143–52. discussion 1153-1155.

41. Phillips JH, Gruss JS, Wells MD, et al. Periosteal suspension of the lower eyelid and cheek following subciliary exposure of facial fractures. Plast Reconstr Surg 1991;88(1):145–8.

42. Garfein E, Doscher M, Tepper O, et al. Reconstruction of the pediatric midface following oncologic resection. J Reconstr Microsurg 2015;31(5):336–42.

43. Abramson Z, Susarla SM, Lawler M, et al. Three-dimensional computed tomographic airway analysis of patients with obstructive sleep apnea treated by maxillomandibular advancement. J Oral Maxillofac Surg 2011;69(3):677–86.

44. Morzycki A, Budden C, Skulsky S, et al. Long term speech and feeding outcomes in patients with pierre robin sequence. J Craniofac Surg 2022;33(2):475.

45. Rai S, Rattan V, Jolly SS, et al. Spontaneous regeneration of bone in segmental mandibular defect. J Maxillofac Oral Surg 2019;18(2):224–8.

46. Kaban LB, Padwa BL, Mulliken JB. Surgical correction of mandibular hypoplasia in hemifacial microsomia: The case for treatment in early childhood. J Oral Maxillofac Surg 1998;56(5):628–38.

47. Chan C, Włodarczyk JR, Wolfswinkel E, et al. Establishing a novel treatment algorithm for pediatric mandibular tumor reconstruction. J Craniofac Surg 2022;33(3):744.

48. Mittal N, Goyal M, Sardana D. Autogenous grafts for reconstruction arthroplasty in temporomandibular joint ankylosis: a systematic review and meta-analysis. Br J Oral Maxillofac Surg 2022;60(9):1151–8.

49. Zavala A, Ore JF, Broggi A, et al. Pediatric mandibular reconstruction using the vascularized fibula free flap: functional outcomes in 34 consecutive patients. Ann Plast Surg 2021;87(6):662.

50. Shih L, Abu-Ghname A, Davis MJ, et al. Applications of fat grafting in pediatric patients. Semin Plast Surg 2020;34(1):53–8.

51. Miloro M, Zuniga JR. Does immediate inferior alveolar nerve allograft reconstruction result in functional sensory recovery in pediatric patients? J Oral Maxillofac Surg 2020;78(11):2073–9.

Moving?

Make sure your subscription moves with you!

To notify us of your new address, find your **Clinics Account Number** (located on your mailing label above your name), and contact customer service at:

Email: journalscustomerservice-usa@elsevier.com

800-654-2452 (subscribers in the U.S. & Canada)
314-447-8871 (subscribers outside of the U.S. & Canada)

Fax number: 314-447-8029

Elsevier Health Sciences Division
Subscription Customer Service
3251 Riverport Lane
Maryland Heights, MO 63043

*To ensure uninterrupted delivery of your subscription, please notify us at least 4 weeks in advance of move.

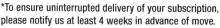

Printed and bound by CPI Group (UK) Ltd, Croydon, CR0 4YY

08/05/2025

01864750-0020